244
Advances in Polymer Science

Editorial Board:
A. Abe · A.-C. Albertsson · K. Dušek · J. Genzer
W.H. de Jeu · S. Kobayashi · K.-S. Lee · L. Leibler
T.E. Long · I. Manners · M. Möller · E.M. Terentjev
M. Vicent · B. Voit · G. Wegner · U. Wiesner

Advances in Polymer Science

Recently Published and Forthcoming Volumes

Chitosan for Biomaterials II
Volume Editors: Jayakumar, R.,
Prabaharan, M., Muzzarelli, R.A.A.
Vol. 244, 2011

Chitosan for Biomaterials I
Volume Editors: Jayakumar, R.,
Prabaharan, M., Muzzarelli, R.A.A.
Vol. 243, 2011

**Self Organized Nanostructures
of Amphiphilic Block Copolymers II**
Volume Editors: Müller, A.H.E., Borisov, O.
Vol. 242, 2011

**Self Organized Nanostructures
of Amphiphilic Block Copolymers I**
Volume Editors: Müller, A.H.E., Borisov, O.
Vol. 241, 2011

Bioactive Surfaces
Volume Editors: Börner, H.G., Lutz, J.-F.
Vol. 240, 2011

Advanced Rubber Composites
Volume Editor: Heinrich, G.
Vol. 239, 2011

Polymer Thermodynamics
Volume Editors: Enders, S., Wolf, B.A.
Vol. 238, 2011

Enzymatic Polymerisation
Volume Editors: Palmans, A.R.A., Heise, A.
Vol. 237, 2010

High Solid Dispersion
Volume Editor: Cloitre, M.
Vol. 236, 2010

Silicon Polymers
Volume Editor: Muzafarov, A.
Vol. 235, 2011

Chemical Design of Responsive Microgels
Volume Editors: Pich, A., Richtering, W.
Vol. 234, 2010

**Hybrid Latex Particles – Preparation
with Emulsion**
Volume Editors: van Herk, A.M.,
Landfester, K.
Vol. 233, 2010

Biopolymers
Volume Editors: Abe, A., Dušek, K.,
Kobayashi, S.
Vol. 232, 2010

Polymer Materials
Volume Editors: Lee, K.-S., Kobayashi, S.
Vol. 231, 2010

Polymer Characterization
Volume Editors: Dušek, K., Joanny, J.-F.
Vol. 230, 2010

**Modern Techniques for Nano-
and Microreactors/-reactions**
Volume Editor: Caruso, F.
Vol. 229, 2010

Complex Macromolecular Systems II
Volume Editors: Müller, A.H.E.,
Schmidt, H.-W.
Vol. 228, 2010

Complex Macromolecular Systems I
Volume Editors: Müller, A.H.E.,
Schmidt, H.-W.
Vol. 227, 2010

Shape-Memory Polymers
Volume Editor: Lendlein, A.
Vol. 226, 2010

Polymer Libraries
Volume Editors: Meier, M.A.R.,
Webster, D.C.
Vol. 225, 2010

Polymer Membranes/Biomembranes
Volume Editors: Meier, W.P., Knoll, W.
Vol. 224, 2010

Organic Electronics
Volume Editors: Meller, G., Grasser, T.
Vol. 223, 2010

Inclusion Polymers
Volume Editor: Wenz, G.
Vol. 222, 2009

**Advanced Computer Simulation
Approaches for Soft Matter Sciences III**
Volume Editors: Holm, C., Kremer, K.
Vol. 221, 2009

Chitosan for Biomaterials II

Volume Editors: R. Jayakumar
M. Prabaharan
R.A.A. Muzzarelli

With contributions by

J.D. Bumgardner · A. des Rieux · N. Duhem · J. Dutta ·
P.K. Dutta · T. Furuike · C. Gao · W.O. Haggard ·
R. Jayakumar · J.A. Jennings · C. Jérôme · M.R. Leedy ·
X. Liu · L. Ma · Z. Mao · H.J. Martin · R.A.A. Muzzarelli ·
P.A. Norowski · N. Nwe · M. Prabaharan · V. Préat ·
H. Ragelle · K. Rinki · R. Riva · H. Tamura

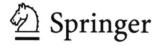

Editors
Prof. R. Jayakumar
Amrita Center for Nanosciences
and Molecular Medicine
Amrita Institute of Medical Sciences
and Research Centre
Amrita Vishwa Vidyapeetham
Kochi 682 041
India
rjayakumar@aims.amrita.edu

Prof. M. Prabaharan
Department of Chemistry
Faculty of Engineering and Technology
SRM University
Kattankulathur 603 203
India
mprabaharan@yahoo.com

Prof. Riccardo A. A. Muzzarelli
University of Ancona
Faculty of Medicine
Institute of Biochemistry
Ancona
Italy
muzzarelli.raa@gmail.com

ISSN 0065-3195 e-ISSN 1436-5030
ISBN 978-3-642-24060-7 e-ISBN 978-3-642-24061-4
DOI 10.1007/978-3-642-24061-4
Springer Heidelberg Dordrecht London New York

Library Control Congress Number: 2011934438

© Springer-Verlag Berlin Heidelberg 2011
This work is subject to copyright. All rights are reserved, whether the whole or part of the material is concerned, specifically the rights of translation, reprinting, reuse of illustrations, recitation, broadcasting, reproduction on microfilm or in any other way, and storage in data banks. Duplication of this publication or parts thereof is permitted only under the provisions of the German Copyright Law of September 9, 1965, in its current version, and permission for use must always be obtained from Springer. Violations are liable to prosecution under the German Copyright Law.
The use of general descriptive names, registered names, trademarks, etc. in this publication does not imply, even in the absence of a specific statement, that such names are exempt from the relevant protective laws and regulations and therefore free for general use.

Printed on acid-free paper

Springer is part of Springer Science+Business Media (www.springer.com)

Volume Editors

Prof. R. Jayakumar
Amrita Center for Nanosciences
and Molecular Medicine
Amrita Institute of Medical Sciences
and Research Centre
Amrita Vishwa Vidyapeetham
Kochi 682 041
India
rjayakumar@aims.amrita.edu

Prof. Riccardo A. A. Muzzarelli
University of Ancona
Faculty of Medicine
Institute of Biochemistry
Ancona
Italy
muzzarelli.raa@gmail.com

Prof. M. Prabaharan
Department of Chemistry
Faculty of Engineering and Technology
SRM University
Kattankulathur 603 203
India
mprabaharan@yahoo.com

Editorial Board

Prof. Akihiro Abe

Professor Emeritus
Tokyo Institute of Technology
6-27-12 Hiyoshi-Honcho, Kohoku-ku
Yokohama 223-0062, Japan
aabe34@xc4.so-net.ne.jp

Prof. A.-C. Albertsson

Department of Polymer Technology
The Royal Institute of Technology
10044 Stockholm, Sweden
aila@polymer.kth.se

Prof. Karel Dušek

Institute of Macromolecular Chemistry
Czech Academy of Sciences
of the Czech Republic
Heyrovský Sq. 2
16206 Prague 6, Czech Republic
dusek@imc.cas.cz

Prof. Jan Genzer

Department of Chemical &
Biomolecular Engineering
North Carolina State University
911 Partners Way
27695-7905 Raleigh, North Carolina, USA

Prof. Dr. Wim H. de Jeu

DWI an der RWTH Aachen eV
Pauwelsstraße 8
D-52056 Aachen, Germany
dejeu@dwi.rwth-aachen.de

Prof. Shiro Kobayashi

R & D Center for Bio-based Materials
Kyoto Institute of Technology
Matsugasaki, Sakyo-ku
Kyoto 606-8585, Japan
kobayash@kit.ac.jp

Prof. Kwang-Sup Lee
Department of Advanced Materials
Hannam University
561-6 Jeonmin-Dong
Yuseong-Gu 305-811
Daejeon, South Korea
kslee@hnu.kr

Prof. L. Leibler
Matière Molle et Chimie
Ecole Supérieure de Physique
et Chimie Industrielles (ESPCI)
10 rue Vauquelin
75231 Paris Cedex 05, France
ludwik.leibler@espci.fr

Prof. Timothy E. Long
Department of Chemistry
and Research Institute
Virginia Tech
2110 Hahn Hall (0344)
Blacksburg, VA 24061, USA
telong@vt.edu

Prof. Ian Manners
School of Chemistry
University of Bristol
Cantock's Close
BS8 1TS Bristol, UK
ian.manners@bristol.ac.uk

Prof. Martin Möller
Deutsches Wollforschungsinstitut
an der RWTH Aachen e.V.
Pauwelsstraße 8
52056 Aachen, Germany
moeller@dwi.rwth-aachen.de

Prof. E.M. Terentjev
Cavendish Laboratory
Madingley Road
Cambridge CB 3 OHE, UK
emt1000@cam.ac.uk

Prof. Dr. Maria Jesus Vicent
Centro de Investigacion Principe Felipe
Medicinal Chemistry Unit
Polymer Therapeutics Laboratory
Av. Autopista del Saler, 16
46012 Valencia, Spain
mjvicent@cipf.es

Prof. Brigitte Voit
Leibniz-Institut für Polymerforschung
Dresden
Hohe Straße 6
01069 Dresden, Germany
voit@ipfdd.de

Prof. Gerhard Wegner
Max-Planck-Institut
für Polymerforschung
Ackermannweg 10
55128 Mainz, Germany
wegner@mpip-mainz.mpg.de

Prof. Ulrich Wiesner
Materials Science & Engineering
Cornell University
329 Bard Hall
Ithaca, NY 14853, USA
ubw1@cornell.edu

Advances in Polymer Sciences
Also Available Electronically

Advances in Polymer Sciences is included in Springer's eBook package *Chemistry and Materials Science*. If a library does not opt for the whole package the book series may be bought on a subscription basis. Also, all back volumes are available electronically.

For all customers who have a standing order to the print version of *Advances in Polymer Sciences*, we offer free access to the electronic volumes of the Series published in the current year via SpringerLink.

If you do not have access, you can still view the table of contents of each volume and the abstract of each article by going to the SpringerLink homepage, clicking on "Browse by Online Libraries", then "Chemical Sciences", and finally choose *Advances in Polymer Science*.

You will find information about the

– Editorial Board
– Aims and Scope
– Instructions for Authors
– Sample Contribution

at springer.com using the search function by typing in *Advances in Polymer Sciences*.

Color figures are published in full color in the electronic version on SpringerLink.

Aims and Scope

The series *Advances in Polymer Science* presents critical reviews of the present and future trends in polymer and biopolymer science including chemistry, physical chemistry, physics and material science. It is addressed to all scientists at universities and in industry who wish to keep abreast of advances in the topics covered.

Review articles for the topical volumes are invited by the volume editors. As a rule, single contributions are also specially commissioned. The editors and publishers will, however, always be pleased to receive suggestions and supplementary information. Papers are accepted for *Advances in Polymer Science* in English.

In references *Advances in Polymer Sciences* is abbreviated as *Adv Polym Sci* and is cited as a journal.

Special volumes are edited by well known guest editors who invite reputed authors for the review articles in their volumes.

Impact Factor in 2010: 6.723; Section "Polymer Science": Rank 3 of 79

Preface

Chitin and chitosan are known for their excellent biological properties, among which the biocompatibility with human cells, the ordered regeneration of wounded tissues, the immunoenhancing activity, the induction of immediate hemostasis, the radical scavenging activity, and the antimicrobial activity. Recent studies indicate that chitin and chitosan are most versatile in drug and gene delivery, elaborated diagnostics, devices for selective recognition of tumor cells, and surgical aids ranging from anti-adhesion gels to coated sterile stents.

The present volumes entitled "Chitosan for Biomaterials I and II" were conceived to provide broad and thorough knowledge for highly advanced applications of chitosan and its derivatives in the form of micro- and nanoparticles, nanocomposites, membranes, and scaffolds. The books consist of 15 chapters written in a manner that meets the expectations of scientists in various disciplines.

Chapter 1 deals with the use of chitosan and its derivatives in gene therapy. The effect of several parameters on transfection efficiency of DNA (or gene silencing of siRNA) has been discussed. Moreover, specific ligand and pH-sensitive modifications of chitosan for improvement of cell specificity and transfection efficiency (or gene silencing) are explained. Chapter 2 discusses the recent applications of chitosan nano/microparticles in oral/buccal delivery, stomach-specific drug delivery, intestinal delivery, colon-specific drug delivery, and gene delivery. Chapter 3 is focused on the recent developments of chitosan nanoparticles in bladder, breast, colon, lung, melanoma, prostate, pancreatic, and ovarian cancer therapy. Chapter 4 reviews the design of chitosan-based thiomers and their mechanism of adhesion. In addition, delivery systems comprising of thiolated chitosans and their in vivo performance are discussed. The importance of chitosan in particulate systems for vaccine delivery is emphasized in Chap. 5 according to administration routes, particularly the noninvasive routes involving the oral and pulmonary mucosae. Chapter 6 explains various multifunctional chitosan nanoparticles and their recent applications in tumor diagnosis and therapy. Chapter 7 discusses the current advances and challenges in the synthesis of chitosan-coated iron oxide nanoparticles, and their subsequent surface modifications for applications in cancer diagnosis and therapy. Chapter 8 reviews the recent updates of chemical modifications of chitosan matrices using the cross-linking agents and their applications as drug-eluting devices such as vascular stents, artificial skin, bone grafts, and nerve guidance conduits. Chapter 9 discusses current efforts and key research challenges in the development of chitosan and other polymeric bio-nanocomposite materials for use in drug delivery applications. Chapter 10 provides an overview of chitosan and its derivatives as drug delivery carriers. Here, a special emphasis has been given on the chemical modifications of chitosan in order to achieve a specific application in biomedical fields. Chapter 11 highlights different fabrication methods to produce chitosan-based scaffolds. Moreover, the suitability of chitosan-based scaffolds for bone, cartilage, skin, liver, cornea, and nerve tissue engineering applications is discussed in this chapter. Chapter 12 discusses about chitosan and its derivatives as biomaterials for tissue repair and regeneration. In addition, integration with cell growth factors, genes, and stem cells, applications of the chitosan-based biomaterials in the repair of skin, cartilage, bone, and other tissues are dealt with. Chapter 13 examines the different mechanisms and bond strengths of chitosan coatings to implant alloys, coating composition and physiochemical properties, degradation, delivery of therapeutic agents such as growth factors and antibiotics, and in vitro and in vivo compatibilities. Chapter 14 highlights the beneficial activities of chitosan, and then it directs attention to the important developments of certain technologies capable to expand the surface area of chitosans, with impressive performance improvements in various applications such as drug delivery and orthopedic scaffolds. Finally, Chap. 15 discusses production, properties, and applications of fungal cell wall polysaccharides such as chitosan and glucan.

Summer 2011

R. Jayakumar
R.A.A. Muzzarelli
M. Prabaharan

Contents

Polymeric Bionanocomposites as Promising Materials
for Controlled Drug Delivery 1
M. Prabaharan and R. Jayakumar

Chitosan and Chitosan Derivatives in Drug Delivery
and Tissue Engineering 19
Raphaël Riva, Héloïse Ragelle, Anne des Rieux, Nicolas Duhem,
Christine Jérôme, and Véronique Préat

Chitosan: A Promising Biomaterial for Tissue Engineering Scaffolds ... 45
P.K. Dutta, Kumari Rinki, and Joydeep Dutta

Chitosan-Based Biomaterials for Tissue Repair and Regeneration 81
Xing Liu, Lie Ma, Zhengwei Mao, and Changyou Gao

Use of Chitosan as a Bioactive Implant Coating
for Bone-Implant Applications 129
Megan R. Leedy, Holly J. Martin, P. Andrew Norowski, J. Amber Jennings,
Warren O. Haggard, and Joel D. Bumgardner

New Techniques for Optimization of Surface Area and Porosity
in Nanochitins and Nanochitosans 167
Riccardo A. A. Muzzarelli

Production, Properties and Applications of Fungal Cell Wall
Polysaccharides: Chitosan and Glucan 187
Nitar Nwe, Tetsuya Furuike, and Hiroshi Tamura

Index 209

Polymeric Bionanocomposites as Promising Materials for Controlled Drug Delivery

M. Prabaharan and R. Jayakumar

Abstract Polymeric bionanocomposites (PBNCs) have established themselves as a promising class of hybrid materials derived from natural and synthetic biodegradable polymers and organic/inorganic fillers. A critical factor underlying biomedical nanocomposite properties is the interaction between the chosen matrix and the filler. This chapter discusses current efforts and key research challenges in the development of these composite materials for use in potential drug delivery applications. PBNCs discussed here include layered PBNCs, quantum-dot-loaded PBNCs, clay-dispersed PBNCs, carbon-nanotube-loaded PBNCs, core–shell PBNCs, hydrogel-based PBNCs, and magnetic PBNCs. We conclude that PBNCs are promising materials for drug delivery applications.

Keywords Bionanocomposites · Drug delivery · Polymers · Hydrogels · Quantum dot

Contents

1. Introduction 2
2. Drug Delivery 3
   - 2.1 Layered PBNCs 3
   - 2.2 Quantum-Dot-Loaded PBNCs 7
   - 2.3 Clay-Dispersed PBNCs 8
   - 2.4 CNT-Loaded PBNCs 9
   - 2.5 Core–Shell PBNCs 11

M. Prabaharan (✉)
Department of Chemistry, Faculty of Engineering and Technology, SRM University, Kattankulathur 603 203, India
e-mail: mprabaharan@yahoo.com

R. Jayakumar
Amrita Center for Nanosciences and Molecular Medicine, Amrita Institute of Medical Sciences and Research Centre, Amrita Vishwa Vidyapeetham, Kochi 682 041, India

2.6 Hydrogel-Based PBNCs 13
2.7 Magnetic PBNCs 15
3 Conclusions 16
References 17

1 Introduction

Polymeric bionanocomposites (PBNCs) form a fascinating interdisciplinary area that brings together biology, materials science, and nanotechnology. New PBNCs are impacting diverse areas, in particular, biomedical science. Generally, PBNCs are the result of the combination of biodegradable polymers and inorganic/organic fillers at the nanometer scale. The extraordinary versatility of these new materials springs from the large selection of biopolymers and fillers available to researchers. Existing biopolymers include polysaccharides, aliphatic polyesters, polypeptides and proteins, and polynucleic acids; fillers include clays, hydroxyapatite, and metal nanoparticles [1].

The interaction between filler components of nanocomposites at the nanometer scale enables them to act as molecular bridges in the polymer matrix. This is the basis for the enhanced mechanical properties of the nanocomposite as compared to conventional microcomposites [2]. PBNCs add a new dimension to these enhanced properties in that they are biocompatible and/or biodegradable materials. For the sake of this review, biodegradable materials can be described as materials that are degraded and gradually absorbed and/or eliminated by the body, whether degradation is caused mainly by hydrolysis or mediated by metabolic processes [3]. Therefore, these PBNCs are of immense interest for biomedical technologies such as tissue engineering, bone replacement and repair, dental applications, and controlled drug delivery.

Current opportunities for PBNCs in the biomedical arena arise from the multitude of applications and the vastly different functional requirements for each of these applications. For example, the screws and rods that are used for internal bone fixation bring the bone surfaces in close proximity to promote healing. This stabilization must persist for weeks to months without loosening or breaking. The modulus of the implant must be close to that of the bone for efficient load transfer [4, 5]. The screws and rods must be noncorrosive, nontoxic, and easy to remove if necessary [6]. Thus, a PBNC implant must meet certain design and functional criteria regarding biocompatibility, biodegradability, mechanical properties, and, in some cases, aesthetic demands. The underlying solution to the use of PBNCs in vastly differing applications is the correct choice of matrix polymer chemistry, filler type, and matrix–filler interaction.

This article discusses current efforts and focuses on key research challenges in the emerging usage of PBNCs for potential drug delivery applications. In drug therapy, it is important to provide therapeutic levels of pharmaceutically active agents to the site of action and maintain them during the treatment. Furthermore, it is necessary to minimize temporal variations in drug concentration that can lead to periods of overdosing. Modified release technologies are employed to deliver active ingredients in a controlled manner, providing some actual therapeutic temporal and/or spatial control of drug release. In this respect, PBNCs could be potential carriers for controlled drug delivery due to their enhanced functionality and multifunctional properties, in contrast to their more-limited single-component counterparts.

2 Drug Delivery

2.1 Layered PBNCs

For the past four decades, polymer-layered silicate nanocomposites have attracted intense research interest with the promise of applications across many industries. However, the proposed widespread commercial use of this technology has not been fully realized, with a few notable exceptions in automotive, barrier (packaging), fire retardant, and structural applications. This slow progress is in part due to the difficulties in melt-blending nanoclays and polymers at elevated temperatures to achieve a homogeneous dispersion of nanoclay platelets in the polymer matrix without degradation of both polymer and nanoclay. This constraint is in part eliminated for low melting point biodegradable polymer/biopolymer layered silicate nanocomposites, such as those with poly(caprolactone) [7, 8], poly(ethylene glycol) PEG [9], poly (ethylene-oxide) PEO [10], polylactides [11, 12] and poly(4-vinylpyrrolidone) P4VP [13], where improved mechanical and functional stability of biopolymers can be achieved. Concomitant with the development of polymer nanocomposites, there has been renewed interest in the area of hot-melt extrusion as a technique for the preparation of polymer/biomolecule composite materials for drug delivery [14]. The main advantage of using extrusion technology is the ability to move from the batch processing normally used for polymer and drug manufacture to a continuous process. This enables consistent product flow at relatively high throughput rates, such that a drug-loaded polymer can be extruded, for example, into a sheet or thin film for patches or into a tube for catheters or other medical tubing. Furthermore, the bioactive-molecule-loaded extrudate can be pelletized followed by secondary melt processing, such as injection molding to make heart valves.

A number of researchers have examined the use of hot-melt extrusion to prepare biomedical polymer–drug mixtures, e.g., hydroxypropylcellulose [15], PEO [16], and a commercially available melt-extruded formulation called Kaletra [17]. Other groups have used solution cast methods to produce drug-loaded polymer nanocomposites in the form of hydrogels [18], nanoparticles [19], and solution cast nanocomposites [20] although the latter has limitations with regard scale-up of the process and is not environmentally friendly. Drug release from polymeric matrices has been modeled by different researchers [21], and the mechanism of drug release from solid dispersions in water-soluble polymers has been reviewed by Craig [22]. Molecular interactions between the drug molecule and polymer chains also affect the mechanism of drug release. Layered silicates alone have also been used in pharmaceutical applications as adsorbents, thickeners, and excipients [23]. Recent

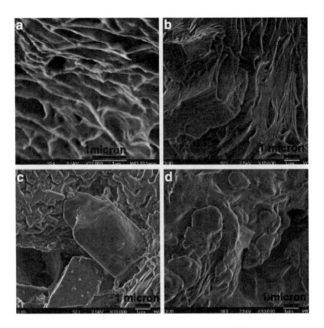

Fig. 1 FE-SEM images of fractured surfaces of (**a**) PEG, (**b**) PEG loaded with paracetamol and montmorillonite, PEGP5M1, (**c**) PEGP5M1 and (**d**) PEG loaded with paracetamol and fluoromica, PEGP5S5 [27]

research has outlined the use of layered silicates [24], mesoporous silicates [25], and double-layered hydroxides as drug and gene delivery vehicles [26].

Recently, composites of paracetamol-loaded PEG with a naturally derived and partially synthetic layered silicate (nanoclay) were prepared using hot-melt extrusion [27]. The extent of dispersion and distribution of the paracetamol and nanoclay in the PEG matrix was examined using a combination of field emission scanning electron microscopy (FE-SEM) (Fig. 1), high resolution transmission electron microscopy (HR-TEM) and wide-angle X-ray diffraction (WAXD). The paracetamol polymorph was shown to be well dispersed in the PEG matrix, and the nanocomposite to have a predominately intercalated and partially exfoliated morphology. The form 1 monoclinic polymorph of the paracetamol was unaltered after the melt mixing process. The crystalline behavior of the PEG on addition of both paracetamol and nanoclay was investigated using differential scanning calorimetry (DSC) and polarized hot-stage optical microscopy. The crystalline content of PEG decreased by up to 20% when both drug and nanoclay were melt-blended with PEG, but the average PEG spherulite size increased by a factor of 4. The time taken for 100% release of paracetamol from the PEG matrix and corresponding diffusion coefficients were significantly retarded on addition of low loadings of both naturally occurring and partially synthetic nanoclays. The dispersed layered silicate platelets encase the paracetamol molecules, retarding diffusion and altering the dissolution behavior of the drug molecule in the PEG matrix.

Kevadia et al. reported the intercalation of procainamide hydrochloride (PA), an antiarrythmia drug in montmorillonite (MMT), as a new drug delivery device

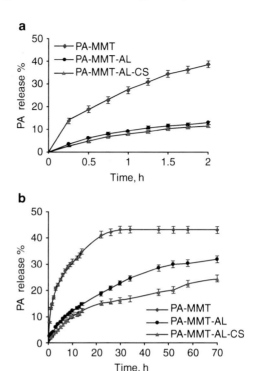

Fig. 2 Release profiles of PA in (a) gastric (pH 2.2) and (b) intestinal fluid (pH 7.4) at 37 ± 0.5°C

[28]. Optimum intercalation of PA molecules within the interlayer space of MMT was achieved by means of different reaction conditions. Intercalation of PA in the MMT galleries was confirmed by X-ray diffraction, FT-IR, and thermal analysis (DSC). In order to retard the quantity of drug release in the gastric environment, the prepared PA–MMT composite was compounded with alginate (AL), and further coated with chitosan (CS). The surface morphology of the PA–MMT–AL and PA–MMT–AL–CS nanocomposites beads was analyzed by SEM. The in vitro release experiments revealed that AL and CS were able to retard the drug release in gastric environments, and release the drug in the intestinal environments in a controlled manner (Fig. 2). The release profiles of PA from composites were best fitted in Higuchi kinetic model, and Korsmeyer–Peppas model suggested diffusion controlled release mechanism.

Thin films and coatings that sustain the release of DNA from surfaces could play an important role in the development of localized approaches to gene therapy [29]. For example, polymer-coated intravascular stents have been used to localize the delivery of DNA to the vascular wall and could lead to innovative gene-based treatments for vascular diseases or related conditions [30]. Likewise, plasmid-eluting polymer matrices have been applied to the localized delivery of DNA to cells in the context of tissue engineering [31]. Although degradable polymer matrices can be used to sustain the release of encapsulated DNA, general methods for the localized, efficient, and sequential delivery of DNA from thin films and

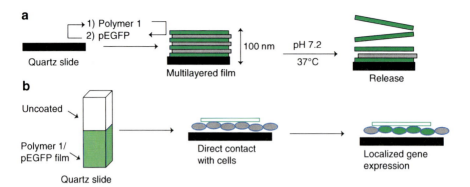

Fig. 3 (**a**) Layer-by-layer fabrication of a multilayered film from alternating layers of degradable polymer 1 (*gray*) and a plasmid DNA encoding enhanced green fluorescent protein (*pEGFP*, *dark gray*). Incubation of this material under physiological conditions results in the gradual release of DNA. (**b**) Direct and localized transfection of cells using a quartz slide coated with a multilayer polymer 1/DNA film. Coated quartz slides are placed manually on top of cells growing on the surface of a tissue culture dish

surfaces do not yet exist. Recently, multilayered polyelectrolyte assemblies 100 nm thick fabricated from alternating layers of a degradable cationic polymer and plasmid DNA were used to localize the delivery of DNA to cells growing in contact with or in the vicinity of macroscopic film-coated objects (Fig. 3) [32]. In addition to the localization of DNA at the surface of film-coated substrates, it was found that these films present DNA in a condensed form that may influence and enhance the internalization and processing of DNA by cells. The layer-by-layer assembly approach used in this study provides control over the location and distribution of plasmid DNA in thin, nanostructured films that can be fabricated onto a variety of complex macroscopic substrates. As such, the materials and approaches reported here could represent an attractive framework for the local or non-invasive delivery of DNA from the surfaces of implantable materials or biomedical devices. The design principles outlined above introduce new opportunities for design of more advanced layered materials that enhance or influence further the mechanisms through which DNA and other biological materials are internalized.

Recently, layered double hydroxide (LDH) biopolymer nanocomposites were prepared using new hybrid materials based on the combination of LDH and two biopolymers (a protein and a polysaccharide) as an effective drug delivery material [33]. In this study, Ibuprofen (IBU) was chosen as a model drug, being intercalated in a Mg–Al LDH matrix. The resulting hybrid was used to prepare bionanocomposite materials by association with two biopolymers: zein, a highly hydrophobic protein, and alginate, a polysaccharide widely applied for encapsulating drugs. Preliminary kinetic studies of IBU liberation from PBNCs processed as beads showed a better protection against drug release at the stomach pH and a controlled liberation in the intestinal tract conditions. This effect can be attributed to the hydrophobic nature of zein, which limits the passage of water and swelling of biocomposite beads prepared with such systems, delaying the release of the drug.

2.2 Quantum-Dot-Loaded PBNCs

Natural biodegradable polymers such as dextran and chitosan have been considered for targeted drug delivery [34], and quantum dots (QDs) are being explored for imaging the distribution of drug in vivo [35]. The unique integration of drug targeting and visualization has high potential to address the current challenges in cancer therapy. Thus, it is attractive to consider the possibility of investigating a system that combines the biodegradable material, chitosan, and the semiconductor QDs. Monodispersed ZnO QDs of size 2–4 nm were successfully synthesized by a chemical hydrolysis method and exhibited a strong blue emission at ~440 nm [36]. The experimental scheme depicted in Fig. 4 enabled fabrication of water-dispersed ZnO-QD-chitosan-folate carrier loaded with the anticancer drug, doxorubicin. The experimentally observed drug loading efficiency was ~75%. Chitosan enhances the stability of the QDs because of the hydrophilicity and cationic charge characteristics of chitosan. The drug release response of doxorubicin hydrochloride (DOX)-loaded ZnO-QD-chitosan-folate carrier was characterized by an initial rapid drug release followed by a controlled release.

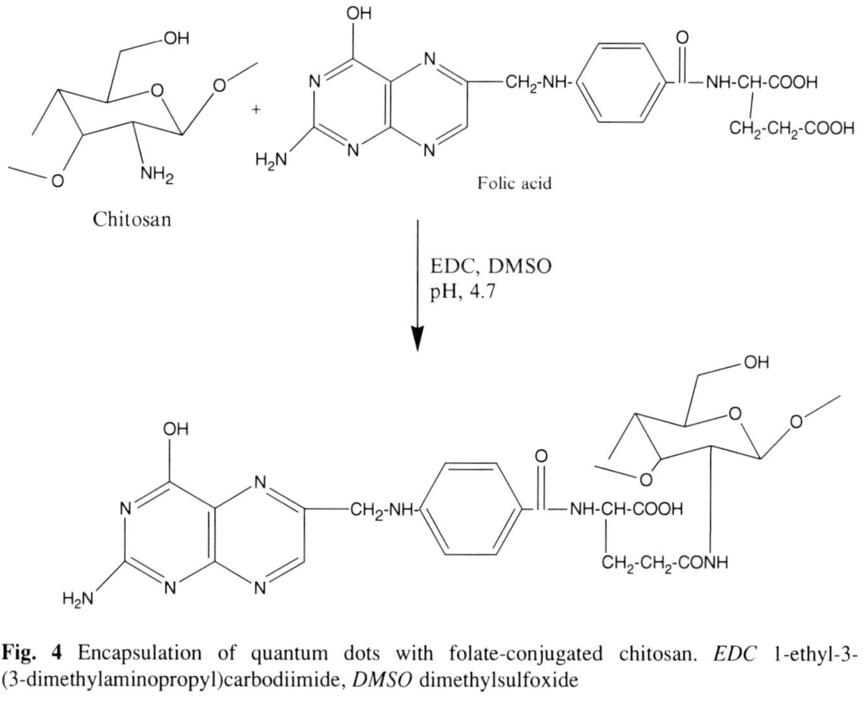

Fig. 4 Encapsulation of quantum dots with folate-conjugated chitosan. *EDC* 1-ethyl-3-(3-dimethylaminopropyl)carbodiimide, *DMSO* dimethylsulfoxide

2.3 Clay-Dispersed PBNCs

In the last few decades, hybrid systems composed of clay particles dispersed in a polymer matrix have been designed to obtain polymer–clay nanocomposites (PCNC) with new and interesting properties. In these systems, the dispersed particles have at least one dimension in the nanometer range and, consequently, there are strong interfacial interactions between the polymer matrix and clay particles as opposed to conventional composites. PCNC have attracted great interest due to the wide range of advantageous properties compared to the free polymers, such as increased mechanical strength, thixotropy, reduced gaseous permeability, and higher heat resistance, even though the quantity of clay might be 5% or less. As a result of these advantageous properties, PCNC have been proposed for several applications in biochemical and pharmaceutical fields [37].

Both biopolymers and clay minerals have been proposed as adequate supports for new drug delivery systems. The use of PCNC for drug delivery purposes appears to be an interesting strategy for improving the features of both clays and polymers [38]. The properties of the drug delivery systems based on PCNC can be modulated by suitable choice of nanocomposite component materials (i.e., the polymers and clays used) and/or manufacturing conditions. Several methods have been described for loading the drug into PCNC. For example, the drug can be adsorbed on the composite surface by suspending the nanocomposites in an active solution and allowing the drug molecules to interact with the PCNC [39]. Another possible loading process could be provided by preparing the polymer–clay nanocomposite in the presence of the active ingredient, i.e., by mixing the polymer matrix, clay particles, and the active ingredient [19]. Coating methods are an interesting possibility for obtaining the modified drug delivery PCNC systems. For example, drug granules of pellets can be partially or completely coated with a solution of the PCNC by using a piece of fluid bed equipment [40]. The release pattern of the encapsulated drug particles can be controlled by the thickness of the PCNC coating and the size of the active ingredient particles. Otherwise, nanoparticles can be obtained by coating of inert particles with a first drug layer (reservoir) and then with a PCNC layer (diffusion layer).

Regarding the mechanisms of drug release from the PCNC, diffusion of the drug molecules through the PCNC matrices, swelling or erosion of the PCNC, and ionic interaction between the drug molecules and the polymer and/or clay have been proposed. Frequently, drug release results have been explained on the basis of different mechanisms. For example, the complexation of magnesium aluminum silicate (MAS) with alginate beads improved the entrapment efficiency of diclofenac. The release rate of the beads followed different kinetics depending on the release medium, being controlled by interaction between the clay and the polymer, which led to an increase in the tortuosity of the swollen beads. Additionally, this interaction caused a stronger gel matrix and a slower disintegration of the beads, compared to non-clay-reinforced beads, which led to the slower release rate of diclofenac. In a recent work, Lu and Mai examined most of the existing models for interpreting the permeability of PCNC and proposed a tortuosity-based model, taking into account the possible PCNC morphologies, i.e., intercalating, flocculating, and exfoliating and modifying the previous models to consider the random motion of gas and/or liquid molecules in the constrained environment of the PCNC [41].

2.4 CNT-Loaded PBNCs

In recent years, there has been intense interest in carbon nanotubes (CNTs) because of their unusual physical properties and large application potential, covering a broad range, in nanotechnology [42]. With their remarkable tensile strength, high resilience, flexibility, and other superlative electrical, and physico-chemical properties, CNTs have been of paramount importance to researchers in recent years [43]. The large surface area together with the above-mentioned properties has also made CNTs and their derivatives attractive and potential candidates for nanoelectronics, nanolithography, composite materials, sensors, optical actuators, biomolecular recognition, and biomedical applications including DNA modification, drug delivery, and gene delivery [44]. In general, it is widely acknowledged that the chemical modification of CNT surfaces with functional monomers and polymers or physical wrapping of the polymers over the surface of the nanotubes are the methods for making CNT–polymer hybrid materials with tailor-made properties and functionalities [45]. Kumar et al. reported a simple method for the functionalization of multiwalled carbon nanotubes (MWNTs) with a biomedically important polymer, poly(2-hydroxyethyl methacrylate) [poly(HEMA)], by chemical grafting of HEMA monomer followed by free radical polymerization (Fig. 5). The nanotubes were first oxidized with a mixture of concentrated nitric acid and sulfuric acid (1:3), in order to obtain carboxylic acid functionalized MWNTs. Then, the grafting of HEMA on to the surface of MWNTs was carried by chemical functionalization of HEMA with acid chloride-bound nanotubes by esterification reaction [46]. FT-IR was used to identify functionalization of –COOH and HEMA groups attached to the surface of the nanotubes. The presence of poly(HEMA) on the nanotubes was confirmed by FE-SEM, TEM, and thermogravimetric analyses. Additionally, the dispersibility of the polymer-functionalized nanotubes in methanol was also demonstrated. Considering the biomedical importance of poly(HEMA) and the recent successful in vivo studies on CNTs, these materials are expected to be useful in the pharmaceutical industry as novel biomaterials composites with potential applications in drug delivery.

A specially designed CNT has been developed for use in the early detection and treatment of cancer. The key functionalities for biomedical diagnosis and drug delivery are incorporated into the CNTs. Guo et al. assembled the nanotubes with different properties and functionalities based on a unique nanoscale design [47]. An idealized representation of the nanostructure design for in vivo imaging and drug storage is schematically illustrated in Fig. 6. The hollow core and polymer-coated surfaces of the nanotube can be used to store antitumor agents such as paclitaxel as

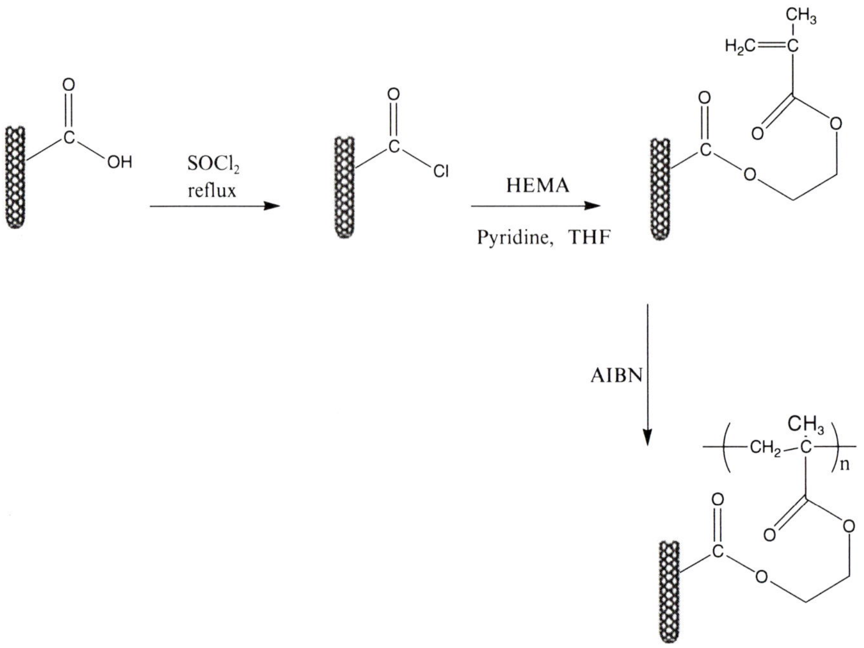

Fig. 5 Reaction scheme for the synthesis and preparation of polyHEMA-functionalized MWNTs. *AIBN* azobis iso butyronitrile

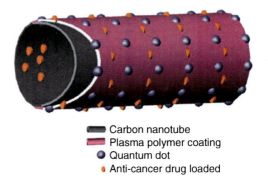

Fig. 6 Concept of a CNT functionalized with a plasma polymer coating, luminescent QDs, and loaded with anticancer drugs. The functionalized CNTs can be used as biomarkers and drug carriers

a consequence of non-covalent adsorption. For deep tissue imaging, the outer surface of the nanotube is conjugated with luminescent materials such as QD. In this study, in vivo imaging of live mice is achieved by intravenously injecting QD-conjugated CNTs. With near-IR emission around 752 nm, the CNTs with surface-conjugated QDs (CNT-QD) exhibit a strong luminescence for non-invasive optical in vivo imaging. CNT surface modification is achieved by a plasma polymerization approach that deposits ultrathin acrylic acid or poly(lactic-*co*-glycolic acid) (PLGA) films (~3 nm) onto the nanotubes. The anticancer agent paclitaxel is loaded at 112.5 ± 5.8 mg mg^{-1} to PLGA-coated CNT. Cytotoxicity of this novel drug delivery system is evaluated in vitro using PC-3MM2 human prostate carcinoma cells and quantified by the 3-(4,5-dimethylthiazol-2-yl)-2,5-diphenyltetrazolium bromide (MTT) assay. The in vivo distribution determined by inductively coupled plasma mass spectrometry (ICP-MS) indicates CNT-QD uptake in various organs of live animals.

2.5 Core–Shell PBNCs

For most biomedical applications, it is necessary to use biomacromolecules to impart biological functionality and biocompatibility [48]. However, it remains a challenge to incorporate biomacromolecules, such as proteins, into core–shell nanoassemblies due to their fragility. On the other hand, bionanoparticles (BNPs), such as viruses and virus-like biogenic assemblies, are promising building blocks for materials development because they are monodisperse in size and shape, and can be functionalized in a robust, well-defined manner [49]. Various functional structures can be obtained through hierarchical self-assembly of BNPs [50]. Recently, a versatile strategy based on noncovalent interactions of BNPs and polymers has been developed to obtain raspberry-like core–shell biocomposites [51]. To enhance the polymer/oligomer–virus interactions, functional groups promoting hydrogen bonding and electrostatic interactions are necessary. Therefore, P4VP was employed in this study because it is well known that P4VP and block copolymers comprising P4VP can assemble with other polymers or nanoparticles to form various morphologies. As shown in Fig. 7, the Cow Pea mosaic virus (CPMV)-co-P4VP nanocomposite was obtained by mixing aqueous solutions of CPMV and P4VP to prepare biocomposite spheres. The structures have very good coverage of the NPs on the surface of polymeric spheres, as characterized by TEM and FE-SEM analyses. Since BNPs, such as viruses and virus-like particles, ferritins, heat shock protein cages, and enzyme complexes, are highly organized scaffolds with robust chemical and physical properties and fascinating structural symmetries, myriad BNPs have drawn attention in the past decade in functional materials development [52]. This method allows the synthesis of hierarchically assembled composite colloids using BNPs as building blocks, which will lead

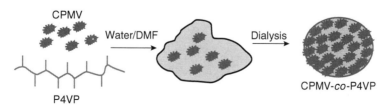

Fig. 7 Formation of CPMV-co-P4VP raspberry-like nanocomposites through noncovalent interactions

to broad potential applications including drug delivery and tissue engineering. Moreover, this approach should be applicable to other types of polymers and biomacromolecules.

Micro- and nanoparticles of biocompatible and biodegradable polymers such as poly(lactic-*co*-glycolic acid) (PLGA) are widely used as delivery devices for the administration of sensitive biopharmaceuticals such as proteins, peptides, and genes. PLGA composite particles combine at least two different materials, i.e., the polymeric excipient PLGA and one or more active pharmaceutical ingredients. This leads therefore to a number of quality criteria, e.g., drug loading (i.e., the drug fraction in the drug–polymer co-formulation), encapsulation efficiency (i.e., the fraction of the drug used in the process that is encapsulated in PLGA), or homogeneity and stability of the produced co-formulations. Finally, there are further aspects of product quality related to pharmaceutical activity that can be assessed in specific testings, either in vitro or in vivo. Kluge et al. prepared PLGA micro/nanocomposite using supercritical fluid extraction of emulsion process [53]. By variation of PLGA concentration and stirring rate during emulsion preparation, particles of pure PLGA with average sizes ranging between 100 nm and a few micrometers with very narrow size distributions have been produced in a controlled and reproducible manner (Fig. 8). Moreover, lysozyme has been used for the formation of composite particles with PLGA. Three different encapsulation methods have been investigated

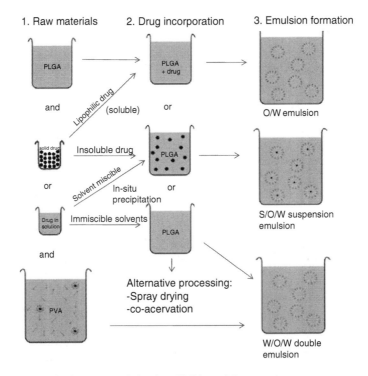

Fig. 8 Strategies for drug encapsulation into PLGA particles

and evaluated by determining the corresponding encapsulation efficiencies. With the method of in situ suspension emulsions, an encapsulation efficiency of up to 48.5% has been achieved. The current study highlights the potential of supercritical fluid extraction of emulsion as an attractive and scalable process for the manufacturing of drug–PLGA composite particles for pharmaceutical applications.

2.6 Hydrogel-Based PBNCs

Chitosan, a polysaccharide derived from naturally abundant chitin, is currently receiving a great deal of interest for biomedical application because of good biocompatibility, biodegradability, and bioactivities [54]. Chitosan-based thermosensitive hydrogel systems have been extensively studied for biomedical applications, e.g., drug delivery [55] and tissue engineering [56]. All of them are injectable liquids at low temperature and transform to semisolid hydrogels at body temperature. This is mainly because the temperature-responsive hydrogels do not require organic solvents, copolymerization agents, or externally applied trigger for gelation suitable for biomaterial applications [57].

Chenite et al. [58] first developed a novel approach for production of thermosensitive neutral hydrogel based on chitosan/polyol salt combinations that could undergo sol–gel transition at a temperature close to 37°C. Other researchers also evaluated the hydrogel for use in pharmaceutical applications [59] and cartilage repair [60]. Many modified chitosan polymers also have thermosensitive characteristics, such as PEG-grafted chitosan [61], hydroxybutyl chitosan [62], N-isopropylacrylamide-grafted chitosan [63] and quaternized chitosan [64]. All of them are injectable liquid at low temperature and transform to semisolid hydrogels at body temperature. Therefore, they have a broad range of medical applications, particularly for sustained in vivo drug release and tissue engineering. However, the burst delivery of drug-loaded gels is obvious. This disadvantage can restrict their application as biomaterials. Nanoparticles have been proposed as drug delivery systems with potential applications such as prolonging the residence time of drugs in the blood circulation [65] or improving transmucosal transport of macromolecular bioactive compounds [66]. In recent years, nanoparticles based on polyelectrolyte complexes from oppositely charged macromolecules as controlled drug release formulations, especially for peptide and protein drug delivery, have attracted considerable attention [67].

Polyelectrolytes are macromolecules carrying a relatively large number of functional groups that either are charged, or that can become charged under suitable conditions, [68]. The macromolecules may constitute either polycations or polyanions, depending on their functional group type. Polyelectrolyte complexes are therefore formed by the reaction of one polyelectrolyte with another oppositely charged polyelectrolyte in an aqueous solution. The process is simple, feasible, and usually performed under mild conditions. Another advantage of this system is that since preparation of the complex is through physical crosslinking by electrostatic interactions instead of chemical crosslinking; the possibility of toxicity associated with crosslinking reagents involved in chemical crosslinking processes can be eliminated. Among these polymers, polysaccharides have been frequently studied for drug delivery and medical applications. A few papers [69, 70] also reported the quaternized chitosan nanoparticles were biocompatible and nontoxic according to cytotoxicity assay and have been used as an antibacterial agent, drug, and gene delivery system. Through the electrostatic effect of $-N^+(CH_3)_3$ and $-COO^-$, the nanoparticles of N-(2-hydroxyl) propyl-3-trimethyl ammonium chitosan chloride–carboxymethyl chitosan were prepared. The nanoparticles with different charges were obtained by the different ratio of $-N^+(CH_3)_3$ and $-COO^-$, which were suitable for drug delivery with opposite charges, such as propranolol and diclofenac sodium. Recently, the synthesis and characterization of a thermosensitive chitosan/poly(vinyl alcohol) (PVA) composite hydrogel containing nanoparticles with different charges for drug delivery were reported [71]. The release of the positive drug was slowest with hydrogels containing negative nanoparticles. Similarly, the release of the negative drug was slowest with hydrogels containing positive nanoparticles. However, the releases of the two drugs were both the fastest with the pure hydrogels. This indicated that the addition of nanoparticles was helpful in slowing the suitable drug release. Though the nanoparticles did not reinforce the gel strength, the electrostatic effect between nanoparticles and drugs reduced the burst release. Therefore, the composite gels are attractive for application as carriers for drug delivery.

Triggered delivery of drugs can also be achieved with nanocomposites by using polymers that respond to external stimuli such as temperature. In one example, Wu et al. reported on the temperature-dependent sol–gel transitions in thermosensitive nanocomposite hydrogels made from Laponite nanoplatelets and Pluronic-type polymers [72]. Pluronics are thermosensitive triblock copolymers composed of poly (ethylene oxide)-poly(propylene oxide)-poly(ethylene oxide) (PEO-PPO-PEO), and are important in injectable applications. The fast dissolution properties of pure Pluronic hydrogels hinder their use for long-term drug release applications. The addition of silicate nanoparticles was found to shift the phase transition temperature and to enhance the dissolution resistant properties of the hydrogels. As a consequence, the release of a macromolecular model drug, albumin, could be significantly lengthened.

A study by Lee and Chen described how to deliver model drugs from hydrogels made of acrylic acid-poly(ethylene glycol) methyl ether acrylate and natural Bentonite clay nanoparticles [73]. These authors found that the elution kinetics are strongly dependent on the interactions between the surface charges of the clay and the drug. Vitamin B12 (zwitter ionic), vitamin B2 (uncharged), crystal violet (cationic), and phenol red (anionic) were used as model drugs. Attractive interactions between the negatively charged silicate surfaces and the drug resulted in slower release rates, whereas repulsive interactions between the two increased the rate of drug elution. The authors highlighted the mucoadhesive properties of their hydrogels that increase the efficiency of drug delivery. Another similar study by Takahashi et al. described the ability of a PEO-polyamide blockcopolymer-Laponite nanocomposite to deliver an uncharged hydrophobic model drug, pyrene [74]. The molecular interactions between the Laponite and the pyrene resulted in sustained release drug delivery profiles of a period of weeks.

2.7 Magnetic PBNCs

With the growing interest in nanocomposites and their applications in biology and medicine, studies examining the biocompatibility of those materials are crucial. Magnetic hydrogel nanocomposites based on poly (*N*-isopropylacrylamide) and iron oxide nanoparticles were fabricated via UV-polymerization with tetra(ethylene glycol) dimethacrylate acting as the crosslinking agent [75]. In vitro biocompatibility analysis via NIH 3T3 murine fibroblast cytotoxicity was investigated. The fibroblasts in both direct and indirect contact with the hydrogels exhibited favorable cell viability, indicating minimal cytotoxicity of the systems. In addition, swelling studies indicated that hydrogels with lower crosslink densities yield higher swelling ratios and that the presence of magnetic nanoparticles did not affect the swelling response of the hydrogel systems. Upon exposure to an alternating magnetic field, the hydrogel nanocomposites with iron oxide nanoparticles showed the capability of remote heating (Fig. 9). This evaluation shows that these hydrogels have the potential to be used in biomedical applications such as drug delivery and hyperthermia for cancer treatment.

Surface control of magnetic nanoparticles is gaining in importance because surface modification has been proven useful in a wide range of technological applications, including electronics and photonics, heterogeneous catalysis, chemical sensing, water remediation, information storage, and medical diagnosis [76]. Compared to polymer coatings, silica-coated nanoparticles represent one alternative for increasing relaxivity and expanding modularity through different chemistries [77].

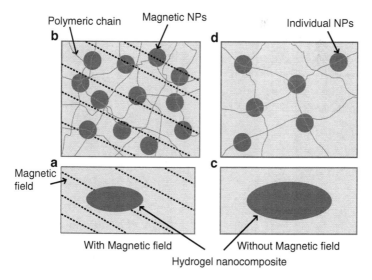

Fig. 9 Effect of an alternating magnetic field on a NIPAAm/iron oxide-based hydrogel nanocomposite. (a, b) The collapsing response of the hydrogel system upon the increase in temperature from the heating of the magnetic particles in the AC magnetic fields and (c, d) NIPAAm/iron oxide-based hydrogel nanocomposite without magnetic field

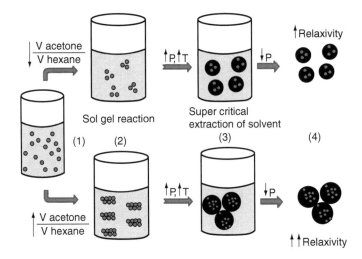

Fig. 10 Processing pathway for obtaining nanocomposite material. (*1*) Colloidal dispersion of γ-Fe$_2$O$_3$ nanoparticles in hexane. (*2*) Initial sol with silicon precursor, water, solvents, and iron oxide NPs at ambient conditions. (*3*) Expanded sol under supercritical conditions with gel composite particles. (*4*) Dry composite particles. *V* volume, *P* pressure, *T* temperature

Recently, monodisperse iron oxide/microporous silica core–shell composite nanoparticles [core(γ-Fe$_2$O$_3$)/shell(SiO$_2$)] with a diameter of approximately 100 nm and a high magnetization were synthesized by combining sol–gel chemistry and supercritical fluid technology [78]. The chemical process to fabricate the material is shown in Fig. 10. This one-step processing method, which is easily scalable, allows quick fabrication of materials with controlled properties and in high yield. The particles have a specific magnetic moment (per kg of iron) comparable to that of the bulk maghemite and show superparamagnetic behavior at room temperature. The nanocomposites are proven to be useful as T2 magnetic resonance imaging agents. They also have potential to be used in nuclear magnetic resonance (NMR) proximity sensing, theranostic drug delivery, and bioseparation.

3 Conclusions

In this chapter, we have discussed an emerging group of PBNCs based on various natural as well as synthetic polymers and nanofillers that are either used extensively or show promise in biomedical fields. These novel materials vary from inorganic/ceramic-reinforced nanocomposites for magnetic and mechanical enhancement to peptide-based nanomaterials in which peptides are both the filler and the matrix, with the chemistry designed to render the entire material biocompatible. Interest in these PBNCs varies from application-oriented design to understanding a multitude of structure–property relations. Requisite functional criteria include mechanical strength, biocompatibility, biodegradability, morphology, and a host of other parameters, depending on end use. However, at the basis of the performance of these PBNCs are interactions between the polymer and the filler, which can be tuned and perfected to suit specific needs. We hope that further research into these interactions will prove valuable in contemplating the design of novel PBNCs for biomedical applications.

Acknowledgments One of the authors, R. Jayakumar, is grateful to SERC Division, Department of Science and Technology (DST), India, for providing the fund under the scheme of "Fast Track Scheme for Young Investigators" (Ref. No. SR/FT/CS-005/2008). The authors are thankful to Department of Biotechnology (DBT), Government of India for providing financial support to carry out research work under the Bioengineering Program (Ref. No. BT/PR13885/MED/32/145/2010).

References

1. Ruiz-Hitzky E, Darder M, Aranda P (2005) J Mater Chem 15:3650
2. Alivisatos AP (1996) Science 271:933
3. Daniels AU, Chang MKO, Andriano KP (1990) J Appl Biomater 1:57
4. Bradley GW (1979) J Bone Joint Surg 61:866
5. Terjesen T, Apalset K (1988) J Orthop Res 6:293
6. Gillett N, Brown SA, Dumbleton JH, Pool RP (1985) Biomaterials 6(2):113
7. Calberg C, Jerome R, Grandjean J (2004) Langmuir 20:2039
8. Chen B, Evans JRG (2006) Macromolecules 39:747
9. Chen B, Evans JRG (2005) Polym Int 54:807
10. Zhao Q, Samulski ET (2003) Macromolecules 36:6967
11. Chang JH, An YU, Cho D, Giannelis EP (2003) Polymer 44:3715
12. Nam JY, Ray SS, Okamato M (2003) Macromolecules 36:7126
13. Koo CM, Ham HT, Choi MH, Kim SO, Chung IJ (2003) Polymer 44:681
14. Brietenbach J (2002) Eur J Pharm Biopharm 54:107
15. Repka MA, Gutta K, Prodduturi S, Munjal M, Stodghill SP (2005) Eur J Pharm Sci 59:189
16. Crowley MM, Zhang F, Koleng JJ, McGinity JW (2002) Biomaterials 23:4241
17. Rosenburg J, Ulrich R, Liepold B, Berngl G, Brientenbach J, Alani LI (2005) USA Patent 20,050,143,404, 30 June
18. Lee WF, Chen YC (2004) J Appl Polym Sci 94:692
19. Dong Y, Feng SS (2005) Biomaterials 26:6068
20. Cypes SH, Saltzman WM, Giannelis EP (2003) J Control Release 90:163
21. Siepmann J, Streubel A, Peppas NA (2002) Pharm Res 19:306
22. Craig DQM (2002) Int J Pharm 231:131
23. Carretero MI (2002) Appl Clay Sci 21:155
24. Lin FH, Chen CH, Cheng WTK, Kuo TF (2006) Biomaterials 27:3333
25. Cavallaro G, Pierro P, Palumbo FS, Testa F, Pasqua L, Aiello R (2004) Drug Deliv 11:41
26. Desigaux L, Belkacem MB, Richard P, Cellier J, Leone P, Cario L, Leroux F, Taviot-Gueho C, Pitard B (2006) Nano Lett 6:199
27. Campbell K, Craig DQM, McNally T (2008) Int J Pharm 363:126
28. Kevadiya BD, Joshi GV, Bajaj HC (2010) Int J Pharm 388:280. doi:10.1016/j.ijpharm.2010.01.002
29. Saltzman WM, Olbricht WL (2002) Nat Rev Drug Discov 1:177
30. Klugherz BD, Jones PL, Cui X, Chen W, Meneveau NF (2000) Nat Biotechnol 18:1181
31. Saltzman WM (1999) Nat Biotechnol 17:534

32. Jewell CM, Zhang J, Fredin NJ, Lynn DM (2005) J Control Release 106:214
33. Alcantara ACS, Aranda P, Darder M, Ruiz-Hitzky E (2010) J Mater Chem 20:9495
34. Yuan Q, Venkatasubramanian R, Hein S, Misra RDK (2008) Acta Biomater 4:1024
35. Jaiswai JK, Mattoussi H, Mauro JM, Simon SM (2003) Nat Biotechnol 21:47
36. Yuan Q, Hein S, Misra RDK (2010) Acta Biomater 6(7):2732–2739. doi:10.1016/j.actbio. 2010.01.025
37. Viseras C, Aguzzi C, Cerezo P, Bedmar MC (2008) Mater Sci Technol 24:1020
38. Odidi I, Odidi A (2007) Int Pat Appl WO 2007131357, p 84
39. An J, Dultz S (2007) Appl Clay Sci 36:256
40. Greenblatt D, Hughes L, Whitman DW (2004) Eur Pat Appl EP1470823, p 13
41. Lu C, Mai Y (2007) Compos Sci Technol 67:2895
42. Baughman RH, Zakhidov AA, de Heer WA (2002) Science 297:787
43. Rao CNR, Satishkumar BC, Govindaraj A, Nath M (2001) Chem Phys Chem 2:78
44. Ajayan PM (1999) Chem Rev 99:1787
45. Lin Y, Meziani MJ, Sun YP (2007) J Mater Chem 17:1143
46. Kumar NA, Ganapathy HS, Kim JS, Jeong YS, Jeong YT (2008) Eur Polym J 44:579
47. Guo Y, Shi D, Cho H, Dong Z, Kulkarni A, Pauletti GM et al (2008) Adv Funct Mater 18:2489
48. Vriezema DM, Aragones MC, Elemans JAAW, Cornelissen JJLM, Rowan AE, Nolte RJM (2005) Chem Rev 105:1445
49. Wang Q, Lin T, Tang L, Johnson JE, Finn MG (2002) Angew Chem 114:477
50. Douglas T, Yong M (1998) Nature 393:152
51. Li T, Niu Z, Emrick T, Russell TP, Wang Q (2008) Small 4:1624
52. Douglas T, Dickson DPE, Betteridge S, Charnock J, Garner CD, Mann S (1995) Science 269:54
53. Kluge J, Fusaro F, Casas N, Mazzotti M, Muhrer G (2009) J Supercrit Fluids 50:327
54. Rinaudo M (2006) Prog Polym Sci 31:603
55. Hsiue GH, Chang RW, Wang CH, Lee SH (2003) Biomaterials 24:2423
56. Shu XZ, Liu YC, Palumbo FS, Luo Y, Prestwich GD (2004) Biomaterials 25:1339
57. Jeong B, Kim SW, Baeb YH (2002) Adv Drug Deliv Rev 54:37
58. Chenite A, Chaput C, Wang D, Combes C, Buschmann MD, Hoemann CD, Leroux JC, Atkinson BL, Binette F, Selmani A (2000) Biomaterials 21:2155
59. Gariepy ER, Leclair G, Hildgen P, Gupta A, Leroux JC (2002) J Control Release 82:373
60. Hoemann CD, Sun J, Legare A, McKee MD, Ranger P, Buschmann MD (2001) Trans Orthop Res Soc 26:626
61. Bhattarai N, Ramay HR, Gunn J, Matsen FA, Zhang MQ (2005) J Control Release 103:609
62. Dang JM, Sun DN, Ya YS, Sieber AN, Kostuik JP, Leong KW (2006) Biomaterials 27:406
63. Chung HJ, Bae JW, Park HD, Lee JW, Park KD (2005) Macromol Symp 224:275
64. Wu J, Su ZG, Ma GH (2006) Int J Pharm 315:1
65. Gref R, Minamitake Y, Peracchia MT, Trubetskoy V (1994) Science 263:1600
66. Mathiowitz E, Jacob JS, Jong YS, Carino GP, Chickering DE, Chaturvedi P, Santos CA, Vijayaraghavan K, Montgomery S, Bassett M, Morrel C (1997) Nature 386:410
67. Xu YM, Du YM, Huang RH, Gao LP (2003) Biomaterials 24:5015
68. Spalla O (2002) Curr Opin Colloid Interface Sci 7:179
69. Shi ZL, Neoha KG, Kanga ET, Wang W (2006) Biomaterials 27:2440
70. Wang XY, Du YM, Luo JW (2008) Nanotechnology 19(6):65707
71. Tang Y, Zhao Y, Li Y, Du Y (2010) Polym Bull 64:791
72. Wu CJ, Schmidt G (2009) Macromol Rapid Commun 30:1492
73. Lee WF, Chen YC (2004) J Appl Polym Sci 91:2934
74. Takahashi T, Yamada Y, Kataoka K, Nagasaki Y (2005) J Control Release 107:408
75. Meenach SA, Anderson AA, Suthar M, Anderson KW, Hilt JZ (2009) J Biomed Mater Res 91A:903
76. Jeong U, Teng XW, Wang Y, Yang H, Xia YN (2007) Adv Mater 19:33
77. Barbe C, Bartlett J, Kong L, Finnie K, Lin HQ, Larkin M, Calleja S, Bush A, Calleja G (2004) Adv Mater 16:1959
78. Taboada E, Solanas R, Rodriguez E, Weissleder R, Roig A (2009) Adv Funct Mater 19:2319

Chitosan and Chitosan Derivatives in Drug Delivery and Tissue Engineering

Raphaël Riva, Héloïse Ragelle, Anne des Rieux, Nicolas Duhem, Christine Jérôme, and Véronique Préat

Abstract Chitosan is a nontoxic, biodegradable, and biocompatible polysaccharide of β(1-4)-linked D-glucosamine and N-acetyl-D-glucosamine. This derivative of natural chitin presents remarkable properties that have paved the way for the introduction of chitosan in the biomedical and pharmaceutical fields. Nevertheless, the properties of chitosan, such as its poor solubility in water or in organic solvents, can limit its utilization for a specific application. An elegant way to improve or to impart new properties to chitosan is the chemical modification of the chain, generally by grafting of functional groups, without modification of the initial skeleton in order to conserve the original properties. The functionalization is carried out on the primary amine group, generally by quaternization, or on the hydroxyl group. This review aims to provide an overview of chitosan and chitosan derivatives used for drug delivery, with a special emphasis on chemical modifications of chitosan to achieve specific biomedical purpose. The synthesis of the main chitosan derivatives will be reviewed. The applications of chitosan and these chitosan derivatives will be illustrated.

Keywords Chitosan · Chitosan derivatives · Drug delivery

R. Riva, and C. Jérôme
Centre for Education and Research on Macromolecules, University of Liège, Sart-Tilman, Building B6a, 4000 Liège, Belgium

H. Ragelle, A. des Rieux, N. Duhem, and V. Préat (✉)
Louvain Drug Research Institute, Université catholique de Louvain, Avenue Mounier, 73 B1 7312, 1200 Brussels, Belgium
e-mail: veronique.preat@uclouvain.be

Contents

1 Introduction 20
2 Production and Properties of Chitosan 21
3 Chemical Modifications of Chitosan 22
   3.1 Quaternized Chitosan Derivatives 22
   3.2 Amphiphilic Chitosan Derivatives 24
   3.3 Chitosan-Based Hydrogels 28
4 Biomedical Applications of Chitosan and Chitosan Derivatives 28
   4.1 Gene Delivery by Chitosan and Chitosan Derivatives 29
   4.2 Chitosan Derivatives for the Delivery of Poorly Soluble Drugs 31
   4.3 Chitosan and Chitosan Derivatives in Tissue Engineering 34
5 Conclusion 36
References 37

1 Introduction

Polymers are extensively used for the delivery of an active pharmaceutical ingredient. They can form a matrix or membrane that can control the release of a drug over a prolonged period, thus avoiding repetitive dosing. They can also be used to form (nano)carriers to deliver drugs, in particular poorly soluble drugs or biotechnology-based drugs. Both systems can protect the drug from degradation. Moreover, when the carrier is functionalized by a targeting agent, the encapsulated drug may be selectively released inside or near a specific tissue or organ. Polymeric delivery systems can modify the pharmacokinetics of a drug, leading to a higher therapeutic index by decreasing the side effects and/or increasing efficacy. Several polymeric drug delivery systems such as nanoparticles, micelles, hydrogels, or matrices are being studied worldwide. Generally, these systems are composed of a biocompatible polymer, degradable or not, and of an active pharmaceutical ingredient dispersed or covalently bound to the polymer. The release of the drug usually occurs by diffusion through the polymer, by degradation of the polymer, or by disorganization of the supramolecular structure of the carrier.

Among all the polymers available to be used for drug delivery systems, (bio) degradable polymers are highly recommended. Indeed, one of the key points of this kind of system is the removal of the carrier after the release of the active pharmaceutical ingredients. Moreover, to avoid side effects, in particular when the carrier is injected, the polymer must be biocompatible. For all of these reasons, natural polymers such as polysaccharides, polypeptides, or phospholipids are generally used as building blocks for the formulations [1].

This paper will focus on chitosan and chitosan derivatives developed for biomedical applications. In the first section, the remarkable properties of chitosan will be exposed. The main chemical modifications used to adapt this material for biomedical applications will be reviewed. Their applications in drug delivery systems and tissue engineering will then be discussed.

2 Production and Properties of Chitosan

Chitosan is a nontoxic, semicrystalline [2], biodegradable [3, 4], and biocompatible [5, 6] linear polysaccharide of randomly distributed N-acetyl glucosamine and glucosamine units (Fig. 1).

Chitosan is not widely present as such in nature and thus cannot be directly extracted from natural resources. Indeed, chitosan is a derivative of natural chitin, the second most abundant polysaccharide in nature after cellulose [2]. Typically, chitosan is obtained by deacetylation of the N-acetyl glucosamine units of chitin, generally by hydrolysis under alkali conditions at high temperature. The deacetylation of chitin is rarely complete. When the degree of acetylation falls below the value of 60 mol%, chitin becomes chitosan. In nature, chitin is present in life forms and more particularly in insects and crustaceans where it represents the major component of their exoskeleton. Chitin is also present in the cell wall of some mushrooms [7, 8]. Generally, chitosans produced from mushrooms present a narrow molecular weight distribution compared to chitosan produced from shrimps, and a non-animal source is considered to be safer for biomedical and healthcare uses.

Chitosan offers remarkable biological properties, which have paved the way for its application in the pharmaceutical and biomedical fields [9, 10] in new drug delivery systems [1, 11, 12] or as a scaffold for tissue engineering [13]. Indeed, chitosan has good mucoadhesive properties due to its positive charge [14], which increases the adhesion to mucosa and so the time of contact for drug penetration. Its haemostatic properties makes chitosan a good candidate for wound dressing [15, 16]. Moreover, the antibacterial property of chitosan also limits the risk of infection [17, 18].

Chitosan is a polycation whose charge density depends on the degree of acetylation and pH. So, chitosan chains are able to interact by electrostatic interactions with negatively charged molecules. It can form nanoparticles by ionic gelation with polyphosphates [19] and with nucleic acids [20–22].

However, chitosan suffers from a poor solubility in water, which is a major drawback for drug formulations. Indeed, chitosan is only soluble in acidic solutions of pH below 6.5, required to insure the protonation of the primary amine. In such cases, the presence of positive charges on the chitosan skeleton increases the repulsion between the different polymer chains, facilitating their solubilization.

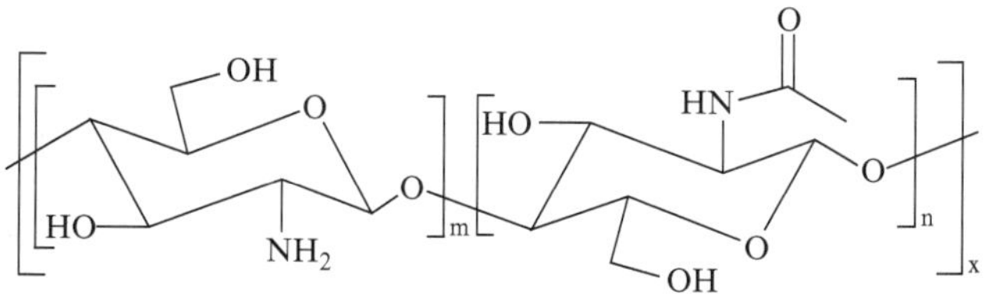

Fig. 1 Chemical structure of chitosan

As far as organic solvents are concerned, chitosan is slightly soluble in dimethyl sulfoxide (DMSO) and *p*-toluene sulfonic acid [23]. This poor solubility is a limitation for the processing of chitosan and is also a brake in its chemical modification. In order to tackle this drawback, chitosan oligomers are sometimes preferred. These oligomers (polymerization degree of around 20) are much more soluble into water compared to their polymer counterpart, even at physiological pH. Several methods for the synthesis of chitosan oligomers are reported that are mainly based on an acidic hydrolysis at high temperature. Nevertheless, final hydrolysis yields are often low and lead to a mixture of products (oligomers, glucosamine monomers) that must be purified [24, 25].

An important aspect for the application of chitosan in drug delivery systems is the fate of the chitosan in the body after absorption or injection. Generally, chitosan is eliminated by renal clearance but if the molecular weight is too large a degradation step by enzymes is required [26]. In the human body, three chitinases showed an activity leading to the formation of smaller chains [26]. Nevertheless, the rate of degradation depends on the molecular weight and the acetylation degree of the starting material [27].

3 Chemical Modifications of Chitosan

In order to improve or impart new properties to chitosan, chemical modification of the chitosan chains, generally by either grafting of small molecules or polymer chains onto the chitosan backbone or by quaternization of the amino groups, has been investigated. Chitosan chains possess three attractive reactive sites for chemical modification: two hydroxyl groups (primary or secondary) and one primary amine. The site of modification is dictated by the desired application of the final chitosan derivative. For example, the preservation of the primary amine is highly desirable for transfection application. Some chitosan derivatives having potential application in drug delivery and tissue regeneration are presented in Sects. 3.1–3.3.

3.1 Quaternized Chitosan Derivatives

Several chemical modifications of chitosan have been tested to make the solubility and/or positive charge of chitosan independent of pH.

The quaternization of the primary amine was investigated [28, 29]. This chemical modification increased the solubility of chitosan in water [30], keeping chitosan soluble over a wide pH range. In addition, the cationic character [23] can be controlled and kept pH-independent, which is desirable for improving the stability of ionic complexes [31, 32]. Typically, the reaction of chitosan with methyl iodide under basic conditions is the most straightforward route for quaternizing chitosan [33].

Among all the quaternized chitosans described into literature, N,N,N-trimethyl chitosan chloride (TMC) is the most widely applied for gene therapy applications [28, 33, 34]. The quaternization maintained and improved the muco-adhesive properties of chitosan, depending on the quaternization degree, which makes this chitosan derivative an ideal candidate for gene delivery [23]. Typically, TMC can be synthesized by reaction of chitosan with methyl iodide in the presence of sodium hydroxide into N-methyl-2-pyrrolidinone at 60 °C. In a second step, the iodide ion is substituted by chloride by an ion exchange process [34] (Fig. 2).

To enhance the delivery properties of TMC, Verheul and coworkers developed a synthetic route for the preparation of thiol-bearing TMC [35, 36]. Indeed, the presence of thiol increased the muco-adhesion of chitosan derivatives by formation of a disulfide bond with mucin proteins of the cell membrane [37, 38].

To increase the water solubility of chitosan, Toh et al. grafted succinic acid onto chitosan and demonstrated, by measurement of the cloud point, a higher solubility in water at pH 7.3 when 20 mol% of primary amine are converted into carboxylic acid [39]. Moreover, the grafting of carboxylic acids onto chitosan chains improved the transfection efficiency compared to pure chitosan but led to the formation of a weaker complex with DNA.

To improve the transfection efficiency of chitosan, the grafting of cationic polymer chains onto chitosan was also investigated [40–42]. Jere et al. successfully grafted low molecular weight poly(ethylene imine) (PEI) chains onto chitosan with formation of the corresponding chitosan-g-PEI copolymer [43]. The grafting of the PEI occurred in two steps. First, chitosan was reacted with potassium periodate in an acetate buffer leading to opening of the glucosamine ring with formation of two aldehyde groups. The reaction of the pendant primary amine of PEI oligomers with these aldehyde groups allowed the grafting with formation of an imine, which was

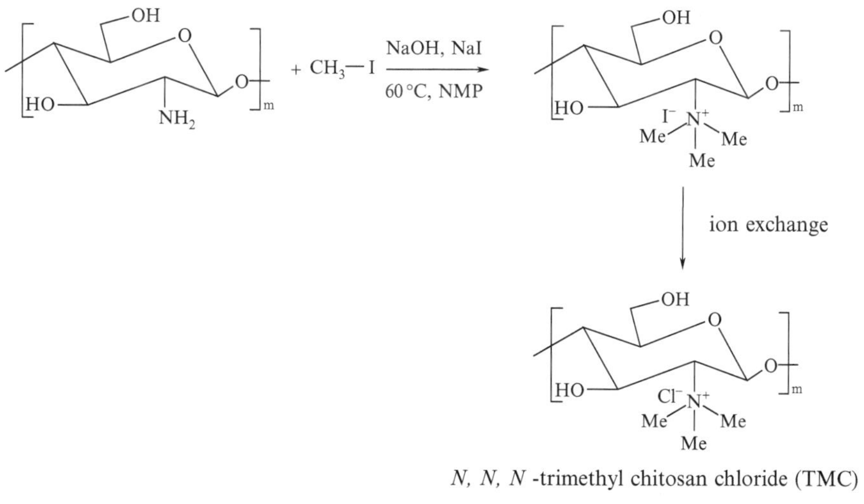

Fig. 2 General synthesis of N,N,N-trimethyl chitosan chloride

rapidly converted into amine by reduction with NaBH$_4$ during the second step. A one-step alternative strategy was proposed by Gao et al. based on the use of carbonyldiimidazole as coupling agent [44]. The grafting of poly(L-arginine) (PLR) chains was proposed by Noh et al. via formation of an amide bond between the primary amine of chitosan on the carboxyl acid of the PLR [45].

Another approach based on the introduction of amine groups onto chitosan was also proposed. Ghosn et al. investigated the introduction of secondary and tertiary amines to improve the transfection efficiency of chitosan [46]. This one-step synthesis was based on the grafting of a carboxylic acid-bearing imidazole onto chitosan by amide formation, mediated by 1-ethyl-3-(3-dimethylaminopropyl) carbodiimide (EDC), and was simple and reproducible and improved the solubility and the buffering capacity of the chitosan derivatives.

3.2 Amphiphilic Chitosan Derivatives

To synthesize amphiphilic chitosan derivatives, the grafting of hydrophobic molecules was investigated. Initially, the grafting of hydrophobic alkyl chains onto chitosan is the most straightforward way to impart amphiphilic properties to chitosan. For this purpose, alkyl aldehydes or alkyl ketones were selectively grafted onto the primary amino groups of chitosan with formation of the corresponding Schiff base [47–49]. A reduction step mediated by sodium/potassium borohydride (NaBH$_4$/KBH$_4$) or sodium cyanoborohydride (NaBH$_3$CN) converted the imine group into the more stable amine with formation of the corresponding N-alkyl chitosan derivatives (Fig. 3).

For biomedical applications, the use of NaBH$_3$CN, able to generate toxic side products (e.g., HCN), is not acceptable. The synthesis and application in drug

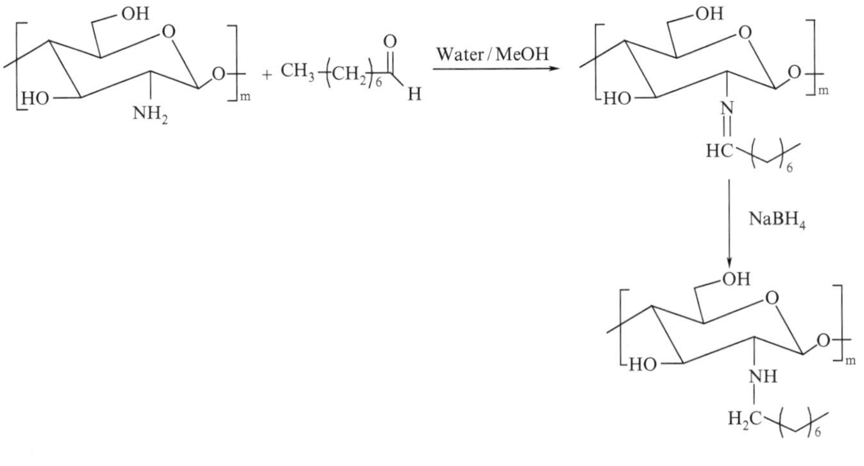

Fig. 3 Grafting of alkyl chain by reductive amination

delivery of *N*-alkyl chitosan derivatives with different chain lengths (C3, C5, C6, C8, C10, and C12) are reported in the literature [50–52]. Nevertheless, these *N*-alkyl-chitosan derivatives did not show optimum properties for the formulation of nanoparticles for drug delivery systems. In most cases, a double functionalization is proposed based on the grafting of both hydrophobic and hydrophilic moieties to improve the amphiphilic property of chitosan derivatives. As a representative example, Zhang et al. sequentially grafted octyl chains by reductive amination followed by the addition of sulfate groups onto chitosan chains [53, 54]. Typically, the reaction occurred in a water/methanol mixture in order to solubilize both hydrosoluble chitosan and liposoluble alkyl aldehyde. After reduction of the imine group, the primary hydroxyl groups of chitosan were selectively converted into sulfates by reaction of the *N*-octyl-chitosan with chlorosulfonic acid. Note the triple functionalization of chitosan by an octyl chain on some of the primary amines, by a poly(ethylene glycol) (PEG) chain on the remaining primary amines, and by a sulfate on some hydroxyl groups of chitosan chains. This provided both hydrophobic and hydrophilic character enhancement as proposed by Yao and coworkers [55, 56]. Another example was proposed by Zhang et al. who synthesized amphiphilic quaternized *N*-octyl-*N*-trimethyl chitosan chloride derivative by reaction of *N*-octyl-chitosan with iodomethane [49]. Huo et al. synthesized *N*-octyl-*O*-glycol-chitosan by successive reaction of chitosan chains with *N*-octyl-aldehyde followed by the ring opening of ethylene oxide under basic conditions [48]. Xiangyang successfully converted the remaining amino group of *N*-octyl-chitosan into carboxylic acid by reaction with succinic anhydride [57]. Li et al. proposed a similar strategy, but based on the use of phtalic anhydride [58]. An interesting approach was proposed by Liu et al. [59] whereby hexahydroxyphtalic acid was grafted onto *N*-octyl-chitosan by opening of acid anhydride by the remaining primary amine. Surprisingly, the hexahydroxyphtalic group was easily removed under acidic conditions leading to the precipitation of *N*-octyl-chitosan. The grafting of alkyl chains is not limited to reductive amination. Ercelen et al. grafted 2-(dodecen-1-yl)succinic anhydride onto oligo-chitosan chains by opening of the cyclic anhydride by the nucleophilic primary amine [47]. Lao et al. proposed the grafting of a C18 alkyl chain terminated by an epoxide followed by conversion of both remaining primary amines and hydroxyl groups into sulfate [60].

The grafting of aromatic groups as hydrophobic moieties was also investigated. Koutroumanis et al. grafted a 2-carboxybenzyl group by reductive amination [61]. Opnasasopit et al. reacted chitosan chains with phtalimic anhydride with formation of hydrophobic phtalimide-chitosan. The amphiphilic property was obtained by the grafting of poly(vinyl pyrrolidone) polymer chains terminated by a carboxylic acid group onto the primary amine, mediated by the crosslinker EDC [62]. Opnasasopit and coworkers extended this strategy by replacing poly(vinyl pyrrolidone) chains by PEG chains [63].

With the purpose of preparing chitosan-based amphiphilic copolymer with only natural and renewable compounds, the grafting of fatty acids was investigated by several research groups [64–67]. Generally, the grafting occurred by formation of an amide bond between the primary amine of chitosan and the terminal carboxylic acid of the fatty acid, mediated by EDC in a water/alcohol mixture under vigorous stirring (Fig. 4).

Saturated stearic acid [65, 68–70] and unsaturated lineoic acid [66, 67] are two examples of fatty acids successfully grafted onto chitosan oligomers by this strategy. With this purpose, Zhang et al. preferred to first convert the carboxylic acid of oleic acid into acid chloride before it was reacted with chitosan in chloroform in the presence of pyridine [71]. Using a similar strategy, stearic, palmitic, or octanoic anhydride were grafted onto chitosan by Jiang et al. [64].

Steroid derivatives were also employed as natural compounds able to confer amphiphilic properties to chitosan. Several examples of grafting of 5β-cholanic acid [72–75] and cholesterol [76] onto O-glycol-chitosan are reported in the literature (Fig. 5). For steroids, the strategy relies on the activation of the carboxylic acid by N-hydrosuccinimide in order to favor the grafting efficiency on the primary amine of glycol chitosan, mediated by EDC.

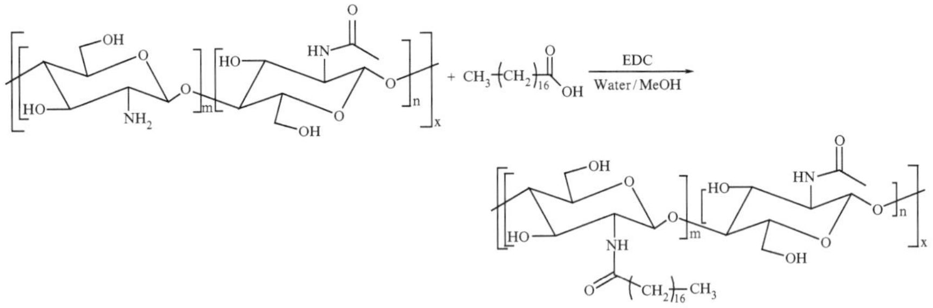

Fig. 4 Grafting of stearic acid onto chitosan

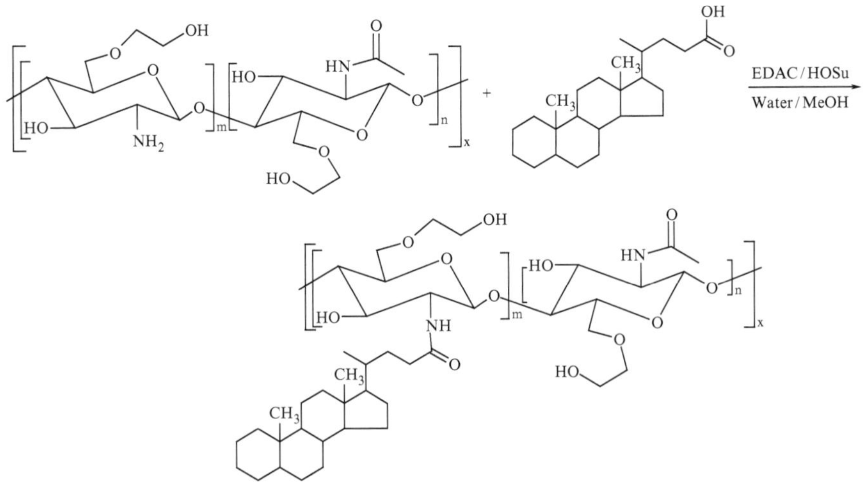

Fig. 5 Grafting of cholanic acid onto O-glycol chitosan

The grafting of hydrophobic biodegradable and biocompatible aliphatic polyester chains [77], and more particularly poly(ε-caprolactone) (PCL) chains [78–80], was investigated for the preparation of biocompatible and biodegradable chitosan-based amphiphilic grafted copolymers for nanoparticles formulation. For this purpose, two grafting strategies were investigated: the "grafting from" and the "grafting onto" techniques [81, 82] (Fig. 6).

In the "grafting from" technique, PCL chains are synthesized by the initiation of polymerization of ε-caprolactone directly by the primary amine, or the hydroxyl groups, present on the chitosan chain. A selective initiation of the polymerization exclusively by the hydroxyl groups can be reached if the primary amines are protected before polymerization and deprotected afterwards [80, 83, 84]. The grafting of PCL by "grafting from" initiated by the hydroxyl group was reported by Duan et al. [80]. Typically, the primary amines were protected by formation of a stable electrostatic complex with methylsulfonic acid, which is easily removed by precipitation in a phosphate buffer after polymerization. In the case of the "grafting onto" technique, polymer chains bearing an appropriate functional group at one chain-end were grafted onto the primary amine or hydroxyl groups of chitosan [85]. In the same way as for the "grafting from" technique, no selectivity on the grafting site was possible if the primary amines were not protected, e.g., by reaction with phtalic anhydride with formation of phtalimide-chitosan [78]. Moreover, the protection of the primary amine was also very helpful to solubilize chitosan in organic media. Ester or urethane links are two examples of organic functions used for the grafting of PCL terminated by a carboxylic acid [86] or an isocyanate group [78], respectively, onto hydroxyl groups of phtalimide-chitosan. Compared to the "grafting from", the "grafting onto" technique allowed a better control of the number and molecular weight of the PCL grafts onto chitosan. The grafting of polymer chain onto chitosan is not limited to PCL. The grafting of PEG chains onto chitosan is widely described in the literature [87–91]. Recently, Casettari et al. grafted carboxylic acid-terminated PEG chains onto the primary amines of chitosan and compared the toxicity of the resulting grafted copolymer to chitosan [85]. However, the grafting of hydrophilic PEG chains was not enough to confer amphiphilic properties but can be coupled with the grafting of PCL chains. So, a heterografted chitosan bearing PCL and PEG chains was synthesized by Liu et al. by simultaneous grafting of carboxylic acid-terminated PEG and PCL onto the hydroxyl group of phtalimide-chitosan [92].

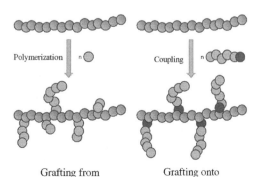

Fig. 6 The "grafting from" and the "grafting onto" techniques

3.3 Chitosan-Based Hydrogels

Due to its remarkable properties, chitosan has been applied to the synthesis of scaffolds or hydrogels dedicated to tissue engineering. A hydrogel is defined as a polymer network able to absorb an important quantity of water. These hydrogels are called physical gels if the origin of the network is due to physical phenomena (phase separation, sol–gel transition, etc.) and called chemical gels if the network is due to the formation of covalent links between the polymers chains. By its hydrophilic nature, chitosan can be applied as starting material for the elaboration of biodegradable and biocompatible hydrogels. Nevertheless, the properties of these chitosan-based hydrogels are not satisfying enough for specific applications [93]. In order to increase the mechanical properties of chitosan, Madhumathi prepared hydroxyapatite/chitosan composite [94]. Chitosan derivatives were then used for the synthesis of improved chitosan-based hydrogels. So, chitosan-g-PEG graft copolymer, synthesized by nucleophilic attack of the primary amine of chitosan onto chloride-terminated PEG, was able to form a stable physical hydrogel [95]. Chemical chitosan-based hydrogel was successfully prepared by Michael addition of a thiol-terminated six-armed star-shaped PEG onto acrylate-bearing chitosan [96]. Photopolymerizable chitosan-g-PEG was synthesized by Poon et al. for layer-by-layer cell encapsulation [97]. N-[(2-Hydroxy-3-trimethylammonium)propyl] chitosan chloride (HTCC) was chemically modified using glycidyltrimethylammonium chloride (GTMAC) by Shi et al. [98].

Another approach to improve the properties of chitosan hydrogels is via the preparation of polymer composites. Porous hydrogels of N-carboxymethyl chitosan/polyvinyl alcohol were prepared by Lee et al. [99]. Hydroxypropyl chitosan was combined with sodium alginate for the formation of biodegradable hydrogels [100]. Chitosan–hyaluronic acid composite was prepared by Tan et al. [101].

With the purpose of conferring thermosensitivity to chitosan-based hydrogels, Park et al. proposed the grafting of carboxylic acid-terminated poly(ethylene oxide-b-propylene oxide) block copolymer (Pluronic) onto the primary amine of chitosan, mediated by EDC coupling agent [102]. With the same purpose, Wang et al. grafted poly(N-isopropyl acrylamide) (NiPAM) chains onto chitosan by the copolymerization of acrylic acid-derivatized chitosan and N-isopropylacrylamide (NIPAAm) in aqueous solution [103].

4 Biomedical Applications of Chitosan and Chitosan Derivatives

Chitosan and chitosan derivatives have been extensively studied for drug delivery and other biomedical applications due to (1) their biocompatibility and low toxicity, (2) their possible formulation in nanoparticles or in gels, and (3) their cationic properties. An overview of their use in biomedical applications will be given for gene delivery, solubilization of poorly soluble drugs, tissue engineering, and protein/vaccine delivery. These examples are not exhaustive but clearly demonstrate the benefit of chitosan derivatives in drug delivery.

4.1 Gene Delivery by Chitosan and Chitosan Derivatives

4.1.1 Chitosan as Carrier for Gene Delivery

Over the past few decades, many studies have reported the potential of gene therapy for purposes such as (1) silencing a gene (siRNA, shRNA), (2) compensating for defective genes, and (3) producing beneficial proteins or vaccines (DNA). However, the delivery of nucleic acids is confronted by many hurdles, like degradation by nuclease or lack of efficiency because their negative charges impair crossing over cellular membranes. For this purpose, viral vectors have been widely used for encapsulation of the genes. Nevertheless, these vectors present some immunogenic, cytotoxic, and oncogenic side effects [104, 105]. The substitution of these viral vectors by synthetic vectors made of polycationic polymers is an alternative way to protect the nucleic acids and to allow them to reach their therapeutic targets: the cytoplasm for siRNA or the nucleus for DNA.

Chitosan is one of the most commonly studied polymers in nonviral gene delivery [106]. Indeed, its positive charges under slightly acidic conditions allow its interaction with nucleic acids such as DNA or siRNA and the condensation of the nucleic acids into nanoparticles. In addition, the biocompatibility and low toxicity of chitosan enable its in vivo use [107]. However, the poor buffering capacity and poor solubility in water [46] make chitosan less efficient than other cationic synthetic polymers, such as PEI or PLL.

Two major formulation methods for nucleic acid-loaded nanoparticles are described in the literature. The simple complexation method consists in mixing chitosan and nucleic acids without any purification of the nanoparticles [108]. Using this process, Howard et al. obtained 78% of gene silencing on EGFP-H1299 cells [108]. However, as the obtained product might contain nucleic acid/chitosan complexes coexisting with free chitosan and free nucleic acids, this method could result in lower efficiency after intravenous administration. An alternative method, which ensures the entrapment of the nucleic acid into the nanoparticles, is ionic gelation involving the addition of a crosslinking agent. Therefore, in this method, formation of nanoparticles is based not only on electrostatic interactions but also on physical entrapment, resulting in stronger connections between the components. The most commonly used crosslinking agent is tripolyphosphate [109, 110]. Some authors used also polymers like alginate and polyguluronate as crosslinking agents [99].

The ability of chitosan to form complexes with nucleic acids is highly dependent on its structural characteristics. Indeed, the deacetylation degree (i.e., the percentage of deacetylated primary amine groups along the macromolecular chain) determines the positive charge density of the polymer and, consequently, influences the electrostatic interactions with nucleic acids. To ensure a good complexation, the deacetylation degree must be higher than 65% [32]. Thibault et al. also reported that complexes with a greater degree of deacetylation showed a higher level of binding to cells, resulting in enhanced uptake [111].

Another physical characteristic to be considered is the molecular weight of chitosan, which influences the size and the stability of the nanoparticles. High molecular weight chitosan allows a better stability of the nanoparticles, which is advantageous for the protection of the nucleic acids but can also be an obstacle to the intracellular dissociation of complexes and therefore for nucleic acid release. Thus, the most efficient chitosans showed an intermediate stability and a kinetics of dissociation that occurred in synchrony with lysosomal escape [111]. For optimum DNA delivery and to ensure high transfection level, chitosan should have a molecular weight of between 10 and 50 kDa [106]. In contrast, for siRNA (13.4 kDa), higher molecular weight chitosan (65–170 kDa) can form stable nanocomplexes and induce a higher silencing efficacy [112]. Indeed, longer DNA strands may be able to compensate for the shorter chitosan chains in the assembly process.

The formation of nanoparticles also depends on the N:P ratio, defined as the molar ratio of chitosan amino groups to nucleic acid phosphate groups. The N:P ratio is different depending on the type of nucleic acid used, but in both cases an excess of chitosan is required to ensure good complexation of nucleic acids. For DNA, a ratio of between 3:1 and 5:1 is optimal [106], whereas higher ratios are necessary for siRNA. Indeed, Liu et al. showed that 50% and 80% EGFP (enhanced green fluorescent protein) silencing was obtained in H1299 cells at siRNA N:P ratios of 50 and 150, respectively, whereas only 10% knockdown occurred at N:P ratios of 2 and 10 [112].

4.1.2 Gene Delivery with Chitosan Derivatives

Although a few authors have reported good gene delivery efficiency using native chitosan, several publications demonstrate the limitations of this polymer. Indeed, one of the first restrictions is the poor solubility of the chitosan at physiological pH because of the partial protonation of the amino groups. This pH-dependence influences nucleic acid binding capacity and therefore the transfection effectiveness. Indeed, Zhao et al. obtained the highest transfection level on chondrocytes using chitosan/pEGFP complexes at pH 6.8 and 7 whereas a remarkable decrease was observed at pH 7.4, which may be due to the decondensation of the complex [113]. Therefore, decreasing the pH sensitivity of chitosan could be advantageous. Hence, among the chitosan derivatives used in gene delivery, TMC (Fig. 2) has been the most studied [114].

Moreover, in comparison to other cationic polymers like PEI, chitosan showed restricted transfection efficiency. This might be caused by the insufficient endosomal release of the complexes, due to the weak buffering capacity of chitosan [115]. Based on these findings, new strategies were developed like the elaboration of innovative multicomponent formulations or the synthesis of new chitosan derivatives, e.g., a chitosan-g-PEI carrier efficiently and safely delivered siRNA to lung cancer cells [43].

Targeting function can also be grafted onto chitosan to achieve specific targeting. For example, RGD (arginine–glycine–aspartic acid) peptide has been conjugated with chitosan using a thiolation reaction. RGD enhances selective intratumoral delivery of siRNA loaded in RGD-chitosan nanoparticles and induces significant antitumoral activity [107]. Mannosylated chitosan-g-PEI has also been designed as a targeted gene carrier [40].

4.2 Chitosan Derivatives for the Delivery of Poorly Soluble Drugs

Amphiphilic copolymers present a double affinity for both hydrophilic and hydrophobic environments and are able to self-organize in water to form, in most cases, specific architectures such as micelles or vesicles, which can be used as carrier in drug delivery systems. The supramolecular organization in water generates small hydrophobic domains well-dispersed inside the solution. The self-assembled nanosized colloidal particles display a hydrophobic core surrounded by a hydrophilic outer shell in aqueous conditions, which allows the solubilization of hydrophobic drugs. Indeed, the inner core can serve as a nanocontainer for poorly soluble drugs. Micelles as drug carriers provide a set of advantages, i.e., increase water-solubility of sparingly soluble drug, improvement of bioavailability, reduction of toxicity, enhancement of permeability across the physiological barriers, and changes in drug biodistribution [116]. Because intravenous injection of a micellar solution induces extreme dilution by blood, polymer micelles could disassemble and release the loaded drug. However, their critical micellar concentration and kinetic stability was usually higher than those of surfactant micelles [68].

Hydrophobically modified chitosan derivatives have been designed to increase the solubility of poorly soluble drugs. However, chitosan is not optimal as the hydrophilic part of an amphiphilic self-assembling polymer because it is only soluble in acidic aqueous solutions with pH values lower than its pKa value (6.5). Hence, glycol chitosan has been used to synthesize new amphiphilic chitosan-based polymers. These amphiphilic glycol chitosan derivatives are expected to self-aggregate and to ensure the solubility of poorly soluble drugs with a better stability in physiological conditions than chitosan derivatives.

Four major groups of hydrophobically modified chitosan have been used as potential drug delivery carrier for poorly soluble drugs: (1) steroid derivatives, (2) fatty acids derivatives, (3) aryl and alkyl derivatives, and (4) carboxymethyl derivatives of chitosan (Figs. 3–6). Others types of modified chitosan have also been synthesized [117–119]

Many of the poorly soluble drugs included in amphiphilic chitosan-based nanocarriers are anticancer drugs, e.g., paclitaxel, doxorubicine, camptothecin, and Mytomycin C. Besides increasing their solubility, the polymeric micelles allow passive targeting in the tumor by the enhanced permeability and retention (EPR) effect. This is a form of selective delivery termed as "passive targeting" [116]. In addition to the size, the stability of the nanoparticles is an important parameter for a successful passive targeting. If the particles circulate in the bloodstream for longer periods, they can reach tumor sites more effectively. Some other therapeutics agents were also studied, e.g., anti-HIV, antifungal, and nonsteroidal anti-inflammatory agents, as well as corticosteroids and proteins.

Drug loading in the polymeric nanocarriers is generally achieved by a method requiring the use of organic solvent to dissolve the drug, dialysis, oil-in-water emulsion solvent evaporation, and solid dispersion. Drug incorporation can modify various physicochemical parameters of the carrier like size or surface charge.

4.2.1 Steroid Derivatives of Chitosan

The main steroids used to hydrophobically modify chitosan are 5β-cholanic acid [72, 120], cholic acid [121], and cholesterol [76, 122] (Fig. 5).

Hydrophobically modified glycol chitosan (HGC) with 5β cholanic acid has been extensively studied both in vitro and in vivo. This polymer was developed as a new Cremophor EL-free alternative carrier systems for docetaxel [74] and paclitaxel. Physical characteristics of the nanoparticules such as size, hydrophobic core, and stability depend on the degree of 5-β cholanic acid substitution. The maximum loading content of paclitaxel into HGC nanoparticles was 10 wt% and the loading efficiency was above 90% [120]. Cytotoxicity studies on MCF7 breast cancer cells showed that HGC nanoparticles were less toxic than Cremophor EL, and allowed a higher dose of paclitaxel administration. The survival rate of mice that received 50 mg/kg paclitaxel in HGC nanoparticles increased substantially compared to 20 mg/kg PTX in Cremophor EL–ethanol solutions [120].

4.2.2 Fatty Acid Derivatives of Chitosan

Different fatty acids were used to generate amphiphilic chitosan derivatives: linoleic acid [66, 67], stearic acid [68, 70], and oleic acid [71] (Fig. 4).

The stability of the micellar structure can be controlled by adjusting the balance between hydrophobic acyl groups and hydrophilic chitosan in an N-acyl chitosan. The critical micellar concentration of chitosan modified with the smaller acyl chain length like octanoyl was weaker than that using a longer chain length like stearoyl because the hydrophobicity of the chitosan derivative was poorer [64]. Hence, the most studied fatty acid grafted on chitosan is stearic acid, especially stearic acid-grafted chitosan oligosaccharides (CSO-SAs). CSO-SA has been studied for the solubilization of several molecules, including lamivudine stearate [69], 10-hydroxycamptothecin [123], mytomycin [70], doxorubicine [71], and DNA [65]. As CSO-SA can rapidly release the drug by dilution, stearic acid was solubilized into the core of CSO-SA micelles and was shown to significantly reduced doxorubicine release. This was because the enhanced hydrophobic interaction between stearic acid and stearic acid segments in CSO-SA forms a tightly packed hydrophobic core, and because of the ionic interaction between stearic acid and doxorubicine [68]. A second way to reduce the initial burst of drug release from CSO-SA micelles is to crosslink the shell of CSO-SA micelles using glutaraldehyde. The drug release could be highly controlled by the shell crosslinking of the micelles without affecting the cellular uptake and drug encapsulation efficiency of CSO-SA micelles [70]. PEGylation of CSO-SA did not affect the cellular uptake of the micelles by cancer cells, and significantly reduced the internalization of the CSO-SA micelles into macrophages [124].

4.2.3 Aryl and Alkyl Derivatives of Chitosan

N-mPEG-*N*-octyl-*O*-sulfate chitosan (mPEGOSC) was synthesized with various PEG chain lengths and various degrees of substitution. One of the derivatives was able to increase the concentration of entrapped paclitaxel by three orders of magnitude. Solubilization performance was influenced by crystallinity: the lower the degree of crystallinity, the higher the entrapment efficiency [55]. Micelle dissociation in plasma proceeded very rapidly for the first 5 min and then slowed down. The micelles based on PEGylated chitosan greatly decreased the accumulation in the liver and the spleen and slowed down the elimination of paclitaxel in the later stage of intravenous injection [56]. Paclitaxel-loaded *N*-octyl-*O*-glycol chitosan micelles showed lower toxicity and higher maximum tolerated dose than Taxol [48]. Other alkyl chitosans like *N*-succinyl-*N*-octyl chitosan [57] and *N*-octyl-*N*-trimethyl chitosan have been studied [49].

N-Phthaloylchitosan (PLC) is a typical aryl-modified chitosan developed to improve the solubility of poorly soluble drugs like camptothecin [63], retinoic acid [62], or prednisone acetate [125]. PLC showed concentration-dependent cytotoxicity in Hela cells, whereas none of the PLC-grafted poly(ethylene glycol) methyl ether (PLC-*g*-mPEG) micelles were cytotoxic in vitro [63]. PLC-*g*-mPEG improved the stability of a light-sensitive drug, all-*trans* retinoic acid from photodegradation [62].

4.2.4 Polycaproloactone Derivatives of Chitosan

Functionalization of chitosan with polycaprolactone (PCL) led to the synthesis of chitosan-PCL and a ternary derivative, chitosan-*g*-PCL-mPEG (CPP) [79, 80, 126]. Spherical micelles were formed through self-assembly of CPP in aqueous media. Encapsulation efficiency higher than 5% could be achieved. The micelles can be subjected to glutaraldehyde treatment to prolong the release of the incorporated drugs [126]. The importance of substituent grafting was again highlighted as an important factor for the morphology and the behavior of the nanoparticles [127, 128].

4.3 Chitosan and Chitosan Derivatives in Tissue Engineering

Tissue engineering aims to develop functional substitutes for damaged or diseased tissues through complex constructs of living cells, bioactive molecules, and 3D porous scaffolds that support cell attachment, proliferation, and differentiation. Such constructs can be formed either by seeding cells within a preformed scaffold or through injection of a mixture of living cells and solidifiable precursor to the defective tissue. As cell and bioactive molecule carriers, injectable scaffolds are appealing, particularly from the clinical point of view, because they offer the possibility of homogeneously distributing cells and molecular signals throughout the scaffold and can be injected directly into cavities with minimally invasive surgery. After injection and solidification, an in situ scaffold provides a temporary 3D matrix on which the cells can adhere, proliferate, and differentiate to form new, functional tissue [129].

Due to its properties, the natural biopolymer chitosan is an excellent candidate for the preparation of wound dressings and hydrogel scaffolds for tissue engineering. There are different ways to form hydrogels from chitosan. Chitosan could be used alone but this is rarely the case because pure chitosan hydrogel is fragile and has low mechanical strength, which limits its application in tissue engineering [130]. Chitosan has therefore been combined with other compounds or chemically modified to improve its properties for tissue engineering applications, in particular to create thermosensitive hydrogels that will gel in situ.

4.3.1 Chitosan Hydrogels for Tissue Engineering

Chitosan has been mainly combined with β-glycerophosphate [131–134] to make thermosensitive chitosan solutions. If highly deacetylated chitosan is mixed with β-glycerophosphate [135], it gels at 37 °C. The major function of β-glycerophosphate is to lower the surface electrostatic charge of chitosan and thus elevate the pH of the system [130]. By increasing the ratio of β-glycerophosphate in the hydrogel, the pH of the resulting solution was higher and the gelation time decreased [136]. The underlying mechanism is that the poly-alcohol group of β-glycerophosphate cuts off the chitosan chain, accelerating the formation of a hydrophilic shell around the chitosan molecule, and thus improving the chitosan chain protective hydration, which prevents the associative effects at low temperatures and neutral pH. However, with an increase in temperature, hydrophilic interactions and hydrogen bonding start playing an important role and trigger physical crosslinking throughout the whole solution, starting the gelation process [136].

However, the hydrogels obtained are weak and some toxicity has been reported, mainly due to the high osmolarity (781 mOsm for 0.8 w/v% chitosan/glycerophosphate [137]) induced by the addition of glycerophosphate [138, 139]. This is the reason why Kim et al. [134] dialyzed the chitosan solution to reduce the glycerophosphate concentration required to make chitosan gels at 37 °C. Others combined chitosan/glycerophosphate solutions with other compounds to increase the hydrogel modulus.

Collagen displays low immunogenicity, biocompatibility, and biological degradability. However, collagen has a unique molecular identifying signal system that can improve cellular adhesion, proliferation, and differentiation, hence providing a suitable scaffold bed for cellular expansion and differentiation. Collagen gels at body temperature, although with the disadvantages of having a fast degradation rate and a relatively low mechanical strength [136]. Chitosan/glycerophosphate/collagen hydrogels possess an excellent cellular compatibility. Chitosan/glycerophosphate has also been complemented with hydroxyethylcellulose [129] for cartilage reconstruction or for improving the myocardial performance in infarcted heart [140, 141], or with ethylcellulose [142] for neural repair. For each study, the hydrogels were biocompatible and improved significantly the function for which they were developed. Starch has also been added to chitosan/glycerophosphate [143]. The physical properties, including flexibility, of crosslinked chitosan hydrogels can be improved by blending chitosan with pregelatinized starch. The presence of starch in the system increased the water absorption of the hydrogel when compared to the system without starch.

Chitosan was also complemented with polyvinyl alcohol (PVA) for wound-healing [144] and bone regeneration [145]. The chitosan/PVA wound dressing was more swellable, flexible, and elastic because of its crosslinking interaction with PVA. The hydrogel significantly improved the wound healing effect compared with a gauze control and the conventional product. For bone regeneration, the chitosan/PVA blend was supplemented with hydroxyapatite, which significantly enhanced the gel strength. The authors reported that the weak chitosan chain association with phosphate resulted in an increase in gelation speed and an enhancement of gel strength. The early burst of drug release was minimized or avoided in comparison with the pure chitosan/PVA gel.

4.3.2 Chitosan Derivatives for Tissue Engineering

Chitosan has three types of reactive functional groups that allow modifications of chitosan to produce various useful hydrogels for tissue engineering applications [146].

Poon et al. [97] developed a chitosan-g-PEG-g-methacrylate copolymer that was both thermoresponsive and UV-curable. Cells remained mostly viable when they were encapsulated inside this gel and suffered little damage from the single brief UV exposure.

N-[(2-Hydroxy-3-trimethylammonium)propyl] chitosan chloride (HTCC) shows better water solubility, moisture retentiveness, antimicrobial activity, absorptive property, and cell proliferative capacity than chitosan [98]. To form a gel, HTCC was mixed with glycerophosphate. The mechanical and swelling properties of the hydrogel were readily controlled by pH, the content of HTCC, and the content of glycerophosphate. The gel could easily incorporate drug in the solution state, which was stable below or at room temperature and became transparent at 37 °C. In addition, these hydrogels possessed good biocompatibility, and the cells could adhere and migrate inside the hydrogel networks.

Park et al. [102] designed an injectable cell delivery chitosan–Pluronic hydrogel for articular cartilage regeneration. The chitosan–Pluronic solution underwent a sol–gel transition at around 25 °C. The chitosan–Pluronic hydrogel showed effective chondrocyte proliferation and promoted extracellular matrix expression compared with alginate hydrogel.

Tan et al. [101] proposed a new class of biocompatible and biodegradable composite hydrogels derived from water-soluble chitosan and oxidized hyaluronic acid upon mixing, without the addition of a chemical crosslinking agent. The gelation is attributed to the Schiff base reaction between amino and aldehyde groups of polysaccharide derivatives. N-Succinyl-chitosan and aldehyde hyaluronic acid were synthesized for preparation of the composite hydrogels. The results demonstrated that the composite hydrogel supported cell survival and that the cells retained chondrocytic morphology.

Thermosensitive chitosan hydrogels were also obtained through grafting with well-known thermosensitive synthetic polymers like poly(NIPAAm) [103]. Hydrogels were synthesized by the copolymerization of acrylic acid-derivatized chitosan (CSA) and NIPAAm in aqueous solution. Cell adhesion and spreading was higher on the surface of poly(NIPAAm-*co*-CSA) hydrogels than that of PNIPAAm hydrogel. These hydrogels showed more rapid detachment of cell sheets. When the temperature decreased, the poly(NIPAAm-*co*-CSA) hydrogel showed hydrophilicity and the cells spontaneously detached along with their deposited extracellular matrix.

As chemical crosslinking can cause toxicity, chitosan was chemically modified using N-acetyl-L-cysteine (NAC), with the degree of substitution of thiol groups kept below 50% to minimize interference with biological function, and then crosslinked by disulfide bond formation in air [147]. Disulfide-crosslinked chitosan hydrogels were rapidly formed, their mechanical and swelling properties being controlled by the content of free thiol, concentration of thiol, and the molecular weight of chitosan. In vitro release of insulin and bovine serum albumin (BSA) was dependent on loading efficiency, composition of thiolated chitosan, and the drug entrapped, but the drug bioactivity was not affected during formation of the hydrogels. These hydrogels exhibited good compatibility and cells could adhere and migrate inside the hydrogel networks.

For corneal regeneration, Liang et al. [148] describe an in situ-formed hydrogel based on a water-soluble derivative of chitosan, hydroxypropyl chitosan, and sodium alginate dialdehyde. The composite hydrogel was both nontoxic and biodegradable and showed that corneal endothelial cells transplanted using the composite hydrogel could survive and retain normal morphology.

5 Conclusion

Chitosan has received considerable attention as a functional biopolymer for diverse pharmaceutical and biomedical applications. It is a nontoxic, biocompatible, and biodegradable polymer. Chitosans can be formulated as nanocarriers mainly by ionic interactions, leading to drug-loaded colloidal systems with mucoadhesive and controversial permeation-enhancer properties. They can also be formulated as hydrogels.

However, for most applications, practical use of chitosan has been limited by its physicochemical properties, in particular its low solubility above pH 6.5 and the pH-dependence of the ionic interactions in the formulations. Hence, chitosan derivatives have been recently developed to widen and improve the potential biomedical applications of chitosan.

Due to its cationic properties, chitosan has been extensively used for gene delivery. However, due to its low buffering capacity and the low stability of nucleic acid-loaded chitosan nanoparticles, several chemical modifications have been introduced to improve transfection efficiency in vivo: (1) quaternization to improve solubility and stability of the nanoparticles, (2) grafting of polymer chains such as PEI to improve endosomal escape, or (3) grafting of ligands for specific cell targeting.

When a hydrophobic moiety is conjugated to chitosan, the resulting polymer can self-assemble and encapsulate poorly soluble drugs. Grafting a steroid, fatty acid, or PCL onto chitosan or glycol chitosan leads to nanocarriers that are useful for drug delivery, in particular passive or active targeting of anticancer drugs to tumors.

Chitosan can form 3D scaffold that are too weak to be useful in tissue engineering. Hence, inclusion in the chitosan matrix and/or grafting onto chitosan of other substances such as collagen, other biopolymers, or hydroxyapatite has been achieved to improve the mechanical properties of the scaffold and to mimic the nanostructure of the tissue for a better cell adhesion/infiltration and/or to provide thermosensitivity for in situ gelation.

The chemical modifications of chitosan described are not exhaustive but clearly demonstrate their benefit for drug delivery. Similarly, besides the described improvements in delivery of genes or poorly soluble drugs and in scaffolds for tissue engineering, other improvements in the delivery of therapeutic peptide and proteins or vaccines using chitosan-based systems have also been reported.

However, before the translation can be made to a marketed product containing modified chitosan as an excipient, extensive preclinical studies, including toxicological studies, as well as clinical studies are required. Moreover, scaling up of the chemical synthesis and precise physicochemical characterization of the novel polymers will be needed.

References

1. Park JH, Saravanakumar G et al (2010) Targeted delivery of low molecular drugs using chitosan and its derivatives. Adv Drug Deliv Rev 62:28–41
2. Rinaudo M (2006) Chitin and chitosan: properties and applications. Prog Polym Sci 31:603–632
3. Bagheri-Khoulenjani S, Taghizadeh SM et al (2009) An investigation on the short-term biodegradability of chitosan with various molecular weights and degrees of deacetylation. Carbohydr Polym 78:773–778

4. Varum KM, Myhr MM et al (1997) In vitro degradation rates of partially N-acetylated chitosans in human serum. Carbohydr Res 299:99–101
5. VandeVord PJ, Matthew HWT et al (2002) Evaluation of the biocompatibility of a chitosan scaffold in mice. J Biomed Mater Res 59:585–590
6. Sashiwa H, Aiba SI (2004) Chemically modified chitin and chitosan as biomaterials. Prog Polym Sci 29:887–908
7. Rane KD, Hoover DG (1993) Production of chitosan by funghi. Food Biotechnol 7:11–33
8. Aranaz I, Harris R et al (2010) Chitosan amphiphilic derivatives. Chemistry and applications. Curr Org Chem 14:308–330
9. Illum L (1998) Chitosan and its use as a pharmaceutical excipient. Pharm Res 15:1326–1331
10. Kumar M, Muzzarelli RAA et al (2004) Chitosan chemistry and pharmaceutical perspectives. Chem Rev 104:6017–6084
11. Paños I, Acosta N et al (2008) New drug delivery systems based on chitosan. Curr Drug Discov Technol 5:333–341
12. Varshosaz J (2007) The promise of chitosan microspheres in drug delivery systems. Expert Opin Drug Deliv 4:263–273
13. Madihally SV, Matthew HWT (1999) Porous chitosan scaffolds for tissue engineering. Biomaterials 20:1133–1142
14. Lehr C-M, Bouwstra JA et al (1992) In vitro evaluation of mucoadhesive properties of chitosan and some other natural polymers. Int J Pharm 78:43–48
15. Yang J, Tian F et al (2008) Effect of chitosan molecular weight and deacetylation degree on hemostasis. J Biomed Mater Res B Appl Biomater 84B:131–137
16. Minagawa T, Okamura Y et al (2007) Effects of molecular weight and deacetylation degree of chitin/chitosan on wound healing. Carbohydr Polym 67:640–644
17. Sudarshan NR, Hoover DG et al (1992) Antibacterial action of chitosan. Food Biotechnol 6:257–272
18. Ong SY, Wu J et al (2008) Development of a chitosan-based wound dressing with improved hemostatic and antimicrobial properties. Biomaterials 29:4323–4332
19. Calvo P, Remunan-López C, Vila-Jato JL, Alonso MJ (1997) Novel hydrophilic chitosan-polyethylene oxide nanoparticles as protein carriers. J Appl Polym Sci 63:125–132
20. Lee KY (2007) Chitosan and its derivatives for gene delivery. Macromol Res 15:195–201
21. Guliyeva Ü, Öner F et al (2006) Chitosan microparticles containing plasmid DNA as potential oral gene delivery system. Eur J Pharm Biopharm 62:17–25
22. Erbacher P, Zou SM et al (1998) Chitosan-based vector/DNA complexes for gene delivery: biophysical characteristics and transfection ability. Pharm Res 15:1332–1339
23. Mourya VK, Inamdar NN (2008) Chitosan-modifications and applications: opportunities galore. React Funct Polym 68:1013–1051
24. Kim S-K, Rajapakse N (2005) Enzymatic production and biological activities of chitosan oligosaccharides (COS): a review. Carbohydr Polym 62:357–368
25. Einbu A, Grasdalen H et al (2007) Kinetics of hydrolysis of chitin/chitosan oligomers in concentrated hydrochloric acid. Carbohydr Res 342:1055–1062
26. Kean T, Thanou M (2010) Biodegradation, biodistribution and toxicity of chitosan. Adv Drug Deliv Rev 62:3–11
27. Yang YM, Hu W et al (2007) The controlling biodegradation of chitosan fibers by N-acetylation in vitro and in vivo. J Mater Sci Mater Med 18:2117–2121
28. Thanou MM, Kotze AF et al (2000) Effect of degree of quaternization of N-trimethyl chitosan chloride for enhanced transport of hydrophilic compounds across intestinal Caco-2 cell monolayers. J Control Release 64:15–25
29. Kotze AF, Thanou MM et al (1999) Effect of the degree of quaternization of N-trimethyl chitosan chloride on the permeability of intestinal epithelial cells (Caco-2). Eur J Pharm Biopharm 47:269–274
30. Verheul RJ, Amidi M et al (2008) Synthesis, characterization and in vitro biological properties of O-methyl free N, N, N-trimethylated chitosan. Biomaterials 29:3642–3649

31. Lee M, Nah JW et al (2001) Water-soluble and low molecular weight chitosan-based plasmid DNA delivery. Pharm Res 18:427–431
32. Koping-Hoggard M, Tubulekas I et al (2001) Chitosan as a nonviral gene delivery system. Structure-property relationships and characteristics compared with polyethylenimine in vitro and after lung administration in vivo. Gene Ther 8:1108–1121
33. Sieval AB, Thanou M et al (1998) Preparation and NMR characterization of highly substituted N-trimethyl chitosan chloride. Carbohydr Polym 36:157–165
34. Kean T, Roth S et al (2005) Trimethylated chitosans as non-viral gene delivery vectors: cytotoxicity and transfection efficiency. J Control Release 103:643–653
35. Verheul RJ, van der Wal S et al (2010) Tailorable thiolated trimethyl chitosans for covalently stabilized nanoparticles. Biomacromolecules 11:1965–1971
36. Varkouhi AK, Verheul RJ et al (2010) Gene silencing activity of siRNA polyplexes based on thiolated N, N, N-trimethylated chitosan. Bioconjug Chem 21:2339–2346
37. Yin LC, Ding JY et al (2009) Drug permeability and mucoadhesion properties of thiolated trimethyl chitosan nanoparticles in oral insulin delivery. Biomaterials 30:5691–5700
38. Langoth N, Kahlbacher H et al (2006) Thiolated chitosans: design and in vivo evaluation of a mucoadhesive buccal peptide drug delivery system. Pharm Res 23:573–579
39. Toh EK-W, Chen H-Y et al (2011) Succinated chitosan as a gene carrier for improved chitosan solubility and gene transfection. Nanomedicine 7(2):174–183
40. Jiang H-L, Kim Y-K et al (2009) Mannosylated chitosan-graft-polyethylenimine as a gene carrier for Raw 264.7 cell targeting. Int J Pharm 375:133–139
41. Jiang H-L, Kim Y-K et al (2007) Chitosan-graft-polyethylenimine as a gene carrier. J Control Release 117:273–280
42. Li Z-T, Guo J et al (2010) Chitosan-graft-polyethylenimine with improved properties as a potential gene vector. Carbohydr Polym 80:254–259
43. Jere D, Jiang H-L et al (2009) Chitosan-graft-polyethylenimine for Akt1 siRNA delivery to lung cancer cells. Int J Pharm 378:194–200
44. Gao J-Q, Zhao Q-Q et al (2010) Gene-carried chitosan-linked-PEI induced high gene transfection efficiency with low toxicity and significant tumor-suppressive activity. Int J Pharm 387:286–294
45. Noh SM, Park MO et al (2010) Pegylated poly-l-arginine derivatives of chitosan for effective delivery of siRNA. J Control Release 145:159–164
46. Ghosn B, Kasturi SP et al (2008) Enhancing polysaccharide-mediated delivery of nucleic acids through functionalization with secondary and tertiary amines. Curr Top Med Chem 8:331–340
47. Ercelen S, Zhang X et al (2006) Physicochemical properties of low molecular weight alkylated chitosans: a new class of potential nonviral vectors for gene delivery. Colloids Surf B 51:140–148
48. Huo M, Zhang Y et al (2010) Synthesis and characterization of low-toxic amphiphilic chitosan derivatives and their application as micelle carrier for antitumor drug. Int J Pharm 394:162–173
49. Zhang C, Ding Y et al (2007) Polymeric micelle systems of hydroxycamptothecin based on amphiphilic N-alkyl-N-trimethyl chitosan derivatives. Colloids Surf B 55:192–199
50. Desbrieres J, Martinez C et al (1996) Hydrophobic derivatives of chitosan: characterization and rheological behaviour. Int J Biol Macromol 19:21–28
51. Rinaudo M, Auzely R et al (2005) Specific interactions in modified chitosan systems. Biomacromolecules 6:2396–2407
52. Ortona O, D'Errico G et al (2008) The aggregative behavior of hydrophobically modified chitosans with high substitution degree in aqueous solution. Carbohydr Polym 74:16–22
53. Zhang C, Qineng P et al (2004) Self-assembly and characterization of paclitaxel-loaded N-octyl-O-sulfate chitosan micellar system. Colloids Surf B 39:69–75
54. Zhang C, Ping Q et al (2003) Preparation of N-alkyl-O-sulfate chitosan derivatives and micellar solubilization of taxol. Carbohydr Polym 54:137–141

55. Yao Z, Zhang C et al (2007) A series of novel chitosan derivatives: synthesis, characterization and micellar solubilization of paclitaxel. Carbohydr Polym 68:781–792
56. Qu G, Yao Z et al (2009) PEG conjugated N-octyl-O-sulfate chitosan micelles for delivery of paclitaxel: in vitro characterization and in vivo evaluation. Eur J Pharm Sci 37:98–105
57. Xiangyang X, Ling L et al (2007) Preparation and characterization of N-succinyl-N'-octyl chitosan micelles as doxorubicin carriers for effective anti-tumor activity. Colloids Surf B 55:222–228
58. Li H, Liu J et al (2009) Synthesis of novel pH-sensitive chitosan graft copolymers and micellar solubilization of paclitaxel. Int J Biol Macromol 44:249–256
59. Liu J, Li H et al (2010) Novel pH-sensitive chitosan-derived micelles loaded with paclitaxel. Carbohydr Polym 82:432–439
60. Lao S-B, Zhang Z-X et al (2010) Novel amphiphilic chitosan derivatives: synthesis, characterization and micellar solubilization of rotenone. Carbohydr Polym 82:1136–1142
61. Koutroumanis KP, Avgoustakis K et al (2010) Synthesis of cross-linked N-(2-carboxybenzyl) chitosan pH sensitive polyelectrolyte and its use for drug controlled delivery. Carbohydr Polym 82:181–188
62. Opanasopit P, Ngawhirunpat T et al (2007) N-Phthaloylchitosan-g-mPEG design for all-trans retinoic acid-loaded polymeric micelles. Eur J Pharm Sci 30:424–431
63. Opanasopit P, Ngawhirunpat T et al (2007) Camptothecin-incorporating N-phthaloyl-chitosan-g-mPEG self-assembly micellar system: effect of degree of deacetylation. Colloids Surf B 60:117–124
64. Jiang G-B, Quan D et al (2006) Preparation of polymeric micelles based on chitosan bearing a small amount of highly hydrophobic groups. Carbohydr Polym 66:514–520
65. Du Y-Z, Lu P et al (2010) Stearic acid grafted chitosan oligosaccharide micelle as a promising vector for gene delivery system: factors affecting the complexation. Int J Pharm 391:260–266
66. Du Y-Z, Wang L et al (2011) Linoleic acid-grafted chitosan oligosaccharide micelles for intracellular drug delivery and reverse drug resistance of tumor cells. Int J Biol Macromol 48(1):215–222
67. Du Y-Z, Wang L et al (2009) Preparation and characteristics of linoleic acid-grafted chitosan oligosaccharide micelles as a carrier for doxorubicin. Colloids Surf B 69:257–263
68. Ye Y-Q, Yang F-L et al (2008) Core-modified chitosan-based polymeric micelles for controlled release of doxorubicin. Int J Pharm 352:294–301
69. Li Q, Du Y-Z et al (2010) Synthesis of Lamivudine stearate and antiviral activity of stearic acid-g-chitosan oligosaccharide polymeric micelles delivery system. Eur J Pharm Sci 41:498–507
70. Hu F-Q, X-l Wu et al (2008) Cellular uptake and cytotoxicity of shell crosslinked stearic acid-grafted chitosan oligosaccharide micelles encapsulating doxorubicin. Eur J Pharm Biopharm 69:117–125
71. Zhang J, Chen XG et al (2010) Effect of molecular weight on the oleoyl-chitosan nanoparticles as carriers for doxorubicin. Colloids Surf B 77:125–130
72. Park K, Kim JH et al (2007) Effect of polymer molecular weight on the tumor targeting characteristics of self-assembled glycol chitosan nanoparticles. J Control Release 122:305–314
73. Kim JH, Kim YS et al (2008) Antitumor efficacy of cisplatin-loaded glycol chitosan nanoparticles in tumor-bearing mice. J Control Release 127:41–49
74. Hwang HY, Kim IS et al (2008) Tumor targetability and antitumor effect of docetaxel-loaded hydrophobically modified glycol chitosan nanoparticles. J Control Release 128:23–31
75. Park Y, Hong HY et al (2008) A new atherosclerotic lesion probe based on hydrophobically modified chitosan nanoparticles functionalized by the atherosclerotic plaque targeted peptides. J Control Release 128:217–223

76. Yu JM, Li YH et al (2008) Self-aggregated nanoparticles of cholesterol-modified glycol chitosan conjugate: Preparation, characterization, and preliminary assessment as a new drug delivery carrier. Eur Polym J 44:555–565
77. Liu Y, Tian F et al (2004) Synthesis and characterization of a brush-like copolymer of polylactide grafted onto chitosan. Carbohydr Res 339:845–851
78. Liu L, Li Y et al (2004) Synthesis and characterization of chitosan-graft-polycaprolactone copolymers. Eur Polym J 40:2739–2744
79. Wu H, Wang S et al (2011) Chitosan-polycaprolactone copolymer microspheres for transforming growth factor-[beta]1 delivery. Colloids Surf B 82:602–608
80. Duan K, Zhang X et al (2010) Fabrication of cationic nanomicelle from chitosan-graft-polycaprolactone as the carrier of 7-ethyl-10-hydroxy-camptothecin. Colloids Surf B 76:475–482
81. Gnanou Y (1996) Design and synthesis of new model polymers. J Macromol Sci, Rev Macromol Chem Phys C36:77–117
82. Zohuriaan-Mehr MJ (2005) Advances in chitin and chitosan modification through graft copolymerization: a comprehensive review. Iran Polym J 14:235–265
83. Liu L, Chen LX et al (2006) Self-catalysis of phthaloylchitosan for graft copolymerization of epsilon-caprolactone with chitosan. Macromol Rapid Commun 27:1988–1994
84. Liu L, Wang YS et al (2005) Preparation of chitosan-g-polycaprolactone copolymers through ring-opening polymerization of epsilon-caprolactone onto phthaloyl-protected chitosan. Biopolymers 78:163–170
85. Casettari L, Vllasaliu D et al (2010) Effect of PEGylation on the toxicity and permeability enhancement of chitosan. Biomacromolecules 11:2854–2865
86. Cai G, Jiang H et al (2009) A facile route for regioselective conjugation of organo-soluble polymers onto chitosan. Macromol Biosci 9:256–261
87. Yoksan R, Akashi M et al (2003) Controlled hydrophobic/hydrophilicity of chitosan for spheres without specific processing technique. Biopolymers 69:386–390
88. Gorochovceva N, Makuska R (2004) Synthesis and study of water-soluble chitosan-O-poly (ethylene glycol) graft copolymers. Eur Polym J 40:685–691
89. Zhou Y, Liedberg B et al (2007) Chitosan-N-poly (ethylene oxide) brush polymers for reduced nonspecific protein adsorption. J Colloid Interface Sci 305:62–71
90. Saito H, Wu XD et al (1997) Graft copolymers of poly(ethylene glycol) (PEG) and chitosan. Macromol Rapid Commun 18:547–550
91. Ouchi T, Nishizawa H et al (1998) Aggregation phenomenon of PEG-grafted chitosan in aqueous solution. Polymer 39:5171–5175
92. Liu L, Xu X et al (2009) Synthesis and self-assembly of chitosan-based copolymer with a pair of hydrophobic/hydrophilic grafts of polycaprolactone and poly(ethylene glycol). Carbohydr Polym 75:401–407
93. Lee J-Y, Nam S-H et al (2002) Enhanced bone formation by controlled growth factor delivery from chitosan-based biomaterials. J Control Release 78:187–197
94. Madhumathi K, Shalumon KT et al (2009) Wet chemical synthesis of chitosan hydrogel-hydroxyapatite composite membranes for tissue engineering applications. Int J Biol Macromol 45:12–15
95. Bhattarai N, Ramay HR et al (2005) PEG-grafted chitosan as an injectable thermosensitive hydrogel for sustained protein release. J Control Release 103:609–624
96. Kim MS, Choi YJ et al (2007) Synthesis and characterization of in situ chitosan-based hydrogel via grafting of carboxyethyl acrylate. J Biomed Mater Res A 83A:674–682
97. Poon YF, Cao Y et al (2010) Hydrogels based on dual curable chitosan-graft-polyethylene glycol-graft-methacrylate: application to layer-by-layer cell encapsulation. ACS Appl Mater Interfaces 2:2012–2025
98. Shi W, Ji Y et al (2010) Characterization of ph- and thermosensitive hydrogel as a vehicle for controlled protein delivery. J Pharm Sci 100(3):886–895

99. Lee SY, Pereira BP et al (2009) Unconfined compression properties of a porous poly(vinyl alcohol)-chitosan-based hydrogel after hydration. Acta Biomater 5:1919–1925
100. Liang Y, Liu WS et al (2011) An in situ formed biodegradable hydrogel for reconstruction of the corneal endothelium. Colloids Surf B 82:1–7
101. Tan HP, Chu CR et al (2009) Injectable in situ forming biodegradable chitosan-hyaluronic acid based hydrogels for cartilage tissue engineering. Biomaterials 30:2499–2506
102. Park KM, Lee SY et al (2009) Thermosensitive chitosan-pluronic hydrogel as an injectable cell delivery carrier for cartilage regeneration. Acta Biomater 5:1956–1965
103. Wang JY, Chen L et al (2009) Cell adhesion and accelerated detachment on the surface of temperature-sensitive chitosan and poly(N-isopropylacrylamide) hydrogels. J Mater Sci Mater Med 20:583–590
104. Verma IM, Somia N (1997) Gene therapy – promises, problems and prospects. Nature 389:239–242
105. Rolland A, Felgner PL (1998) Non-viral gene delivery systems – preface. Adv Drug Deliv Rev 30:1–3
106. Mao SR, Sun W et al (2010) Chitosan-based formulations for delivery of DNA and siRNA. Adv Drug Deliv Rev 62:12–27
107. Han HD, Mangala LS et al (2010) Targeted gene silencing using RGD-labeled chitosan nanoparticles. Clin Cancer Res 16:3910–3922
108. Howard KA, Rahbek UL et al (2006) RNA interference in vitro and in vivo using a chitosan/siRNA nanoparticle system. Mol Ther 14:476–484
109. Katas H, Alpar HO (2006) Development and characterisation of chitosan nanoparticles for siRNA delivery. J Control Release 115:216–225
110. Csaba N, Koping-Hoggard M et al (2009) Ionically crosslinked chitosan/tripolyphosphate nanoparticles for oligonucleotide and plasmid DNA delivery. Int J Pharm 382:205–214
111. Thibault M, Nimesh S et al (2010) Intracellular trafficking and decondensation kinetics of chitosan-pDNA polyplexes. Mol Ther 18:1787–1795
112. Liu X, Howard KA et al (2007) The influence of polymeric properties on chitosan/siRNA nanoparticle formulation and gene silencing. Biomaterials 28:1280–1288
113. Zhao X, Yu SB et al (2006) Transfection of primary chondrocytes using chitosan-pEGFP nanoparticles. J Control Release 112:223–228
114. Lai WF, Lin MCM (2009) Nucleic acid delivery with chitosan and its derivatives. J Control Release 134:158–168
115. Moreira C, Oliveira H et al (2009) Improving chitosan-mediated gene transfer by the introduction of intracellular buffering moieties into the chitosan backbone. Acta Biomater 5:2995–3006
116. Torchilin VP (2007) Nanocarriers. Pharmaceut Res 24:2333–2334
117. Hombach J, Hoyer H et al (2008) Thiolated chitosans: development and in vitro evaluation of an oral tobramycin sulphate delivery system. Eur J Pharm Sci 33:1–8
118. Saravanakumar G, Min KH et al (2009) Hydrotropic oligomer-conjugated glycol chitosan as a carrier of paclitaxel: Synthesis, characterization, and in vivo biodistribution. J Control Release 140:210–217
119. Rekha MR, Sharma CP (2009) Synthesis and evaluation of lauryl succinyl chitosan particles towards oral insulin delivery and absorption. J Control Release 135:144–151
120. Kim J-H, Kim Y-S et al (2006) Hydrophobically modified glycol chitosan nanoparticles as carriers for paclitaxel. J Control Release 111:228–234
121. Ngawhirunpat T, Wonglertnirant N et al (2009) Incorporation methods for cholic acid chitosan-g-mPEG self-assembly micellar system containing camptothecin. Colloids Surf B 74:253–259
122. Wang Y, Tu S et al (2010) Cholesterol succinyl chitosan anchored liposomes: preparation, characterization, physical stability, and drug release behavior. Nanomed Nanotechnol Biol Med 6:471–477

123. Zhou Y-Y, Du Y-Z et al (2010) Preparation and pharmacodynamics of stearic acid and poly (lactic-co-glycolic acid) grafted chitosan oligosaccharide micelles for 10-hydroxycamptothecin. Int J Pharm 393:144–152
124. Hu F-Q, Meng P et al (2008) PEGylated chitosan-based polymer micelle as an intracellular delivery carrier for anti-tumor targeting therapy. Eur J Pharm Biopharm 70:749–757
125. Bian F, Jia L et al (2009) Self-assembled micelles of N-phthaloylchitosan-g-polyvinylpyrrolidone for drug delivery. Carbohydr Polym 76:454–459
126. Chen C, Cai GQ et al (2011) Chitosan-poly(epsilon-caprolactone)-poly(ethylene glycol) graft copolymers: synthesis, self-assembly, and drug release behavior. J Biomed Mater Res A 96A:116–124
127. Cai G, Jiang H et al (2009) Synthesis, characterization and self-assemble behavior of chitosan-O-poly([epsilon]-caprolactone). Eur Polym J 45:1674–1680
128. Lu Y, Liu L et al (2007) Novel amphiphilic ternary polysaccharide derivates chitosan-g-PCL-b-MPEG: synthesis, characterization, and aggregation in aqueous solution. Biopolymers 86:403–408
129. Yan JH, Yang L et al (2010) Biocompatibility evaluation of chitosan-based injectable hydrogels for the culturing mice mesenchymal stem cells in vitro. J Biomater Appl 24:625–637
130. Qi B, Yu A et al (2010) The preparation and cytocompatibility of injectable thermosensitive chitosan/poly(vinyl alcohol) hydrogel. J Huazhong Univ Sci Technolog Med Sci 30:89–93
131. Crompton KE, Prankerd RJ et al (2005) Morphology and gelation of thermosensitive chitosan hydrogels. Biophys Chem 117:47–53
132. Ruel-Gariepy E, Shive M et al (2004) A thermosensitive chitosan-based hydrogel for the local delivery of paclitaxel. Eur J Pharm Biopharm 57:53–63
133. Ruel-Gariepy E, Chenite A et al (2000) Characterization of thermosensitive chitosan gels for the sustained delivery of drugs. Int J Pharm 203:89–98
134. Kim S, Nishimoto SK et al (2010) A chitosan/beta-glycerophosphate thermo-sensitive gel for the delivery of ellagic acid for the treatment of brain cancer. Biomaterials 31:4157–66
135. Chenite A, Chaput C et al (2000) Novel injectable neutral solutions of chitosan form biodegradable gels in situ. Biomaterials 21:2155–2161
136. Song K, Qiao M et al (2010) Preparation, fabrication and biocompatibility of novel injectable temperature-sensitive chitosan/glycerophosphate/collagen hydrogels. J Mater Sci Mater Med 21:2835–42
137. Crompton KE, Goud JD et al (2007) Polylysine-functionalised thermoresponsive chitosan hydrogel for neural tissue engineering. Biomaterials 28:441–449
138. Crompton KE, Tomas D et al (2006) Inflammatory response on injection of chitosan/GP to the brain. J Mater Sci Mater Med 17:633–9
139. Zheng L, Ao Q et al (2010) Evaluation of the chitosan/glycerol-beta-phosphate disodium salt hydrogel application in peripheral nerve regeneration. Biomed Mater 5:35003
140. Lu S, Wang H et al (2010) Both the transplantation of somatic cell nuclear transfer- and fertilization-derived mouse embryonic stem cells with temperature-responsive chitosan hydrogel improve myocardial performance in infarcted rat hearts. Tissue Eng A 16:1303–15
141. Wang H, Zhang X et al (2010) Improved myocardial performance in infarcted rat heart by co-injection of basic fibroblast growth factor with temperature-responsive chitosan hydrogel. J Heart Lung Transplant 29:881–7
142. Zuidema JM, Pap MM et al (2010) Fabrication and characterization of tunable polysaccharide hydrogel blends for neural repair. Acta Biomater 7(4):1634–1643
143. Ngoenkam J, Faikrua A et al (2010) Potential of an injectable chitosan/starch/beta-glycerol phosphate hydrogel for sustaining normal chondrocyte function. Int J Pharm 391:115–24
144. Sung JH, Hwang MR et al (2010) Gel characterisation and in vivo evaluation of minocycline-loaded wound dressing with enhanced wound healing using polyvinyl alcohol and chitosan. Int J Pharm 392:232–40

145. Tang Y, Du Y et al (2009) A thermosensitive chitosan/poly(vinyl alcohol) hydrogel containing hydroxyapatite for protein delivery. J Biomed Mater Res A 91:953–63
146. Kim IY, Seo SJ et al (2008) Chitosan and its derivatives for tissue engineering applications. Biotechnol Adv 26:1–21
147. Wu ZM, Zhang XG et al (2009) Disulfide-crosslinked chitosan hydrogel for cell viability and controlled protein release. Eur J Pharm Sci 37:198–206
148. Liang Y, Liu W et al (2011) An in situ formed biodegradable hydrogel for reconstruction of the corneal endothelium. Colloids Surf B Biointerfaces 82:1–7

Chitosan: A Promising Biomaterial for Tissue Engineering Scaffolds

P.K. Dutta, Kumari Rinki, and Joydeep Dutta

Abstract The contribution of chitosan as a scaffold material is quite significant in the field of tissue engineering, which is a multidisciplinary field of research and technology development requiring the involvement of chemists, physicists, chemical engineers, biologists, cell-biologists etc. to regenerate injured or damaged tissue. The advantages of using chitosan as a three-dimensional scaffold for tissue engineering applications are due to its versatile physicochemical and biological properties. Further, owing to its easy processability, it can be molded into the desired shape and size. Therefore, it is no exaggeration to say that chitosan is a promising biomaterial for tissue engineering scaffolds. There is an enormous body of work already published in various journals on chitosan as a tissue engineering scaffold but, to our knowledge, this work has not yet been brought together in one chapter. We have used our best efforts to accumulate the research work already done on chitosan in a single place so that chitosan researchers can easily find information and can therefore escalate their research activities. This chapter highlights different methods for the fabrication of scaffolds, the suitability of chitosan as a good scaffolding material, and its application as a scaffold for tissue engineering of bone, cartilage, skin, liver, corneal, vascular, nerve, and cardiac tissue.

Keywords Bone · Chitosan · Nerve · Scaffolds · Skin · Tissue engineering

---

P.K. Dutta (✉) and K. Rinki
Department of Chemistry, Motilal Nehru National Institute of Technology, Allahabad 211004, India
e-mail: pkd_437@yahoo.com

J. Dutta
Department of Chemistry, Disha Institute of Management and Technology, Raipur 492101, India

Contents

1 Introduction 46
2 Scaffolds 47
   2.1 Factors Governing the Design of Scaffolds 47
   2.2 Scaffold Fabrication Techniques 49
3 Chitosan as a Scaffolding Material 52
   3.1 Structural Analysis and Characterization of Chitosan 53
   3.2 Role of Molecular Weight and Degree of Deacetylation 53
4 Application of Chitosan for Regeneration of Various
   Types of Tissue 54
   4.1 Skin Tissue 54
   4.2 Bone and Cartilage Tissue 57
   4.3 Liver Tissue 57
   4.4 Cardiac Tissue 62
   4.5 Vascular Tissue 62
   4.6 Corneal Tissue 68
   4.7 Nerve Tissue 68
   4.8 Some Other Applications 72
5 Conclusions 72
References 72

1 Introduction

A look at the world population reveals that the most common chronic problem associated with man is loss of tissue and organ damage. This can be cured by organ transplantation using tissue engineering techniques. The main problem associated with organ transplantation is shortage of suitable donors. This circumstance demands the need of a suitable scaffold wherein autologous cells can be grown under optimum conditions in vitro and subsequently transplanted back into the human body. This will obviate the need to wait for a donor and, on the other hand, will also increase the patients' comfort and compliance. The very fundamental of tissue engineering is the requirement for a scaffold material with specific characteristics that provides a temporary artificial matrix for cell seeding [1]. One of the most important characteristics of a scaffold material is that it should provide an ideal site for cell attachment and proliferation, leading to further tissue engineering. The extracellular matrix (ECM) not only provides the physical support for cells but also regulates their proliferation and differentiation. Therefore, scaffolds need to be developed for sustaining in vitro tissue reconstruction as well as for in vivo cell-mediated tissue regeneration. Repair of tissue defects can only be possible if the cells are supplied with such an ECM substitute [2]. A scaffold is a support, either natural or artificial, that maintains tissue contour. Substances that are frequently used for scaffold preparation are natural polymers, synthetic polymers, or ceramics with adsorbed proteins or immobilized functional groups [3]. Natural polymers have drawn the attention of various researchers because of their outstanding biocompatibility properties. Biodegradable materials have gained more attention because they have the advantage of allowing new tissue to take over their load-bearing or other functions without creating any potential chronic problems associated with the presence of biostable implants [4]. The paradigm of tissue engineering consists of seeding cells on a scaffold made of either a synthetic or natural polymer blend, maturing the tissue in vitro, and finally implanting the construct at the desired site in the patient as an artificial prosthesis [5, 6]. Overall, the strategy of tissue engineering [7] generally involves the following steps:

1. Identify, isolate, and produce an appropriate cell source in sufficient amount
2. Synthesize a scaffold with the desired shape and dimension, which will subsequently be used as a cell carrier
3. Seed the cells uniformly onto or into the carrier and incubate for a predetermined time in a bioreactor
4. Implant the cell-seeded carrier in a proper animal model. Depending on the site and the structure, vascularization may be necessary

2 Scaffolds

Tissue scaffolds are synthetic bioresorbable polymers that act as functional substitutes for missing or malfunctioning human tissues and organ. The primary role of a scaffold is to provide a temporary substrate to which the transplanted cells can adhere [8]. The most important factors to be considered with respect to nutrient supply to transplanted and regenerated cells are porosity, pore size and pore structure for porous scaffolds with a large surface-area-to volume ratio, and void volume. Optimization of these parameters is desirable for attachment, growth, maximal cell seeding, ECM production, and vascularization. Pores of the same diameter are preferable in scaffolds in order to yield high surface area per volume, provided the pore size is greater than the diameter of a cell in suspension [1, 2].

Thus, scaffolds provide physical support to cells, and pores provide space for remodeling of tissue structures. The major challenge associated with the development of scaffolds is the organization of cells and tissue in a three-dimensional (3D) configuration so that molecular signals are presented in an appropriate spatial and temporal fashion in a common manner that promotes the individual cells to grow and form the desired tissue structures [9, 10].

2.1 Factors Governing the Design of Scaffolds

During design of a scaffold for real-life applications, we must pay attention in choosing the scaffold material, body acceptability, mechanical properties, surface chemistry, and porosity. The porosity, morphology, and mechanical strength of scaffolds are governed by various factors. Some of the factors governing the designing of scaffolds are discussed below.

2.1.1 Materials

During design of scaffolds for tissue engineering applications, one must emphasize the selection of suitable materials. The materials should be biocompatible and biodegradable (i.e., they can be degraded into harmless products, leaving the desired living tissue). Some of the materials used for fabricating scaffolds include natural polymers, synthetic polymers, ceramics, metals, and hybrids of these materials [11]. Metals and ceramics are not a good choice for tissue engineering applications because they are not biodegradable (except for bioceramics such as α-tricalcium phosphate and β-tricalcium phosphate) and because their processability is very limited. For these reasons, natural polymers have gained increased attention because they are biodegradable and biocompatible. One of the major drawbacks exhibited by scaffolds made up of natural polymers is their poor mechanical properties. These problems associated with natural polymers can be circumvented by using synthetic resorbable polymers such as poly(α-hydroxy esters), polyanhydrides, polyorthoesters, and polyphosphazens. Polyglycolic acid (PGA), polylactic acid (PLA), polydioxanone, and copolymers thereof are the only FDA-approved synthetic and degradable polymers.

2.1.2 Porosity and Surface Area

Scaffolds should be highly porous and the pores should be interconnected to favor tissue integration and vascularization. Scaffolds should have appropriate surface chemistry to provide the necessary initial support for the attachment and proliferation of cells, and for the retention of their differentiated functions [12]. The porosity and pore size of the scaffold play crucial roles in the regeneration of a specific tissue. For instance, scaffolds with pore size less than 150 μm have been successfully used for regeneration of skin in burn patients [13]. Angiogenesis is a requirement for some scaffold application scenarios and can be unpleasantly affected by material porosity. Pore morphology can also affect scaffold degradation kinetics and the mechanical properties of the developing tissue [14]. The degree of interconnectivity has a greater influence on osteoconduction than does the actual pore size [15]. Highly porous materials facilitate the easy diffusion of nutrients to, and waste products from, the implant. Similarly, the larger the surface area of the scaffold, the more it favors cell attachment and growth [16].

2.1.3 Mechanical Properties and Processability

The scaffold should possess good mechanical strength so that it can be used for the reconstruction of hard, load-bearing tissues such as bone and cartilage. The biomaterial should be easily processed so that it can be easily fabricated into different shapes and sizes to meet the needs of the desired tissue reconstruction. The scaffold's architecture plays a vital role in maintaining its dimensional stability [15].

The scaffolds should have sufficient structural integrity that matches the mechanical properties of native tissue [17]. The external shape of the scaffold is also extremely important from the clinical point of view because the final anatomical shape of a regenerated tissue is basically dependent on the shape of the associated scaffold [18]. The mechanical properties of scaffold in tissue-engineering applications are of great importance due to the necessity of the structural stability to withstand stress incurred during culturing in vitro and implanting in vivo. In addition, the mechanical properties can significantly affect the specific biological functions of cells within the engineered tissue [19].

2.2 Scaffold Fabrication Techniques

Scaffolds can be fabricated by using different types of methodologies such as fiber bonding, salt leaching, gas-induced foaming, phase separation, electrospinning, solid freeform fabrication, and molecular self assembly [15, 17]. Some of the fabrication techniques are discussed below.

2.2.1 Salt Leaching

Salt leaching is one of the simplest fabrication methods for producing scaffolds with controllable porosity and pore size using various biodegradable polymers. The process for the manufacture of solid polymer–porogen constructs consists of combination of a suitable porogen with a solution of polymer in an appropriate mold. The porogen is then leached out to form porous sponges [20]. The traditional methods generally employ a solid porogen within a 3D polymer matrix to create well-defined pore size, pore structure, and total scaffold porosity. Murphy et al. [21] has introduced a modified method for producing porous, biodegradable tissue engineering scaffolds with improved pore interconnectivity. They fabricated a 3D porous scaffold by using a copolymer of 85:15 poly(lactide-*co*-glycolide) (PLG) via a solvent casting and particulate leaching process. They partially fused the NaCl crystals via treatment in 95% humidity to create the interconnecting pores, prior to the formation of a 3D polymer scaffold. This technique allows scaffolds for tissue engineering to be formed with minimal laboratory equipment and polymer amounts. Several recent modifications to this method demonstrate the tremendous pace of improvement in the manufacture of scaffolds with precise chemical, physical, and biological properties.

2.2.2 Phase Separation

Phase separation is one of the most popular techniques for fabricating porous scaffolds for tissue engineering applications. In this process, phase separation is induced by decreasing the temperature of a polymer solution, which results into two different phases, one having a high polymer concentration (polymer-rich phase) and one having a low polymer concentration (polymer-lean phase). The solvent from the polymer-lean phase is later removed by extraction, evaporation, or sublimation to leave behind open pores. The polymer in the polymer-rich phase solidifies into the skeleton of the polymer foam. This separation can be categorized into two types on the basis of the crystallization temperature of the solvent in the polymer solution. One type is solid–liquid phase separation and the other is liquid–liquid phase separation. When the solvent crystallization temperature is higher than the liquid–liquid phase separation temperature, then it can be separated by lowering the temperature and the process is known as solid–liquid phase separation. This process consists of crystallization of solvent, and the polymer is expelled from the solvent crystallization front. However, when the solvent crystallization temperature is much lower than the phase separation temperature, a liquid–liquid phase separation takes place on decreasing the temperature of the polymer solution. Phase separation is relatively a simple technique for the fabrication of scaffolds having highly organized structures [22].

2.2.3 Solid Freeform Fabrication

Control over internal architecture and interconnectivity is a tough task for researchers. These days, the solid freeform technique (SFF) has attracted the attention of researchers. SFF is a collective term for a group of techniques that can rapidly produce highly complex 3D physical objects using data generated by computer-aided design (CAD) systems, computer-based medical imaging modalities, digitizers, and other data makers. The technique involves in the manufacture of objects in a layer-by-layer fashion from the 3D computer design of the object [23]. Some of the advantages [24] of using SFF technique are listed below:

- In SFF scaffolds, the 3D interconnection of the scaffold can be maintained at a wide porosity level
- Using computerized tomography (CT) or magnetic resonance image (MRI) as the data source, scaffolds can be made with an external geometry conforming to the patients' anatomic structure, and thus the external geometry of the scaffolds can also be designed and customized to fulfill the need of the tissue engineer to construct scaffolds for specific tissues
- Scaffolds with a distinct material and design domain can be fabricated by using SFF techniques

Finite element analysis (FEA) and CAD can be combined with manufacturing technologies such as SFF to allow virtual design, characterization, and production of scaffold that is optimized for tissue replacement. This makes it possible to design and manufacture very complex tissue scaffold structures with functional components that are difficult to fabricate.

2.2.4 Supercritical Fluid Drying

Recently, various types of supercritical fluid processing methods have been developed for the production of microparticles, foams, fibers, and aerogels [25–27]. Fabrication of scaffolds using supercritical fluid has been reported recently by several researchers [28–30]. The rapid expansion of supercritical solutions (RESS) and the gas anti-solvent technique (GAS) are widely used for the formation of microparticles and fibers. In RESS, a supercritical solution is rapidly expanded, which leads to a rapid decrease of the polymer solubility in the supercritical fluid (SCF) and, finally, to the formation of microparticles or nanoparticles with narrow size distribution. In GAS, a polymer solution is expanded into a SCF, which acts as an anti-solvent since it is not miscible with polymer but is miscible with the organic solvent. Because the solvent is miscible with the SCF, it expands, resulting in the reduction of solvent capacity to support polymer dissolution [25]. The author's laboratory [29, 30] have prepared chitosan scaffolds using supercritical carbon dioxide (scCO$_2$). In the first step, the hydrogels were prepared and treated with organic solvent(s) and then placed in the chamber of a supercritical fluid reactor to undergo solvent exchange. Thereafter, the temperature and pressure were raised. Thus, the continuous flow of scCO$_2$ through the sample replaced all the organic solvent with CO$_2$ to obtain a porous chitosan scaffold.

2.2.5 Hydrothermal Preparation

The use of a hydrothermal bomb for preparation of a metal organic framework is a well-known technique in inorganic chemistry [31]. However, the use of a hydrothermal bomb for the preparation of scaffold is very rare. The final mixture with the appropriate composition for scaffold preparation is sealed in a PTFE-lined acid digestion bomb and heated at 40°C for 8 h under autogeneous pressure. After that, the bomb is kept at room temperature to cool the product, which is then frozen at −20°C. Finally, the product is vacuum dried to obtain the desired scaffolds [32–34] (Dutta PK et al., unpublished results).

2.2.6 Electrospinning

Another important scaffold fabrication technique is that of electrospun nanofibers. Electrospun nanofibers could be used to mimic the nanofibrous structure of the ECM in native tissue [35–37]. Electrospinning involves the ejection of a charged polymer fluid onto an oppositely charged surface. This technique is used to create polymeric fibers with diameters in the nanometer range. In electrospinning, a charge is applied to a polymer solution or melt, which is ejected toward an oppositely charged target. The body of the polymer solution or melt becomes charged, and electrostatic repulsion counteracts the surface tension so the droplets become stretched. At a critical point, a stream of liquid erupts from the surface. This point of eruption is known as the "Taylor cone." When the applied voltage is increased beyond a threshold value, the electric forces in the droplet overcome the opposing surface tension forces and a narrow charged jet is ejected from the tip of the Taylor cone [38]. The commonly used polymers for the electrospinning method of fabrication are the aliphatic polyesters [39]. Preparation of chitosan scaffolds by electrospinning has been mentioned by various researchers [37, 40–42]. Duan et al. [43] developed a nanofibrous composite membrane of poly(lactide-*co*-glycolic acid) (PLGA)–chitosan/poly(vinyl alcohol) (PVA) by simultaneous electrospinning of PLGA and chitosan/PVA from two different syringes and mixing on a rotating drum to prepare a nanofibrous composite membrane, which was then crosslinked with glutaraldehyde (GA). The obtained composite membrane was cytocompatible for fibroblastic cells.

3 Chitosan as a Scaffolding Material

Among the naturally derived polymers such as gelatin, collagens, glycosaminoglycan (GAG), starch, and alginate, chitosan, a partially deacetylated derivative of chitin, is chemically similar to GAG and has many desirable properties that make it a suitable candidate for use as a tissue engineering scaffold. Fabricating the hybrid scaffolds by combining natural polymers with synthetic polymers and ceramics is the best method, because the hybrid scaffolds possess both the mechanical strength of synthetic polymers and the biodegradability of natural polymers [15].

The principal derivative of chitin, chitosan, has gained more attention as a scaffold in tissue regeneration due to: (1) the possibility of large scale production and low cost; (2) its positively charged and reactive functional groups that enable it to form complexes with anionic polymers, including proteins that help to regulate cellular activity, [44]; and (3) its antibacterial properties [45]. Apart from this, chitosan is hemocompatible and non-immunogenic, and is degradable into non-toxic oligosaccharides inside the body due to the action of lysozymes. But, chitosan lacks the tensile strength required to match that of several natural tissues [46, 47]. It has been reported that chitosan-based biomaterials do not lead to any inflammatory or allergic reaction following implantation, injection, topical application, or ingestion in the human body [48]. Chitosan possesses wound-healing properties and favors both soft and hard tissue regeneration [49, 50]. By contrast, many synthetic polymers exhibit physicochemical and mechanical properties comparable to those of the biological tissues that they are required to substitute, but are not sufficiently bioactive [51]. Polyesters such as PLA, PLGA, and polycaprolactone (PCL) can be reproduced with specific molecular weights, block structures, degradable linkages, and crosslinking modes, and have excellent mechanical strength [52, 53]. Thus, the lack of mechanical strength of chitosan scaffolds can be resolved by incorporation of inorganic materials so that the hybrid material possesses improved mechanical and biological properties. Many inorganic materials such as calcium carbonate, calcium phosphate, and silica have been studied for the preparation of chitosan–inorganic composites [54].

3.1 Structural Analysis and Characterization of Chitosan

The structure of chitosan plays an important role if it is to serve as a scaffold material for application in tissue engineering. The biocompatibility of chitosan is attributed to its chemical properties. The polysaccharide unit of chitosan resembles the structure of GAGs, which are a major component of ECM of bone and cartilage and, hence, chitosan could be an attractive candidate for an ECM substitute [55]. The cationic nature of chitosan facilitates pH-dependent electrostatic interaction with anionic GAGs, proteoglycans, and other negatively charged molecules. This property is of particular interest in tissue engineering because it makes chitosan suitable in various shapes and sizes, i.e., porous scaffolds [14], planar membranes [56], and hydrogels [57], for specific interactions with growth factors, receptors, and adhesion proteins [58]. The cell adhesion, proliferation, and differentiation properties of chitosan are attributed to its hydrophilic nature, and its compact aggregated polymeric chains are helpful in providing stability to the scaffolds in terms of size and morphology during cell culture [59].

The physical and mechanical properties of chitosan can be ameliorated by using graft copolymerization and crosslinking. Chitosan forms aldimines and ketimines with aldehydes and ketones, respectively. Upon hydrogenation with simple aldehydes, chitosan produces N-alkyl chitosan [60]. The physicochemical and biological properties [61] as well as conformational structures [62] of chitosan are very effective for biomedical applications.

3.2 Role of Molecular Weight and Degree of Deacetylation

The molecular weight (Mw) and degree of deacetylation (DD) of chitosan play pivotal roles in dictating the biological properties of chitosan scaffolds. Notably, the DD itself influences many of the properties of chitosan, namely mechanical properties, biodegradability, immunological activity, wound-healing properties, and osteogenesis enhancement [63–71]. Chitosan scaffolds with higher DD showed higher cell proliferation, lower biodegradation rate, and higher mechanical strength. One of the studies in this direction was done by Hsu et al. [71]. They investigated the role of DD and Mw of chitosan in terms of hydrophilicity, degradation, mechanical properties, and biocompatibility by seeding fibroblastic cells and immortalized rat chondrocytes (IRC) on chitosan films of differing DD and Mw. They observed that in the chitosan films having similar Mw, the higher the DD of chitosan, the smaller was the elongation of chitosan films; with similar DD, a higher Mw led to higher tensile strength. The results of degradation studies showed that for chitosan with the higher average Mw, higher DD led to a higher degradation rate. However, the result for chitosan films with the lower average Mw was found to be opposite, i.e., higher DD led to slower degradation. The average Mw has also some significant effect on degradation rate. For chitosan films having similar DDs, higher average Mw led to the higher degradation rate. The acetyl group, $-NHCOCH_3$ of chitosan plays an important role in deciding the degradation rate. Chitosan with lower DD have more $-NHCOCH_3$ groups and might be more amorphous and degrade faster. The results showed that with the lower average Mw, lower DD led to higher degradation rate of chitosan films. They got the inference from their study that hydrophilicity and biocompatibility of chitosan films were affected by DD. However, the rate of degradation and the mechanical properties were found to be affected by Mw.

Another study in this direction was performed by Chatelet et al. [72]. They investigated the effect of DD on the biological properties of chitosan films by culturing keratinocytes and fibroblasts on chitosan films having different DDs. They found that DD has no significant effect on the in vitro cytocompatibility of chitosan films towards keratinocytes and fibroblasts. They demonstrated that the lower the DD of chitosan, the lower was the cell adhesion on the films, and found that keratinocyte proliferation increases when the DD of chitosan films increases. They concluded from their study that the DD plays a key role in cell adhesion and proliferation, but does not change the cytocompatibility of chitosan.

4 Application of Chitosan for Regeneration of Various Types of Tissue

Chitosan scaffolds may find application in regeneration of skin tissue, liver tissue, bone and cartilage tissue, cardiac tissue, corneal tissue, and vascular tissue to mention a few [73]. A brief account of its application in various branches of tissue engineering is described in this section.

4.1 Skin Tissue

Dermal wounds are very widespread in man. The skin damage can be caused by heat, chemicals, electricity, ultraviolet, nuclear energy, or disease. In the case of wounds that extend entirely through the dermis such as full-thickness burns or deep ulcers, as a result of many skin substitutes such as xenografts, allografts, and autografts have been employed for wound healing. However, the disadvantages of these approaches include the limited availability of skin grafts in severely burned patients and the problems of disease transmission and immune response [52, 53]. One of the good alternatives to skin grafts for curing skin damage is to develop a tissue-engineered skin equivalent. Polymeric tissue scaffolds made of PLGA, collagen, and chitosan are currently being employed for tissue reconstruction [74, 75]. An ideal scaffold for skin tissue engineering should possess the characteristics of excellent biocompatibility, suitable microstructure such as 100–200 μm mean pore size and porosity above 90%, controllable biodegradability, and suitable mechanical properties [76–78]. A brief account of work done by some researchers in the field of skin tissue engineering is given in Table 1.

There are complications in skin tissue engineering for cases of severe burn (third degree burns). Composite skin substitutes are applied to patients suffering from extensive burns, but slow cell ingrowths and insufficient vascularization has made it unreliable for curing the people suffering from third degree burns [81]. Consequently, some researchers are leaning towards the approach of tissue engineering, which utilizes both engineering and life science disciplines, to promote skin regeneration and to sustain and recover skin function [82].

In this direction, some good results-oriented data was reported by Liu et al. [81]. The work demonstrated the fabrication and effect of controlled-release of fibroblast growth factor (bFGF) from chitosan–gelatin microspheres (CGMSs) loaded with bFGF, where human fibroblasts were cultured on the chitosan–gelatin scaffold itself. The comparative study looked at cell morphology, cell proliferation, GAG synthesis, and gene expression with respect to loading of bFGF on the chitosan-gelatin scaffold. The DNA assay result indicated that the DNA content of human fibroblasts seeded on the scaffolds with and without bFGF-CGMS increased with culture time. The cell proliferation was 1.47 times higher over a period of 2 weeks on the scaffolds with bFGF-CGMS than on scaffolds without. GAG production was also higher on scaffolds with bFGF-CGMS than on the chitosan–gelatin scaffolds. Scanning electron microscopy (SEM) observations were also in accordance with the suitability of scaffolds containing bFGF for skin tissue engineering. They indicated that human fibroblasts attached and spread well on the scaffolds with bFGF-CGMS. Overall, the results indicated that chitosan–gelatin scaffolds with bFGF have a good potential as tissue engineering scaffolds to improve skin regeneration efficacy and to promote vascularization.

Very recently, Dhandayuthapani et al. [83] reported the development of novel chitosan–gelatin blend nanofiber systems for skin tissue engineering applications. In this study, they were able to electrospin defect-free chitosan, gelatin, and chitosan-gelatin blend nanofibers with smooth morphology and diameters of 120–200 nm, 100–150 nm, and 120–220 nm, respectively, by optimizing the process and solution parameters. Chitosan and gelatin formed completely miscible blends, as evidenced from differential scanning calorimetry (DSC) and Fourier transform infrared (FTIR) spectroscopy measurements. The tensile strength of the chitosan–gelatin blend nanofibers (37.91 ± 4.42 MPa) was significantly higher than that of the gelatin nanofibers (7.23 ± 1.15 MPa) ($p < 0.05$) and comparable with that of normal human skin.

Table 1 Work done in the field of skin tissue engineering

Matrix and its nature	Study conducted	Culture media	Observation	Conclusion	Name of researchers [Ref]
Nanofibrous composite membrane of PLGA–chitosan/PVA	Morphology, mechanical properties and cytocompatibility of the fibroblast cells	Isolated fibroblast dermal cells from rabbit back skin cultured into the composite membrane of PLGA–chitosan/PVA	Fibroblasts were attached on all the membranes and changed their original round shape to an elongated and spindle-like shape on all membranes. The crosslinked chitosan/PVA membrane showed a little activity	The electrospun PLGA–chitosan/PVA composite membranes combined the advantages of both PLGA and chitosan and would have a great potential for skin tissue engineering	Duan et al. [44]
Collagen/chitosan porous scaffolds prepared using a freeze-drying method	Morphology, the swelling capacity, as well as the in vitro and in vivo degradation of the scaffold crosslinked by different concentrations (0–0.25%) of GA	Human dermal fibroblasts seeded on GA-treated scaffold. In vivo animal tests were performed by embedding the scaffolds subcutaneously on the dorsal surface of rabbit ear	The collagen/chitosan scaffolds can effectively support and accelerate fibroblast infiltration from the surrounding tissue	All the in vitro and in vivo results proved that the GA-crosslinked collagen/chitosan scaffold is suitable for skin tissue engineering	Ma et al. [75]
Chitosan-pectin-TiO$_2$ ternary nanocomposite film	Cytotoxicity	Two cell lines, L929 mouse fibroblast cells and NIH3T3 mouse fibroblast cells, using the MTT assay	The viability assay was measured at 24 h and 48 h after cell seeding. The cell viability was more than 97% for NIH3T3. For L929 it was 100% after 24 h and 97% after 48 h	The MTT assay indicated that the cells grew very well after 48 h of exposure to ternary nanocomposite film. Therefore, ternary film can be considered a biocompatible product for wound healing	Dutta et al. [79]
Chitosan crosslinked with dimethyl 3-3', dithio bis (propionimidate) (CS-DTBP) or glutaraldehyde (CS-GA)	Cytotoxicity test	Human dermal fibroblast cells in the presence of leachate from different chitosan scaffolds (chitosan, CS-GA and CS-DTBP)	The number of cells that grew in the leachate from the CS-DTBP sample was significantly higher than the number of cells in the leachate from the CS-GA sample	DTBP-crosslinked chitosan is less toxic than CS-GA scaffolds	Adekogbe and Ghanem [80]

4.2 Bone and Cartilage Tissue

Scaffold serves as a temporary skeleton inserted into the sites of defective or lost bone to support and stimulate bone tissue regeneration while it gradually degrades and is replaced by new bone tissue [84–87]. Both bioactive ceramics and polymers are used as scaffolding materials. Bioceramics have chemical compositions resembling bone and they also allow osteogenesis. The major drawback of using bioceramics as scaffolding material are its brittle nature and low degradation rates. However, the biodegradation rates and mechanical properties of biopolymers can be tailored to a certain extent for specific applications. Biopolymers are particularly amenable for implantation and can be easily fabricated into desired shapes [15, 88]. Chitosan is widely used as scaffolding for the regeneration of bone tissue because of its osteocompatible and osteoconductive properties, and can enhance bone formation both in vitro and in vivo [51]. The scaffolds should possess excellent mechanical properties. The work done in the field of bone tissue engineering is outlined in Table 2.

As far as chitosan is concerned for cartilage tissue engineering applications, the rate of biodegradation of the scaffold (used to organize cells in vitro) plays a crucial role. The presence of non-biodegradable articles in soft tissue often causes acute foreign body reactions elicited by the body's immune system that can result in severe inflammation and soreness around the implant site. Many studies have reported that chitin and chitosan are biodegradable polymers and that they degrade in vivo mainly through their susceptibility to enzymatic hydrolysis mediated by lysozyme, which is ubiquitous in the human body. However, this action is dependent on factors such as pH, type of chitin or chitosan, and chitosan preparation method. The use of chitosan as scaffolding material for cartilage tissue has been reported by many researchers [2, 101, 102]. Composite chondroitin-6-sulfate/dermatan sulfate/chitosan scaffolds were reported to be used for articular cartilage regeneration [103]. A brief account of work done in cartilage tissue engineering is described in Table 3.

4.3 Liver Tissue

Liver is one of the most important and complex organs, serving several essential functions in the body. A biohybrid artificial liver using isolated hepatocytes and polymer scaffolds is expected to be an alternative method of treatment for liver failure because the shortage of suitable donors and costly surgical procedure has limited the use of liver transplantation. For this approach, various scaffolds have been used and it has been shown that the scaffolding material is crucial for control of cell adhesion, growth, and tissue reconstruction [107]. For the culture of anchorage-dependent cells such as hepatocytes, scaffolds require specific interaction with ECM components, growth factor, and the cell surface receptor to ensure cell survival, differentiation, and function [108]. This must be taken into account during

Table 2 Work done in the field of bone tissue engineering

Matrix and its nature	Study conducted	Culture media	Observation	Conclusion	Name of researchers [Ref]
Chitosan and alginate	Implantation of chitosan–alginate scaffolds into female Sprague-Dawley rats and cell viability test	MG63 osteoblast cells on chitosan–alginate scaffolds	In vitro study showed more calcium deposition after 28 days	The hybrid scaffold showed improved mechanical and biological properties	Li et al. [89]
Chitosan–hydroxyapatite (CS-HA) scaffold	Alkaline phosphate activity (ALP) and total protein content using commercially available kits	Primary human osteoblast (SAOS-2 cell line) incubated for 1 and 3 weeks	The CS-HA scaffold showed much faster cell growth. The cells seeded on the scaffold also expressed a distinct ALP activity	The CS-HA scaffold with excellent biocompatibility has the potential to serve for tissue engineering	Manjubala et al. [90]
Calcium phosphate–chitosan composite scaffold prepared by adding HA and calcium phosphate glass powder to chitosan and keeping it at −20°C for 4 days and then freeze-drying the frozen sample	Cell differentiation as assessed by total protein expression, ALP activity, and osteocalcin release measured spectrophotometrically	Human osteoblast-like MG63 cells on the composite scaffolds	The total protein content of the cells grown on the composite scaffolds increased faster with incubation time than that of the control	Calcium phosphate–chitosan composite scaffolds are suitable for bone tissue engineering	Zhang et al. [91]
3D chitosan/poly(lactic acid-glycolic acid) (PLAGA) composite porous scaffolds	Scaffold fabrication parameter and the cellular responses	Osteoblast-like MC3T3-E1 cells	Good proliferation, increased ALP activity of cells on the composite scaffolds and upregulated gene expression of ALP, osteopontin, and bone sialoprotein	Composite chitosan/PLAGA scaffolds showed excellent mechanical properties and bioactivity. Hence, they may serve as scaffolds for load-bearing bone tissue engineering	Jiang et al. [92]
Macroporous calcium phosphate cement (CPC)	The effect of chitosan on the mechanical properties of	Osteoblast mouse cells (MC3T3-E1)	Cell viability was quantified using an enzymatic assay	MC3T3-E1 cells were able to adhere, spread and	Xu et al. [93]

prepared by incorporating chitosan and mannitol with a series of powder-to-liquid ratios and a wide range of mannitol content	the scaffold and the composite mechanical properties, measured as a function of pore volume fraction up to 80% for the scaffold	on the CPC–chitosan scaffold	proliferate on CPC–chitosan	Kou et al. [94]
Genipin-crosslinked chitin–chitosan scaffolds with hydroxyapatite (HA)	Mechanical properties, various fabrication variables and cellular behavior	Bovine knee chondrocytes (BKC)	Higher chitin content gives larger porosity and Young's modulus, but lower extensibility	More HA deposition has a beneficial effect on the cellular amount, GAG content, and collagen
Genipin-crosslinked collagen–chitosan biodegradable porous scaffolds	Influence of chitosan amount and genipin concentration on the physicochemical properties of the scaffolds	Culture of rabbit chondrocytes in vitro	Good viability of the chondrocytes seeded on the scaffold	The scaffold formulation may be promising for articular cartilage	Yan et al. [95]
HA incorporated into chitosan scaffold by an in situ method	Biomimetic studies leading to cell proliferation	MC 3T3-E1 cells on the apatite layer, as formed on the two kinds of scaffolds	MC3T3-E1 cells on apatite-coated chitosan–nano-HA scaffolds showed better proliferation than on apatite-coated chitosan scaffolds	The addition of nano-HA to the chitosan scaffold improved its bone bioactivity, which could develop the use of chitosan in bone tissue engineering	Kong et al. [96]
Composite scaffolds by incorporating 80 wt% HA in the polyelectrolyte complex matrix of chitosan and poly(acrylic acid) (PAA) in the ratio 40:60	Bioactivity study was performed by seeding Human osteosarcoma (HOS) cells on the composite scaffolds. Cell viability was measured by MTT assay	–	Chitosan–PAA scaffolds incorporating HA showed better viability, cell attachment. and adhesion of HOS cells compared with the chitosan–PAA scaffold	Shailaja et al. [97]

(continued)

Table 2 (continued)

Matrix and its nature	Study conducted	Culture media	Observation	Conclusion	Name of researchers [Ref]
Chitosan sponges were prepared by freeze-drying, and then mineralized with calcium and phosphate solution using the double diffusion method, leading to the formation of HA nanocrystals on the surface of the scaffolds	Growth of osteoblast-like cells on biomimetic apatite-coated chitosan scaffolds and the influence of apatite nanocrystals on cells	Human osteoblast-like cell line (SaOS-2) for a period of 3 weeks on the mineralized scaffolds	The mineralized CS scaffolds and the pure CS scaffolds both showed a similar cell growth trend. The cells seeded on the mineralized scaffold showed a higher total protein content and higher ALP activity after 1 and 3 weeks of culture in comparison to those on the pure CS scaffolds	The presence of apatite nanocrystals in CS scaffolds has a good potential to serve for bone tissue engineering	Manjubala et al. [98]
Biphasic calcium phosphate (BCP) added to chitosan scaffolds	Influence of addition of BCP to porous chitosan scaffolds on the distribution, morphology, and phenotypic expression of osteoblastic cells	D1 ORL UVA mouse mesenchymal stem cells (MSCs) and MC3T3 E1 preosteoblastic cells on chitosan scaffold	Formation of more uniform and complete cells, ECM distribution on the BCP, significantly higher ALP activity and osteocalcin expression, and higher rate of migration for MC3T3 E1cells	Composite scaffolds for culture of MSCs and preosteoblasts enhance bone tissue development in vitro	Sendemir-Urkmez et al. [99]
Chitosan–silica hybrid membrane using a sol–gel process	In vitro cellular activity, in vivo bone regeneration ability, and the in vitro bone bioactivity test by immersing the hybrid and pure chitosan membranes in simulated body fluid	Osteoblastic cells, rat calvarial model to carry out in vivo study	Improved mechanical properties, excellent apatite-forming ability, good cellular responses of the hybrid membrane, and significantly higher rate of new bone regeneration	The enhanced properties of the hybrid membrane were attributed to incorporation of the rigid and bioactive silica xerogel into the hybrid membrane	Lee et al. [100]

Chitosan: A Promising Biomaterial for Tissue Engineering Scaffolds 61

Table 3 Work done in the field of cartilage tissue engineering

Matrix and its nature	Study conducted	Culture media	Observation	Conclusion	Name of researchers [Ref]
Porous poly(DL-lactide) (PDLLA)/chitosan scaffolds	Cell viability was measured using MTT assay	Rabbit chondrocytes seeded onto the PDLLA/chitosan scaffolds	Cells grown on PDLLA/chitosan scaffolds increased on increasing the weight ratio of the chitosan component, were able to preserve the phenotype of chondrocytes, and also supported the production of type II collagen	PDLLA/chitosan scaffolds are able to promote the attachment and proliferation of chondrocytes	Wu et al. [104]
Poly(L-lactide) (PLLA) microspheres using chitosan on the surface	Bioactivity study on control PLLA and the chitosan-coated PLLA microspheres by in vitro culture	Rabbit chondrocytes	Larger amount of chitosan-coated PLLA microspheres exhibited enhanced cell attachment and proliferation	Chitosan-coated PLLA microspheres may serve as injectable cell microcarriers for chondrogenesis in cartilage tissue	Lao et al. [105]
Composite scaffolds prepared by incorporating different amounts of PLGA microspheres into gelatin/chitosan/hyaluronan scaffolds by freeze-drying and crosslinking with 1-ethyl-3-(3-dimethyl aminopropyl) carbodiimide	The effects of incorporation of PLGA microspheres on porosity, compressive modulus, PBS uptake ratio, and weight loss of the scaffolds	In vitro culture of chondrocytes	Composite scaffolds having 50 wt% PLGA microspheres exhibited larger compressive moduli, lower weight loss, and good porosity (>90%). In vitro, these scaffolds had good cell attachment, viability, proliferation, and GAG secretion	Scaffolds with 50 wt% PLGA microspheres have better physical performance and preserved biocompatibility and can be used for chondrogenesis	Tan et al. [106]

the design and selection of polymeric materials for liver tissue-engineering. Calcium alginate sponge has been used for hepatocyte culture [109]. However, the alginate sponge is mechanically unstable due to ion exchange of Ca^{2+} with monovalent cations, and it lacks the cell-adhesive signals that are necessary to preserve long-term hepatocyte function and to suppress apoptosis. Application of chitosan scaffolds in liver tissue engineering is described in Table 4.

4.4 Cardiac Tissue

Myocardial infarction is one of the major public health concerns and the leading cause of death all over the world [118]. Human myocardium lacks the possibility of regeneration after myocardial infarction [119]. This results in a progressive loss of functional myocardium and a successive enlargement of the left ventricular cavity, thus impairing cardiac function [120]. The loss of viable myocardium is irreversible and, if extensive, could result in heart failure. The only available treatment of end-stage heart failure is heart transplantation. Shortage of donor hearts and immunological rejection of the transplanted tissue has limited transplantation to certain patients only. One good alternative for the treatment of heart failure is the replacement of damaged tissue with a tissue-engineered graft generated using cells and biodegradable scaffolds [121]. An ideal scaffold for cardiac tissue engineering should be (1) highly porous with large interconnected pores, (2) hydrophilic, (3) structurally stable, (4) degradable, and (5) elastic (to enable transmission of contractile forces) [122, 123]. The main focus of cardiac tissue engineering is on the development of 3D heart muscle that can be utilized to augment the function of failing myocardium. Table 5 gives glimpses of work done on cardiac tissue engineering applications.

4.5 Vascular Tissue

Vascular diseases, such as blood vessel damage, atherosclerosis, and aneurysms, remain an obstacle for clinicians because of limited donor sites and the immune response to allograft and xenograft. Tissue-engineered blood vessel is an optimal alternative for blood vessel substitution. Vascular transplantation has been commonly used for the treatment of vascular diseases. An ideal scaffold for vascular tissue engineering should use a biocompatible polymer with suitable degradation rate and biological qualities that interact favorably with blood and cells. A variety of biodegradable polymers, like poly(glycerol-sebacate), PLA or PLGA, as well as collagen and chitosan have been evaluated as scaffolds to support the regeneration of tissue-engineered vascular graft. More detail work in this direction is presented in Table 6.

Table 4 Application of chitosan scaffolds to liver tissue engineering

Matrix and its nature	Study made	Culture media	Observation	Conclusion	Name of researchers [Ref]
Hepatocyte-specific porous scaffold by using alginate/galactosylated chitosan (ALG-GC) sponge	Behavior of hepatocytes in ALG-GC sponges	Primary hepatocytes from ICR mouse (5- to 7-week-old male) isolated and seeded in ALG-GC sponge	Albumin secretion and ammonia elimination were higher in ALG-GC sponge than those in the alginate sponge	The ALG-GC sponge may be used as an efficient 3D hepatocyte culture system for liver-tissue engineering	Yang et al. [110]
Porous 3D scaffold of ALG-GC	Viability of hepatocytes in ALG-GC hybrid sponge with respect to the ALG sponge	Primary hepatocytes isolated from ICR mouse (5- to 7-week-old male) into the ALG-GC sponge	High viability of the hepatocytes was obtained for the ALG-GC sponge. However, within the ALG sponge, only a few cells formed spheroids	Hepatocyte enhancement of the scaffold and the mechanical properties of ALG sponge increased	Chung et al. [111]
Hepatocyte attachment into chitosan-alone scaffold and fructose-modified chitosan	Albumin secretion and urea synthesis in both of the scaffolds	Isolated hepatocytes from the liver of male Wistar rats were prepared by two-step collagenase perfusion according to the method of Seglen [112] and cultured on chitosan alone and on fructose-modified chitosan scaffolds	Fructose modification caused an increase in cellular interaction that formed cellular aggregates similar to those in vivo, and was beneficial to cell attachment and the albumin secretion rate. Urea synthesis rate of cells was higher	Fructose-induced surface cellular aggregates enhance liver-specific metabolic activity and improve cell density to a satisfactory level, and so would be helpful in the development of an artificial liver system	Li et al. [113]

(continued)

Table 4 (continued)

Matrix and its nature	Study made	Culture media	Observation	Conclusion	Name of researchers [Ref]
Galactosylated chitosan derivative	Development of synthetic ECM, which could control spreading, adhesion, and proliferation of hepatocyte attachment into chitosan-containing polystyrene (PS) dishes, poly(N-p-vinylbenzyl-4-o-β-D-galactopyranosyl-D-gluconamide) (PVLA)-coated PS dishes, and GC-coated PS dishes	Isolated hepatocytes from ICR mouse (5- to 7-week-old male)	Hepatocyte adhesion in GC-coated PS and PVLA-coated PS was found to be similar (94.7%) after 120 min incubation. Hepatocyte adhesion on the PVLA was facilitated by the galactose-specific interactions between asialoglycoprotein receptors (ASGR) of the hepatocytes and galactose residues of the PVLA	GC showed excellent adhesion and spheroid formation of hepatocytes due to the galactose-specific recognition between GC molecules and ASGR of hepatocytes and provides a good alternative as a synthetic ECM for liver tissue engineering	Park et al. [114]
Matrix composed of collagen and chitosan prepared by using crosslinking agent EDC in N-hydroxysuccinimide (NHS) and a 2-morpholinoethane sulfonic acid (MES) buffer system	Cytotoxicity	–	The cytotoxicity of the urea derivative was found to be quite low compared to that of EDC	Water-soluble EDC is non-toxic and biocompatible. It is not incorporated directly into the crosslinked sponge structure, but is changed to water-soluble urea derivatives	Wang et al. [115]

Highly porous chitosan–gelatin scaffolds by combining three different fabrication techniques, i.e., rapid prototyping, microreplication, and freeze-drying	Hydrophilicity and biodegradability of the scaffolds by performing swelling and degradation studies	Cellular activity of the scaffolds was evaluated by seeding hepatocytes onto the scaffolds	The porous chitosan–gelatin scaffold reveals that the hepatocytes attached well to the matrix and that it has excellent biocompatibility	Jiankang et al. [116]
Natural nanofibrous scaffolds by electrospinning of GC into nanofibers	Mechanical cell culture	Hepatocyte culture studies of nanofibrous scaffolds	Nanofibrous scaffolds showed suitable mechanical properties and slow degradation	
			Albumin secretion and urea synthesis indicated that the well-organized scaffolds were suitable for hepatocyte culture	
			Superior cell bioactivity with higher levels of liver-specific functions like albumin secretion, urea synthesis, and cytochrome P-450 enzyme activity	Feng et al. [117]

Table 5 Work done on cardiac tissue engineering applications

Product developed	Procedure adopted	Evaluation	Conclusion drawn	Name of researchers [Ref]
Functional cell-based cardiac pressure generating construct (CPGC) using chitosan as scaffolding material	Isolated primary cardiac cells from rat heart were plated on the surface of fibrin gels cast in 35-mm tissue culture dishes	CPGC showed intraluminal pressure spikes of 0.08 mm Hg and 0.05 mm Hg without and with electrical stimulation, respectively	The model may provide a pathway towards developing cell-based cardiac pumps	Birla et al. [124]
Porous chitosan scaffolds were prepared using the freeze-drying method and fibrinogen added to the scaffold before cell seeding, resulting in the formation of contractile construct	Chitosan poured into a mold was frozen at −80°C and lyophilized. Fibrinogen was added to the scaffold to begin the gelling process	The lower cell seeding densities, in the range of 1–2 million cells, resulted in the formation of smart material integrated heart muscle	A scaffold thickness of 200 μm was optimal for cardiac cell functionality. Histological results showed a fairly uniform cell distribution throughout the thickness of the scaffold	Blan et al. [125]
Chitosan–collagen composite	Isolated aortic valve endothelial cell (VEC) cultures and preferential adhesion to fibronectin, collagen types IV and I over laminin and osteopontin. Chitosan–collagen type IV films act as protein precoatings	The composite showed improved VEC growth and morphology in comparison to chitosan alone	Certain alteration in the properties of chitosan can improve amenability to valve tissue engineering applications	Cuy et al. [126]

Table 6 Work done in the field of vascular tissue engineering

Product developed	Procedure adopted	Evaluation	Conclusion drawn	Name of researchers [Ref]
PCL membranes modified by deposition of chitosan/heparin multilayer via the electrostatic self-assembly method	A novel ternary polysaccharide derivate, chitosan-g-PCL-b-PEG was prepared in order to immobilize chitosan and provide positive charges onto PCL	Blood compatibility of the control PCL and chitosan-g-PCL-b-PEG/heparin multilayer-deposited PCL membrane was measured using static platelet adhesion and plasma recalcification time experiments	Chitosan/heparin deposition could reduce platelet adhesion and prolong the plasma recalcification. Platelet adhesion and aggregation are thought to be a major mechanism by which biomaterial thrombogenicity is transduced	Liu et al. [127]
A chitosan-based tubular scaffold with a sandwich-like structure for blood vessel tissue engineering	A combination of thermally induced phase separation and an industrial knitting technique was used to produce a porous chitosan–gelatin complex	Cytocompatibity of scaffolds with endothelial cells and vascular smooth muscle cells (vSMCs)	Cellular proliferation studies showed that vSMCs grew and proliferated rapidly on the chitosan-based tubular scaffolds	Zhang et al. [128]
Novel human-like collagen (HLC)/chitosan tubular scaffolds to mimic blood vessel morphologically and mechanically	Scaffold prepared using crosslinking and freeze-drying processes	Human venous fibroblasts onto the HLC/chitosan scaffolds. In vivo, scaffolds were implanted into rabbit liver	Scaffolds provided a more suitable cell environment for cell secretion, more ECM, and showed superior biocompatibility in vitro and in vivo	Zhu et al. [129]
Chitosan/heparin composite	Macroscopically homogeneous chitosan/heparin blended suspension fabricated into composite films and porous scaffolds by an optimized procedure	Immobilization of heparin in the composite matrices (i.e., films and porous scaffolds) showed improved blood compatibility, as well as good mechanical properties and endothelial cell compatibility	Chitosan/heparin composite matrices are promising candidates for blood-contacting tissue engineering	He et al. [130]

4.6 Corneal Tissue

In the human body, the eye is the most delicate and remarkable organ. The cornea is the transparent part of the eye that covers the iris, pupil, and anterior chamber. It has five distinct anatomical layers. From anterior to posterior, the five layers are corneal epithelium, Bowman's layer, corneal stroma, Descemet's membrane, and corneal endothelium. Due to some hereditary diseases, infection, or injury, the cornea becomes opacified and results in loss of vision. According to the World Health Organization, over 10 million individuals are blinded from corneal scarring. Corneal transplantation is the best way to overcome this kind of defect. In the USA, more than 40,000 corneas are transplanted successfully each year. Most patients receiving a corneal transplant suffer from corneal scarring or decompensation due to keratoconus, bullous keratopathy, corneal scars from trauma, Fuchs endothelial dystrophy, and stromal corneal dystrophies such as lattice, granular, or macular dystrophy. In addition to these, in much of the developing world, religious and cultural factors, lack of general education, and the absence of eye banking facilities prevent widespread cadaveric donation for corneal transplantation, leading to the need for an alternative to cadaveric corneal transplantation. Thus, shortage of donor corneal tissue has drawn the attention of researchers towards keratoprosthesis for the treatment of corneal blindness. The ideal keratoprosthesis would be inert and not rejected by the patient's immune system, inexpensive, and maintain long-term clarity. In addition, it would be quick to implant, easy to examine, and allow an excellent view of the retina [131]. Due to its good optical transmittance, chitosan is widely used in corneal tissue engineering scaffolds and corneal regeneration; its transparency is above 85% at 400 nm [132]. Some more details of work in this field are given in Table 7.

4.7 Nerve Tissue

The nervous system plays a vital role in maintaining body functions. Nervous tissue is composed of two main cell types: neurons, which transmit impulses, and the neuralgia, which assist propagation of nerve impulses as well as provide nutrients to the neurons. The nervous system is a complex, sophisticated system that regulates and coordinates the basic functions and activities of our body. Overall, it plays the role of headmaster in giving instructions to all parts of the body. Yet the nervous system is complex and is vulnerable to various disorders. Nervous system disorders cause many diseases such as Alzheimer's disease, brain cancer and brain tumors, Meningitis, Parkinson's disease etc. In recent years, researchers are devoting efforts to cure these diseases by regenerating nervous tissue. Some studies showed that chitosan promotes survival and neurite outgrowth of neural cells in vitro [137–141]. In most of the studies, a nerve guidance conduit is employed for peripheral nerve regeneration. In general, a suitable material for peripheral nerve regeneration should possess the following properties [142, 143]:

Table 7 Work done in the field of corneal tissue engineering

Product developed	Procedure adopted	Evaluation	Conclusion drawn	Name of researchers [Ref]
A chitosan-based membrane made of hydroxypropyl chitosan, gelatin, and chondroitin sulfate	Cellular activity was studied by seeding rabbit corneal endothelial cells onto the hybrid membrane and measuring the biodegradability and biocompatibility (in vivo) by its implantation into rat muscle	Higher glucose permeability than natural human cornea, and the optical transparency of the membrane is similar to that of natural human cornea	The membrane was suitable for corneal endothelial cells to attach and grow. The hybrid membrane also showed good bioabsorption in vivo	Gao et al. [133]
Membranes of poly-D,L-lactic acid (PDLLA), PDLLA modified with collagen (PDLLA/collagen) and PDLLA modified with chitosan (PDLLA/chitosan) were transplanted onto alkali-burned corneas	Reepithelialization of each cornea with fluorescein staining, and histological changes such as corneal wound healing, inflammation, and collagen synthesis	Effect of different biomedical membranes on alkali-burned cornea was studied	Wound healing rate of the PDLLA/chitosan group was higher than in the other groups. PDLLA/chitosan promoted wound healing of alkali-burned corneas in vivo and also decreased scar tissue formation	Du et al. [134]
Hyaluronic-acid-immobilized chitosan (CS-HYA) films crosslinked with EDC	Contact angle, cellular activity of human corneal epithelial cells (HCECs) on films, and cell viability	CS-HYA films had slightly increased transparency and good water absorption capacity for corneal regeneration	CS-HYA films have higher cell viability than the chitosan films. Hence, the CS-HYA films may serve as a potential candidate material for corneal regeneration	Wang et al. [132]
Collagen/chitosan/sodium-hyaluronate (Col-CS-NaHA) complexes	Biocompatibility for corneal tissues on these complexes was measured by cultivating rabbit corneal cells	Feasibility of using Col-CS-NaHA complexes for corneal tissues	Col-CS-NaHA complex may serve as a suitable substrate for cultivating corneal cells and as a scaffold of tissue engineered cornea	Chen et al. [135]
Collagen/chitosan composite hydrogels as corneal implants stabilized by EDC and NHS or a hybrid of poly (ethylene glycol) dibutyraldehyde (PEG-DBA)/EDC/NHS	In vitro, by seeding human corneal epithelial cells (HCECs) and dorsal root ganglia onto the composite hydrogels. In vivo, by implanting the composite hydrogels within the skin of rat and into the pig cornea for 12 months	Optical properties, optimum mechanical properties and suturability, and permeability to glucose and albumin were evaluated	Composite hydrogels had excellent biocompatibility, with successful regeneration of host epithelium, stroma, and nerves	Rafat et al. [136]

1. It must be biocompatible
2. It must allow diffusion transport of nutrients while preventing external cells from entering the conduit
3. The material must be degraded slowly enough to maintain a stable support structure for the entire regeneration process, but it should not remain in the body much longer than needed to prevent later compression of the nerve
4. The material must be able to support cell adhesion and cell spreading on its surface

Chitosans have these biological properties and can serve as the main materials for artificial nerve conduits. Neural stem cells (NSCs) have drawn the interest of researchers because of their potential for neural regeneration [144]. Recently, Scanga et al. [145] reported that chitosan had the greatest surface amine content and the lowest equilibrium water content, which probably contributed to the greater viability of neural precursor cells (NPCs or stem and progenitor cells) as observed over 3 weeks in culture. Plating intact NPC colonies revealed greater cell migration on chitosan relative to the other hydrogels. Importantly, long-term cultures on chitosan showed no significant difference in total cell counts over time, suggesting no net cell growth. Together, these findings reveal chitosan as a promising material for the delivery of adult NPC cell-based therapies. Table 8 focuses on the development of chitosan-based biomaterials for neural tissue regeneration and neural stem cell implantation.

Table 8 Chitosan for neural tissue regeneration and neural stem cell implantation

Product developed	Procedure adopted	Evaluation	Conclusion drawn	Name of researchers [Ref]
Chitin and chitosan tubes	Chitin hydrogel tubes from chitosan solutions using acylation chemistry and mold cast techniques	Lumber dorsal root ganglion dissected from E9 White Rock chicks on chitin and chitosan films separately in a cell culture medium	Chitosan films showed more enhanced neutrite outgrowth than on chitin films	Frier et al. [146]
Porous chitosan scaffolds using different degrees of deacetylation	Buffalo embryonic stem-like (ES-like) cell culture	The polygonal buffalo ES-like cells proliferated well on 88% and 95% DD scaffolds	The scaffolds are promising for neural tissue regeneration and neural stem cell implantation	Thein-Han et al. [147]
Hybrid PCL/chitosan nanofibrous scaffolds	Culture of rat Schwann cells (RT4-D6PT2) on the PCL scaffolds and PCL/chitosan scaffolds	More cell proliferation on the PCL/chitosan scaffolds than on PCL-alone scaffolds	Hybrid scaffolds have more cell proliferation and are thus useful for peripheral nerve regeneration	Prabhakaran et al. [148]

(*continued*)

Table 8 (continued)

Product developed	Procedure adopted	Evaluation	Conclusion drawn	Name of researchers [Ref]
Porous tubular chitosan scaffolds	Novel method for synthesizing porous tubular chitosan scaffolds	Differentiated Neuro-2a cells grew along the oriented macrochannels and the interconnected micropores for beneficial nutrient diffusion and cell ingrowth to the scaffold's interior	Porous chitosan scaffolds with well-defined architectural features may serve as a promising material for nerve tissue engineering	Wang et al. [149]
Chitosan films with different degrees of acetylation (DA)	Neural cell compatibility of chitosan and N-acetylated chitosan using primary chick dorsal root ganglion neurons	Dependency of neural cell compatibility on DA. 0.5% acetylated chitosan films showed the greatest cell viability	Cell compatibility can be adjusted by amine content for the nervous tissue system	Frier et al. [150]
Porous composite nerve conduit of collagen and chitosan prepared by freeze-drying steam extrusion	In vitro culture studies by seeding retinal pigment epithelial cells on composite scaffolds	Cell proliferation study	Composite scaffolds promote the adhesion and proliferation of cells. Increase of chitosan content decreases cell proliferation slightly	Xiangmein et al. [151]
Chitosan as a scaffold for transplantation of bone marrow stromal cell (BMSC)-derived Schwann cells	In vivo studies by transplanting the chitosan sponge containing BMSC-derived Schwann cells into Wistar rats	Faster regeneration of axons in chitosan gel	Chitosan gel sponges with BMSC-derived Schwann cells for regeneration of peripheral nerves	Ishikawa et al. [152]
Chitosan gel sponge	Axonal regeneration of the rat sciatic nerve	–	Sponge may serve as an effective scaffold for axonal regeneration of the rat sciatic nerve	Ishikawa et al. [153]

4.8 Some Other Applications

Apart from the above use of chitosan as scaffolding material in tissue engineering, it also finds application in periodontal tissue engineering [154, 155] and disc tissue engineering [156]. The other uses of chitosan as scaffolding material may find applications in esophageal tissue, dental tissue and breast tissue for organ-specific tissue regeneration.

5 Conclusions

Among other natural polysaccharides, chitosan is a very promising and versatile biomaterial due to the ease with which this material can be manipulated to fit certain circumstances. This discovery has opened several avenues of thought concerning chitosan as a biopolymer for tissue engineering applications. The fundamental principles of tissue engineering are based on living cells, signal molecules, and scaffold. Tissue engineering involves repair of injured body parts and restores their functions by using laboratory-grown tissues, materials, and artificial implants. In this chapter, we have mainly concentrated on the selection of chitosan as scaffolding material and looked at different types of scaffold fabrication techniques as well as the factors governing the design of scaffolds for various tissue engineering applications. It is hoped that this article will act as a research guide for beginners on the use of chitosan as a scaffold for the regeneration of various types of tissues and organs. The description of methods for producing tissue engineering scaffolds may also be useful for practitioners to understand the physicochemical and biological properties of chitosan scaffolds in their real-life application.

Acknowledgments Authors gratefully acknowledged the financial assistance to KR in the form of Institute Research Fellowship from MNNIT, Allahabad and research funding to PKD from UGC, New Delhi. The RSC (London) -Research Fund Grant Award-2009 to PKD is also gratefully acknowledged.

References

1. Dutta J, Dutta PK, Rinki K et al (2008) Current research on chitin and chitosan for tissue engineering applications and future demands on bioproducts. In: Jayakumar R, Prabaharan M (eds) Current research and developments on chitin and chitosan in biomaterials science. Research Signpost, Trivandrum
2. Malafaya PB, Pedro AJ, Peterbauer A et al (2005) Chitosan particles agglomerated scaffolds for cartilage and osteochondral tissue engineering approaches with adipose tissue derived stem cells. J Mater Sci Mater Medicine 16:1077–1085
3. Glowacki J, Mizuno S (2008) Collagen scaffolds for tissue engineering. Biopolymers 89: 338–344

4. Wang M, Chen LJ, Weng J et al (2001) Manufacture and evaluation of bioactive and biodegradable materials and scaffolds for tissue engineering. J Mater Sci Mater Med 12:855–860
5. Hoerstrup SP, Lu L, Lysaght MJ et al (2004) Tissue engineering. In: Ratner BD, Hoffman AS, Schoen FJ et al (eds) Biomaterial science. Elsevier Academic, San Diego
6. Langer R, Vacanti JP (1993) Tissue engineering. Science 260:920–926
7. Ehrenfreund-Kleinman T, Golenser J, Domb AJ (2006) Polysachharide scaffolds for tissue engineering. In: Ma PX, Elisseeff J (eds) Scaffolding in tissue engineering. CRC, Boca Raton
8. Jagur-Grodzinski J (2003) Biomedical applications of polymers. e-polymers 012
9. Thein-Han WW, Kitiyanant Y, Mishra RDK (2008) Chitosan as scaffold matrix for tissue engineering. Mater Sci Technol 24:1062–1075
10. Duarte ARC, Mano JF, Reis RL (2009) Perspectives on supercritical fluid technology for 3D tissue engineering scaffold applications. J Bioact Compat Polym 24:385–400
11. Whang K, Healy E, Elenz DR (1999) Engineering bone regeneration with bioabsorbable scaffolds with novel microarchitecture. Tissue Eng 5:35–51
12. Verma P, Verma V, Ray AR (2005) Chitin and chitosan: chitosan as tissue engineering scaffolds. In: Dutta PK (ed) Chitin and chitosan: opportunities and challenges. SSM International Publication, Midnapore, West Bengal
13. O'Brien FJ, Harley BA, Yannas IV et al (2004) Influence of freezing rate on pore structure in freeze-dried collagen-GAG scaffolds. Biomaterials 25:1077–1086
14. Rinki K, Dutta J, Dutta PK (2007) Chitosan based scaffolds for tissue engineering applications. Asian Chitin J 3:69–78
15. Yang S, Leong K-F, Du Z et al (2001) The design of scaffolds for use in tissue engineering Part I Traditional factors. Tissue Eng 7:679–689
16. Chang BS, Lee C-K, Hong K-S et al (2000) Osteoconduction at porous hydroxyapatite with various pore configurations. Biomaterials 21:1291–1298
17. Shor L, Guceri S, Wen X et al (2007) Fabrication of three-dimensional polycaprolactone/hydroxyapatite tissue scaffolds and osteoblast-scaffold interactions *in vitro*. Biomaterials 28:5291–5297
18. Wu L, Jing D, Ding JA (2006) "room-temperature" injection molding/particulate leaching approach for fabrication of biodegradable three-dimensional porous scaffolds. Biomaterials 27:185–191
19. Ingber D, Karp S, Plopper G et al (1993) Mechanochemical transduction across extracellular matrix and through the cytoskeleton. In: Frangos JA, Ives CL (eds) Physical forces and the mammalian cell. Academic, San Diego
20. Tessmar JKV, Holland TA, Mikos AG (2006) Salt leaching for polymer scaffolds: laboratory-scale manufacture of cell carriers. In: Ma PX, Elisseeff J (eds) Scaffolding in tissue engineering. CRC, Boca Raton
21. Murphy WL, Dennis RG, Kileny JL et al (2002) Salt fusion: an approach to improve pore interconnectivity within tissue engineering scaffolds. Tissue Eng 8:43–52
22. Wang AJ, Cao WL, Gong K et al (2006) Controlling morphology and porosity of 3-D chitosan scaffolds produced by thermally induced phase separation technique. Asian Chitin J 2:69–78
23. Leong KF, Cheah CM, Chua CK (2003) Solid freeform fabrication of three-dimensional scaffolds for engineering replacement tissues and organs. Biomaterials 24:2363–2378
24. Sahai N (2010) Characterization of porous tissue scaffolds using computer aided tissue engineering. M Tech dissertation submitted to MNNIT, Allahabad
25. Partap S, Hebb AK, Rehman I et al (2007) Formation of porous natural-synthetic polymer composites using emulsion templating and supercritical fluid assisted impregnation. Polym Bull 58:849–860
26. Hu X, Lessery AJ (2006) Solid-state processing of polymer in the presence of supercritical carbon Dioxide. J Cell Plast 42:517–527
27. Rinki K, Dutta PK, Hunt AJ et al (2011) Chitosan aerogel exhibiting high surface area for biomedical applications: preparation, characterization and antibacterial study. Int J Polym Mater Article ID 553849 (GPOM-2010–0362.R1)

28. Sachlos E, Wahl DA, Triffitt JT et al (2008) The impact of critical point drying with liquid carbon dioxide on collagen-hydroxyapatite composite scaffolds. Acta Biomater 4: 1322–1331
29. Rinki K, Dutta PK (2008) Preparation of genipin crosslinked chitosan scaffolds using supercritical carbon dioxide (sc. CO_2). Asian Chitin J 4:43–48
30. Rinki K, Dutta PK, Hunt AJ et al (2009) Preparation of chitosan scaffolds using supercritical carbon dioxide. Macromol Symp 277:36–42
31. Wei X, Wang K, Chen J (2011) The functional inorganic composites. Prog Chem 23:42–52
32. Rinki K, Shipra T, Dutta PK et al (2009) Direct chitosan scaffold formation via chitin whiskers by a supercritical carbon dioxide method: a green approach. J Mater Chem 19:8651–8655
33. Rinki K, Dutta PK (2010) Chitosan based scaffolds by lyophilization and sc. CO_2 assisted methods for tissue engineering applications: a benign green chemistry approach. J Macromol Sci Pure Appl Chem A47:429–434
34. Rinki K, Dutta PK (2010) Physicochemical and biological activity study of genipin-crosslinked chitosan scaffolds prepared by using supercritical carbon dioxide for tissue engineering applications. Int J Biol Macromol 46:261–266
35. Jayakumar R, Prabaharan M, Nair SV et al (2010) Novel chitin and chitosan nanofibers in biomedical applications. Biotechnol Adv 28:142–150
36. Li W-J, Laurencin CT, Caterson EJ et al (2002) Electrospun nanofibrous structure: a novel scaffold for tissue engineering. J Biomed Mater Res 60:613–621
37. Mo X, Chen Z, Hans JW (2007) Electrospun nanofibers of collagen-chitosan and P(LLA-CL) for tissue engineering. Front Mater Sci China 1:20–23
38. Kharande TS, Agrawal CM (2008) Functions and requirements of synthetic scaffolds in tissue engineering. In: Laurencin CT, Nair LS (eds) Nanotechnology and tissue engineering: the scaffold. CRC, Boca Raton
39. Kang YM, Lee BN, Ko JH et al (2010) *In vivo* biocompatibility study of electrospun chitosan microfiber for tissue engineering. Int J Mol Sci 11:4140–4148
40. Pillai CKS, Chandra PS (2009) Electrospinning of chitin and chitosan nanofibres. Trends Biomater Artif Organs 22:175–197
41. Liang D, Hsiao BS, Chu B (2007) Functional electrospun nanofibrous scaffolds for biomedical applications. Adv Drug Deliv Rev 59:1392–1412
42. Jia Y-T, Gong J, Xiao-Hua Gu et al (2007) Fabrication and characterization of poly (vinyl alcohol)/chitosan blend nanofibers produced by electrospinning method. Carbohydr Polym 67:403–409
43. Duan B, Yuan X, Zhu Y et al (2006) A nanofibrous composite membrane of PLGA–chitosan/PVA prepared by electrospinning. Eur Polym J 42:2013–2022
44. Chupa JM, Foster AM, Sumner SR et al (2000) Vascular cell responses to polysaccharide materials: *in vitro* and *in vivo* evaluations. Biomaterials 21:2315–2322
45. Dutta PK, Tripathi S, Mehrotra GK et al (2009) Perspectives for chitosan based antimicrobial films for food applications. Food Chem 114:1173–1182
46. Dutta PK, Dutta J, Tripathi VS (2004) Chitin and chitosan: Chemistry, properties and applications. J Sci Ind Res 63:20–31
47. Dutta PK, Dutta J, Chattopadhyaya MC et al (2004) Chitin and chitosan: novel biomaterials waiting for future developments. J Polym Mater 21:321–334
48. Venkatesan J, Kim SK (2010) Chitosan composites for bone tissue engineering – an overview. Mar Drugs 8:2252–2266
49. Muzzarelli RAA (1993) Biochemical significance of exogenous chitins and chitosans in animals and patients. Carbohydr Polym 20:7–16
50. Archana D, Dutta J, Dutta PK (2010) Chitosan-pectin-titanium dioxide nano-composite film: an investigation for wound healing applications. Asian Chitin J 6:45–46
51. Seal BL, Otero TC, Panitch A (2001) Polymeric biomaterials for tissue and organ regeneration. Mater Sci Eng Res 34:147–230

52. Hasirci V, Lewandrowski K, Gresser JD et al (2001) Versatility of biodegradable biopolymers: degradability and an *in vivo* application. J Biotechnol 86:135–150
53. Marler JJ, Upton J, Langer R et al (1998) Transplantation of cells in matrices for tissue regeneration. Adv Drug Deliv Rev 33:165–182
54. Muzzarelli C, Muzzarelli RAA (2002) Natural and artificial chitosan-inorganic composites. J Inorg Biochem 92:89–94
55. Khor E, Lim LY (2003) Implantable applications of chitin and chitosan. Biomaterials 24:2339–2349
56. Mi FL, Shyu SS, Wu YB et al (2001) Fabrication and characterization of a sponge-like asymmetric chitosan membrane as a wound dressing. Biomaterials 22:165–173
57. Jayakumar R, Divyarani VV, Shalumon KT et al (2009) Development of novel α- and β-chitin hydrogel membranes for tissue engineering applications. Asian Chitin J 5:63–70
58. Jiang T, Nair LS, Laurencen CT (2006) Chitosan composites for tissue engineering: bone tissue engineering scaffolds. Asian Chitin J 2:1–10
59. Li J, Pan J, Zhang L, Yu Y (2003) Culture of hepatocytes on fructose-modified chitosan scaffolds. Biomaterials 24:2317–2322
60. Enescu D, Olteanu CE (2008) Functional chitosan and its use in pharmaceutical, biomedical, and biotechnological research. Chem Eng Commun 195:1269–1291
61. Wu T, Zivanovic S, Draughon FA et al (2005) Physicochemical properties and bioactivity of fungal chitin and chitosan. J Agric Food Chem 53:3888–3894
62. Dutta PK, Singh J (2008) Conformational study of chitosan: a review. Proceedings of the National Academy of Sciences India Part IV LXXVIII:255–270
63. Tomihata K, Ikada Y (1997) *In vitro* and *in vivo* degradation of films of chitin and its deacetylated derivatives. Biomaterials 18:567–575
64. Shigemasa Y, Saito K, Sashiwa H et al (1994) Enzymatic degradation of chitins and partially deacetylated chitins. Int J Biol Macromol 16:43–49
65. Hutadilok N, Mochimasu T, Hisamori H et al (1995) The effect of *N*-substitution on the hydrolysis of chitosan by an endo-chitosanase. Carbohydr Res 268:143–149
66. Nordtveit RJ, Varum KM, Smidsrod O (1996) The effect of *N*-substitution on the hydrolysis of chitosan by an endo-chitosanase. Carbohydr Polym 29:163–167
67. Varum KM, Myhr MM, Hjerde RJ et al (1997) *In vitro* degradation rates of partially *N*-acetylated chitosans in human serum. Carbohydr Res 299:99–101
68. Zhang K, Qian Y, Wang H et al (2010) Genipin-crosslinked silk fibroin/hydroxybutyl chitosan nanofibrous scaffolds for tissue-engineering application. J Biomed Mater Res 95A:870–881
69. Sathirakul K, How NC, Stevens WF et al (1996) Application of chitin and chitosan bandages for wound-healing. In: Domard A, Jeauniaux C, Muzzarelli R, Roberts G (eds) Proceedings of the first international conference of the European Chitin Society. Advances in chitin science, vol 1. Jacques Andre Publisher, Lyon
70. Hidaka Y, Ito M, Mori K et al (1999) Histopathological and immunohistochemical studies of membranes of deacetylated chitin derivatives implanted over rat calvaria. J Biomed Mater Res 46:418–423
71. Hsu S, Whu SW, Tsai C et al (2004) Chitosan as scaffold materials: effects of molecular weight and degree of deacetylation. J Polym Res 11:141–147
72. Chatelet C, Damour O, Domard A (2001) Infuence of the degree of acetylation on some biological properties of chitosan films. Biomaterials 22:261–268
73. Kim I-Y, Seo S-J, Moon H-S et al (2008) Chitosan and its derivatives for tissue engineering applications. Biotechnol Adv 26:1–21
74. Chen GP, Sato T, Ohgushi H et al (2005) Culturing of skin fibroblasts in a thin PLGA-collagen hybrid mesh. Biomaterials 26:2559–2566
75. Ma L, Gao CY, Mao ZW et al (2003) Collagen/chitosan porous scaffolds with improved biostability for skin tissue engineering. Biomaterials 24:4833–4841
76. Khnor E, Lim L (2003) Implantated applications of chitin and chitosan. Biomaterials 24:2339–2349

77. Ueno H, Mori T, Fujinaga T (2001) Topical formulations and wound healing applications of chitosan. Adv Drug Deliv Rev 52:105–115
78. Radhika M, Mary B, Sehgal PK (1999) Cellular proliferation on desamidated collagen matrices. Comp Biochem Physiol C Pharmacol Toxicol Endocrinol 124:131–139
79. Archana D, Dutta J, Dutta PK (2010) Synthesis, characterization and bioactivity with improved antibacterial effect of chitosan-pectin-titanium dioxide ternary film for biomedical applications. Asian Chitin J 6:26
80. Adekogbe I, Ghanem A (2005) Fabrication and characterization of DTBP-crosslinked chitosan scaffolds for skin tissue engineering. Biomaterials 26:7241–7250
81. Liu H, Fan H, Cui Y et al (2007) Effects of the controlled-released basic fibroblast growth factor from chitosan-gelatin microspheres on a chitosan-gelatin scaffold. Biomacromolecules 8:1446–1455
82. Powell HM, Boyce ST (2006) EDC cross-linking improves skin substitute strength and stability. Biomaterials 27:5821–5827
83. Dhandayuthapani B, Krishnan UM, Sethuraman S (2010) Fabrication and characterization of chitosan-gelatin blend nanofibers for skin tissue engineering. J Biomed Mater Res 94B:264–272
84. Lu G, Wang G, Sheng B et al (2008) Bimodal carboxymethyl chitosan/collagen nanofiber composite scaffolds for bone tissue engineering. Asian Chitin J 4:49–58
85. Service RF (2000) Tissue engineers build new bone. Science 289:1498–1500
86. Petite H, Viateau V, Bensaid W et al (2000) Tissue-engineered bone regeneration. Nat Biotechnol 18:959–963
87. Muzzarelli RAA (2009) Chitins and chitosans for the repair of wounded skin, nerve, cartilage and bone. Carbohydr Polym 76:167–182
88. Martins AM, Alves CM, Kasper FK et al (2010) Responsive and *in situ*-forming chitosan scaffolds for bone tissue engineering applications: an overview of the last decade. J Mater Chem 20:1638–1645
89. Li Z, Ramay HR, Hauch KD et al (2005) Chitosan–alginate hybrid scaffolds for bone tissue engineering. Biomaterials 26:3919–3928
90. Manjubala I, Ponomarev I, Jandt KD et al (2004) Adhesion and proliferation of osteoblastic cells seeded on chitosan-hydroxyapatite porous scaffold. Eur Cell Mater 7:64
91. Zhang Y, Ni M, Zhang M et al (2003) Calcium phosphate-chitosan composite scaffolds for bone tissue engineering. Tissue Eng 9:337–345
92. Jiang T, Abdel-Fattah WI, Laurencin CT (2006) *In vitro* evaluation of chitosan/poly(lactic acid-glycolic acid) sintered microsphere scaffolds for bone tissue engineering. Biomaterials 27:4894–4903
93. Xu HHK, Simon CG Jr (2005) Fast setting calcium phosphate-chitosan scaffold: mechanical properties and biocompatibility. Biomaterials 26:1337–1348
94. Kuo Y, Lin C (2006) Effect of genipin-crosslinked chitin-chitosan scaffolds with hydroxyapatite modifications on the cultivation of bovine knee chondrocytes. Biotechnol Bioeng 95:132–144
95. Yan LP, Wang YJ, Wu G et al (2010) Genipin-cross-linked collagen/chitosan biomimetic scaffolds for articular cartilage tissue engineering applications. J Biomed Mater Res 95A:465–475
96. Kong L, Gao Y, Lu G et al (2006) A study on the bioactivity of chitosan/nano-hydroxyapatite composite scaffolds for bone tissue engineering. Eur Polym J 42:3171–3179
97. Sailaja GS, Ramesh P, Kumary TV et al (2006) Human osteosarcoma cell adhesion behaviour on hydroxyapatite integrated chitosan–poly(acrylic acid) polyelectrolyte complex. Acta Biomater 2:651–657
98. Manjubala I, Ponomarev I, Wilke I et al (2008) Growth of osteoblast-like cells on biomimetic apatite-coated chitosan scaffolds. J Biomed Mater Res Appl Biomater 84B:7–16
99. Sendemir-Urkmez A, Jamison RD (2006) The addition of biphasic calcium phosphate to porous chitosan scaffolds enhances bone tissue development *in vitro*. J Biomed Mater Res 81A:624–633

100. Lee E, Shin D, Kim H et al (2009) Membrane of hybrid chitosan–silica xerogel for guided bone regeneration. Biomaterials 30:743–750
101. Lee JE, Jeong MH, Ahn HJ et al (2005) Evaluation of chondrogenesis in collagen/chitosan/glycosaminoglycan scaffolds for cartilage tissue engineering. Tissue Eng Regenerative Medicine 2:41–49
102. Yamane S, Iwasaki N, Majima T et al (2005) Feasibility of chitosan-based hyaluronic acid hybrid biomaterial for a novel scaffold in cartilage tissue engineering. Biomaterials 26:611–619
103. Chen YL, Lee HP, Chan HY et al (2007) Composite chondroitin-6-sulfate/dermatan sulphate/chitosan scaffolds for cartilage tissue engineering. Biomaterials 28:2294–2305
104. Wu H, Wan Y, Cao X et al (2008) Proliferation of chondrocytes on porous poly(DL-lactide)/chitosan scaffolds. Acta Biomater 4:76–87
105. Lao L, Tan H, Wang Y et al (2008) Chitosan modified poly(l-lactide) microspheres as cell microcarriers for cartilage tissue engineering. Colloids Surf B Biointerfaces 66:218–225
106. Tan H, Wu J, Lao L (2009) Gelatin/chitosan/hyaluronan scaffold integrated with PLGA microspheres for cartilage tissue engineering. Acta Biomater 5:328–337
107. Putnam AJ, Mooney DJ (1996) Tissue engineering using synthetic extracellular matrices. Nat Med 2:824–826
108. Smentana K (1993) Cell biology of hydrogels. Biomaterials 14:1046–1050
109. Cohen S, Glicklis R, Shapiro L et al (2000) Hepatocyte behavior within three-dimensional porous alginate scaffolds. Biotechnol Bioeng 67:344–353
110. Yang J, Chung TW, Nagaoka M et al (2001) Hepatocyte-specific porous polymer-scaffolds of alginate/galactosylated chitosan sponge for liver-tissue engineering. Biotechnol Lett 23:1385–1389
111. Chung TW, Yang J, Akaike T et al (2002) Preparation of alginate/galactosylated chitosan scaffold for hepatocyte attachment. Biomaterials 23:2827–2834
112. Seglen PO (1972) Preparation of rat liver cells. Exp Cell Res 74:450–454
113. Li J, Pan J, Zhang L et al (2003) Culture of hepatocytes on fructose-modified chitosan scaffolds. Biomaterials 24:2317–2322
114. Park IK, Yang J, Jeong HW et al (2003) Galactosylated chitosan as a synthetic extracellular matrix for hepatocytes attachment. Biomaterials 24:2331–2337
115. Wang XH, Li DP, Wang WJ et al (2003) Crosslinked collagen/chitosan matrix for artificial livers. Biomaterials 24:3213–3220
116. Jiankang H, Dichen L, Yaxiong L et al (2009) Preparation of chitosan–gelatin hybrid scaffolds with well-organized microstructures for hepatic tissue engineering. Acta Biomater 5:453–461
117. Feng ZQ, Chu X, Huang NP et al (2009) The effect of nanofibrous galactosylated chitosan scaffolds on the formation of rat primary hepatocyte aggregates and the maintenance of liver function. Biomaterials 30:2753–2763
118. Sivakumar R, Rajesh R, Buddhan S et al (2007) Antilipidemic effect of chitosan against experimentally induced myocardial infarction in rats. J Cell Animal Biol 1:71–77
119. Wei HJ, Chen CH, Lee WY et al (2008) Bioengineered cardiac patch constructed from multilayered mesenchymal stem cells for myocardial repair. Biomaterials 29:3547–3556
120. Perin EC, Dohmann HF, Borojevic R et al (2003) Transendocardial, autologous bone marrow cell transplantation for severe, chronic ischemic heart failure. Circulation 107:2294–2302
121. Park H, Radisic M, Lim JO et al (2005) A novel composite scaffold for cardiac tissue engineering. In Vitro Cell Dev Biol – Animal 41:188–196
122. Freed LE, Vunjak-Novakovic G (2000) Tissue engineering bioreactors. In: Lanza RP, Langer R, Vacanti JP (eds) Principles of tissue engineering, 2nd edn. Academic, San Diego
123. Radisic M, Obradovic B, Vunjak-Novakovic G (2006) Functional tissue engineering of cartilage and myocardium: bioreactor aspects. In: Ma PX, Elisseeff J (eds) Scaffolding in tissue engineering. CRC, Boca Raton

124. Birla RK, Dow DE, Huang YC et al (2008) Methodology for the formation of functional, cell-based cardiac pressure generation constructs *in vitro*. In Vitro Cell Dev Biol – Animal 44:340–350
125. Blan NR, Birla RK (2008) Design and fabrication of heart muscle using scaffold-based tissue engineering. J Biomed Mater Res 86A:195–208
126. Cuy JL, Beckstead BL, Brown CD et al (2003) Adhesive protein interactions with chitosan: consequences for valve tissue-engineering. J Biomed Mater Res 67A:538–547
127. Liu L, Guo S, Chang J et al (2008) Surface Modification of polycaprolactone membrane via layer-by-layer deposition for promoting blood compatibility. J Biomed Mater Res Appl Biomater 87B:244–250
128. Zhu C, Fan D, Duan Z et al (2009) Initial investigation of novel human-like collagen/chitosan scaffold for vascular tissue engineering. J Biomed Mater Res 89A:829–840
129. Zhang L, Ao Q, Wang A et al (2006) A sandwich tubular scaffold derived from chitosan for blood vessel tissue engineering. J Biomed Mater Res 77A:277–284
130. He Q, Ao Q, Gong K et al (2010) Preparation and characterization of chitosan-heparin composite matrices for blood contacting tissue engineering. Biomed Mater 5:055001
131. Kalayoglu MV. In search of the artificial cornea: recent developments in keratoprostheses. http://www.medcompare.com/spotlight.asp?spotlightid=159
132. Wang Y, Guo L, Ren L et al (2009) A study on the performance of hyaluronic acid immobilized chitosan film. Biomed Mater 4:1–7
133. Gao X, Liu W, Han B et al (2008) Preparation and properties of a chitosan-based carrier of corneal endothelial cells. J Mater Sci Mater Med 19:3611–3619
134. Du LQ, Wu XY, Li MC et al (2008) Effect of different biomedical membranes on alkali-burned cornea. Ophthalmic Res 40:282–290
135. Chen J, Li Q, Xu J et al (2005) Study on biocompatibility of complexes of collagen–chitosan–sodium hyaluronate and cornea. Artif Organs 29:104–113
136. Rafat M, Li F, Fagerholm P et al (2008) PEG-stabilized carbodiimide crosslinked collagen–chitosan hydrogels for corneal tissue engineering. Biomaterials 29:3960–3972
137. Zielinski BA, Aebischer P (1991) Chitosan as a matrix for mammalian cell encapsulation. Biomaterials 15:1049–1056
138. Dillon GP, Yu X, Sridharan A et al (1998) The influence of physical structure and charge on neurite extension in a 3D hydrogel scaffold. J Biomater Sci Polym Edn 9:1049–1069
139. Dillon GP, Yu X, Bellamkonda RV (2000) The polarity and magnitude of ambient charge influences three-dimensional neurite extension from DRGs. J Biomed Mater Res 51A:510–519
140. Gong H, Zhong Y, Li J et al (2000) Studies on nerve cell affinity of chitosan-derived materials. J Biomed Mater Res 52A:285–295
141. Cheng M, Cao W, Gao Y et al (2003) Studies on nerve cell affinity of biodegradable modified chitosan films. J Biomater Sci Polym Edn 14:1155–1167
142. Midha R, Shoichet MS, Dalton PD et al (2001) Tissue engineered alternatives to nerve transplantation for repair of peripheral nervous system injuries. Transplant Proc 33:612
143. Keilhoff G, Stang F, Wolf G et al (2003) Bio-compatibility of type I/III collagen matrix for peripheral nerve reconstruction. Biomaterials 24:2779–2787
144. Ashtona RS, Banerjee A, Punyania S et al (2007) Scaffolds based on degradable alginate hydrogels and poly(lactide-co-glycolide) microspheres for stem cell culture. Biomaterials 28:5518–5525
145. Scanga VI, Goraltchouk A, Nussaiba N et al (2010) Biomaterials for neural-tissue engineering- chitosan supports the survival, migration, and differentiation of adult-derived neural stem and progenitor cells. Can J Chem 88:277–287
146. Frier T, Montenegro KHS et al (2005) Chitin-based tubes for tissue engineering in the nervous system. Biomaterials 26:4624–4632
147. Thein-Han WW, Kitiyanant Y (2007) Chitosan scaffolds for *in vitro* buffalo embryonic stem-like cell culture: an approach to tissue engineering. J Biomed Mater Res Appl Biomater 80B:92–101

148. Prabhakaran MP, Venugopal JR, Chyan TT et al (2008) Electrospun biocomposite nanofibrous scaffolds for neural tissue engineering. Tissue Eng 14:1787–1797
149. Wang AJ, Cao WL, Gong K et al (2006) Development of porous chitosan tubular scaffolds for tissue engineering applications. Asian Chitin J 2:53–60
150. Frier T, Koha HS, Kazaziana K et al (2005) Controlling cell adhesion and degradation of chitosan films by N-acetylation. Biomaterials 26:5872–5878
151. Xiangmei W, Jing Z, Hao C et al (2009) Preparation and characterization of collagen-based composite conduit for peripheral nerve regeneration. J Appl Polymer Sci 112:3652–3662
152. Ishikawa N, Suzuki Y, Dezawa M et al (2009) Peripheral nerve regeneration by transplantation of BMSC-derived Schwann cells. J Biomed mater Res 89A:1118–1124
153. Ishikawa N, Suzuki Y, Ohta M et al (2007) Peripheral nerve regeneration through the space formed by a chitosan gel sponge. J Biomed Mater Res 83A:33–40
154. Peng L, Cheng XR, Wang JW et al (2006) Preparation and evaluation of porous chitosan/collagen scaffolds for periodontal tissue engineering. J Bioactive Compatible Polym 21:207–220
155. Zhang Y, Song J, Shi B et al (2007) Combination of scaffold and adenovirus vectors expressing bone morphogenetic protein-7 for alveolar bone regeneration at dental implant defects. Biomaterials 28:4635–4642
156. Shao X, Hunter CJ (2007) Developing an alginate/chitosan hybrid fiber scaffold for annulus fibrous cells. J Biomed Mater Res 82A:701–710

Chitosan-Based Biomaterials for Tissue Repair and Regeneration

Xing Liu, Lie Ma, Zhengwei Mao, and Changyou Gao

Abstract Tissue repair and regeneration is an interdisciplinary field focusing on development of biological and bioactive substitutes. Chitosan is a natural polysaccharide exhibiting excellent biocompatibility, biodegradability, affinity to biomolecules, and wound-healing activity. It can also be easily modified via chemical and physical reactions to obtain derivatives of various structures, properties, functions, and applications. This paper focuses on chitosan and its derivatives as biomaterials for tissue repair and regeneration. Tuning the structure and properties such as biodegradability, mechanical strength, gelation property, and cell affinity can be achieved through chemical reaction, immobilization of specific ligands such as peptide and sugar molecules, combination with other biomaterials, and chemical or physical crosslinking. To obtain applicable three-dimensional scaffolding materials such as porous sponges, hydrogels, and rods, the formulation and stimuli-responsiveness of this material can also be modified. Moreover, chitosan and its derivatives can function as vectors for delivery of cell growth factors and particularly of functional genes encoding cell growth factors, which are easier to integrate with the formulated materials to obtain scaffolds of higher activity. Recent studies have shown that such scaffolds are of particular importance in mediating the proliferation, migration, and differentiation of stem cells. Finally, integration of chitosan with cell growth factors and associated genes and/or with cells (stem cells) produces chitosan-based biomaterials with applications in repair or regeneration of skin, cartilage, bone, and other tissue.

Keywords Biomaterials · Chitosan · Repair · Regeneration

X. Liu, L. Ma (✉), Z. Mao, and C. Gao (✉)
MOE Key Laboratory of Macromolecular Synthesis and Functionalization, Department of Polymer Science and Engineering, Zhejiang University, Hangzhou 310027, China
e-mail: liema@zju.edu.cn; cygao@mail.hz.zj.cn

Contents

1 Introduction 82
2 Modification of Chitosan for Tissue Repair 85
   2.1 Modification with Functional Groups 85
   2.2 Modification by Specific Ligands 88
   2.3 Modification by Macromolecules 92
   2.4 Crosslinking Modification 94
3 Structures and Functions of Major Importance 96
   3.1 Porous Scaffolds 96
   3.2 Hydrogels 98
   3.3 Rods 100
   3.4 Delivery Systems 102
4 Modulation on Stem Cells 105
   4.1 Two-Dimensional Environments 105
   4.2 Three-Dimensional Environments 106
5 Chitosan-Based Biomaterials for Tissue Repair Applications 108
   5.1 Skin 108
   5.2 Cartilage 112
   5.3 Bone 117
6 Conclusion 121
References 121

1 Introduction

In recent years, advanced surgical therapies including organ transplantation, reconstruction surgery, and use of artificial prosthesis have been applied to treat the loss or failure of organs and tissues. However, they have several therapeutic and methodological drawbacks such as incomplete biological functions, donor shortage, and bacterial or virus infection [1]. Tissue engineering takes the multidisciplinary principles of materials science, medicine, and life science to generate tissues and organs of better biological structures and functions. In a typical therapy based on tissue engineering, cells are seeded into a temporary scaffolding matrix and allowed to remodel the matrix into the desired tissue [2]. It is also possible to implant the matrix materials only, regenerating the tissue following a regenerative medicine strategy based on the recruitment of native cells into the material, and subsequent deposition of extracellular matrix (ECM) [3].

Whether a "cellular" or "acellular" [4] approach is taken, the supporting matrix materials play a crucial role because they act as an artificial ECM to provide a temporary environment for cells to infiltrate, adhere, proliferate, and differentiate. Finally, the matrix guides the repair and regeneration of tissue (Fig. 1). Various forms of material can be considered as the supporting matrix, including three-dimensional (3D) sponges, hydrogels, and microcarriers. For an ideal matrix material, some properties are required that include biocompatibility, suitable microstructure, desired mechanical strength and degradation rate, and most importantly

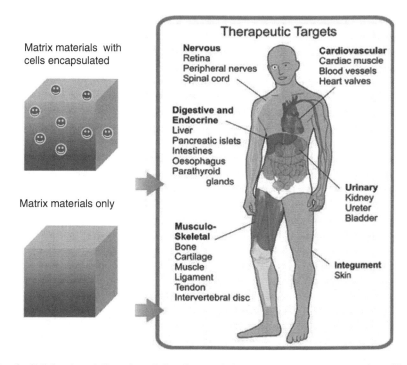

Fig. 1 Cellular (*top left*) and acellular (*bottom left*) tissue engineering approaches. Matrix materials are implanted into patient and act as an artificial ECM for cells to infiltrate, adhere, proliferate, and differentiate, and finally to guide repair and regeneration (modified from [5])

the ability to support cell residence and allow the retention of the metabolic functions [6, 7]. Tissue repair and regeneration is a complicated process. Particularly, many signaling molecules (e.g., growth factors, functional DNAs or siRNAs) are involved in mediating the cell responses and in modulating cell behavior. Therefore, the delivery systems as well as their combination with the various bioactive factors are important, and in many cases take a pivotal role for tissue repair and regeneration.

So far, both natural and synthesized polymers have been used as the supporting matrix for tissue repair and regeneration. Among the synthesized polymers, polyurethane (PU), poly(ethylene glycol) (PEG), poly(vinyl alcohol) (PVA), polycaprolactone (PCL), polylactide (PLA), polyglycolide (PGA), and poly(lactic-*co*-glycolic acid) (PLGA) have been intensively explored [8]. Polymers of natural origin are attractive options, mainly due to their similarities with ECM as well as chemical versatility and biological performance. The widely considered natural polymers include collagen, gelatin, alginate, chitosan, starch, and cellulose.

Chitosan is of particular interest for a broad range of applications as biomaterial and especially as the supporting matrix or delivery system for tissue repair and regeneration. As a linear polysaccharide, chitosan is a partially deacetylated derivative of chitin (an important constituent of the exoskeleton in animals) and is the second most abundant biosynthesized material [9]. Structurally, chitosan is composed of β (1→4)-linked D-glucosamine residues with a variable number of randomly located N-acetyl-glucosamine groups. The ratio of glucosamine to the sum of glucosamine and N-acetyl-glucosamine is defined as the degree of deacetylation (DD) [10]. The average molecular weight (Mw) of chitosan can range from 300–1,000 kDa with a DD of 30–95%, depending on the source and preparation procedure [11, 12]. Mw and DD are the predominant parameters that influence the solubility, mechanical strength, and degradation properties of chitosan and chitosan-based biomaterials. Generally, chitosan is insoluble in neutral or basic conditions, while protonation of free amino groups facilitates solubility of chitosan in dilute acids (pH < 6) [7]. Mw and crystallinity also influence the mechanical properties of chitosan-based materials, although the mechanical strength depends strongly on the material forms and structural parameters such as pore size, porosity, and pore orientation for the porous scaffolds. In vivo degradation of chitosan is mainly attributed to the effect of lysozyme through hydrolysis of acetylated residues [10]. Basically, higher DD not only decreases the number of reactive positions for hydrolysis degradation but also results in larger crystallinity, which further facilitates a slower degradation rate [4]. In addition, the degradation also inherently influences the solubility and mechanical properties owing to the structural changes both at molecular or macroscopic levels.

Due to its outstanding properties in terms of biocompatibility, biodegradability, non-antigenicity, and antibacterial activity, chitosan has become one of the most important biomaterials for diverse applications in drug release, nutrition supplements, wound healing, semipermeable separation etc. [13–16]. Moreover, chitosan possesses some advantages that make it particularly suitable for tissue repair and regeneration. First, it can be easily formulated into matrices of various forms for cell culture and tissue formation. For instance, by a simple freeze-drying method, chitosan-based 3D scaffolds with interconnected porous structures can be prepared [7, 17, 18]. Second, as a result of the protonation of free amino groups under acidic conditions, chitosan exhibits a pH-dependent cationic nature and has the ability to interact with anionic glycosaminoglycans (GAGs), heparin, proteoglycans, and nucleotides like DNA or siRNA. This property is of great importance because a large number of growth factors and cytokines are bound and modulated by GAGs. In addition, delivery systems for DNAs and siRNAs can be obtained through electrostatic interactions between protonated amino groups on chitosan and phosphate groups on nucleotides.

This review firstly focuses on modification of the chitosan molecule to obtain desired properties and functions. The most important material forms (porous scaffolds, hydrogels, and rods) and delivery vectors fabricated from chitosan and its derivatives will be introduced. Particularly, the interaction and modulation of stem cell behavior by chitosan will be discussed. Finally, the applications of chitosan-based materials for repair and regeneration of various tissues and organs such as skin, cartilage, and bone will be summarized.

2 Modification of Chitosan for Tissue Repair

As a kind of renewable resource, unmodified chitosan has been widely used in many fields such as pharmaceutical, agriculture, food, and biomedical applications. In order to realize the full potential of chitosan and bring a breakthrough in its broader utilization, attempts have been made to modify chitosan to obtain various derivatives. For the tissue repair and regeneration applications, chitosan can be functionalized by chemical reaction, coupling with specific ligands or moieties, combining with biomacromolecules, and crosslinking in the presence or absence of crosslinkers.

2.1 Modification with Functional Groups

Chemical modification of chitosan molecules usually occurs at three reactive positions: the amino group at C(2) and the primary and secondary hydroxyl groups at C(3) and C(6), respectively [19]. This is of great significance because the fundamental skeleton of chitosan and its original outstanding physicochemical and biochemical properties as a biomaterial are retained after modification, while achieving desirable structures and functions particularly suitable for tissue repair and regeneration applications. Important chitosan derivatives include sulfated chitosan, trimethyl chitosan, thiolated chitosan, hydroxyalkyl chitosan, carboxyalkyl chitosan, phosphorylated chitosan, and cyclodextrin-linked chitosan.

2.1.1 Sulfated Chitosan

Derivation of chitosan through chemical modification of the amino or hydroxyl group with a sulfate group has been of increasing interest mainly because of the structural similarity of sulfated chitosan to heparin, which displays anticoagulant, antisclerotic, and antiviral activity, and bioaffinity to growth factors [19]. Several techniques have been developed to synthesize sulfated chitosan. For example, Nagasawa et al. [20] used sulfuric acid as sulfating agent in combination with tetrahydrofuran (THF) and phosphorous pentoxide at $-20°C$. In another procedure, 2-chloroethane sulfonic acid sodium salt was applied to obtain sulfoethyl chitosan [21]. It was also feasible to introduce a sulfonic acid function onto chitosan molecules through the reaction with 5-formyl-2-furansulfonic acid, sodium salt [22]. Due to the poor solubility of chitosan in organic solvents in which the sulfation procedure takes place, it can be assumed that the synthesis of sulfated chitosan is performed in heterogeneous conditions and that the constitution of the product is heterogeneous as well.

Structural similarity with heparin endows the sulfated chitosan with high anticoagulant potency. Li et al. [23] used layer-by-layer self-assembly techniques to modify titanium with multilayers of collagen and sulfated chitosan. The coated surface of the multilayers exhibited better anticoagulant property than untreated titanium in terms of platelet adhesion, partial activated thromboplastin time, and prothrombin time. The relationship between Mw and anticoagulant activity of sulfated chitosan has also been studied. It is concluded that the sulfated chitosan with low Mw shows an increased anticoagulant activity, similar to that of heparin [24]. Due to its affinity to many kinds of growth factors, the sulfated chitosan is also applied as a promising component for building of scaffolds or delivery systems for tissue repair and regeneration. Amphiphilic *N*-octyl-*O*-sulfate chitosan can form micelles and has been used as a delivery system for the water-insoluble drug paclitaxel [25]. The PEG monomethyl ether group was conjugated to *N*-octyl-*O*-sulfate chitosan, which further enhanced the biocompatibility and biostability of the system. Our group prepared sulfonated carboxymethyl chitosan (SCC), which was utilized as a component of skin tissue engineering scaffolds [26]. SCC is expected to have the ability of trapping, binding, and protecting growth factors involved in the wound-healing process, such as fibroblast growth factor (FGF) and vascular endothelial growth factor (VEGF), leading to enhanced repairing activity.

2.1.2 Trimethyl Chitosan

It has been known that the protonated form of chitosan in acid conditions exhibits bioadhesion and permeation properties by transiently opening the tight junctions in cell membrane, which is of great significance in drug or gene delivery [27]. However, the poor solubility of chitosan at neutral and basic pH limits its biomedical applications, especially in physiological environments. Attempts have been made to boost the positive charge density, resulting in an enhanced solubility of chitosan over a broader range of pH. Development of trimethyl chitosan (TMC) was an effort in this regard. Methylation of chitosan can be achieved via the reaction of methyl iodide and amino groups (Fig. 2) [28]. A strong alkaline environment is required in order to neutralize the acidic products and avoid protonation of the unreacted primary amino groups. The physicochemical and biological properties of TMC are strongly determined by the degree of quaternization (DQ), which is controlled by the time and route of the reaction.

TMC is supposed to possess the property of permeation enhancement, and therefore has been studied as a delivery vector for proteins and genes. For example, TMC nanoparticles were prepared by ionic crosslinking with tripolyphosphate (TPP) and used as a delivery system for ovalbumin [30]. The loading efficiency and capacity of the protein were up to 95% and 50%, respectively, with an improved integrity. Most importantly, transportation of the protein-loaded particles across nasal mucosa was confirmed by an in vivo uptake test. In another study, the influence of DQ on the property of protein-loaded TMC/TPP nanoparticles was investigated [31]. A lower DQ leads to an increased particle size and a slower release rate of protein.

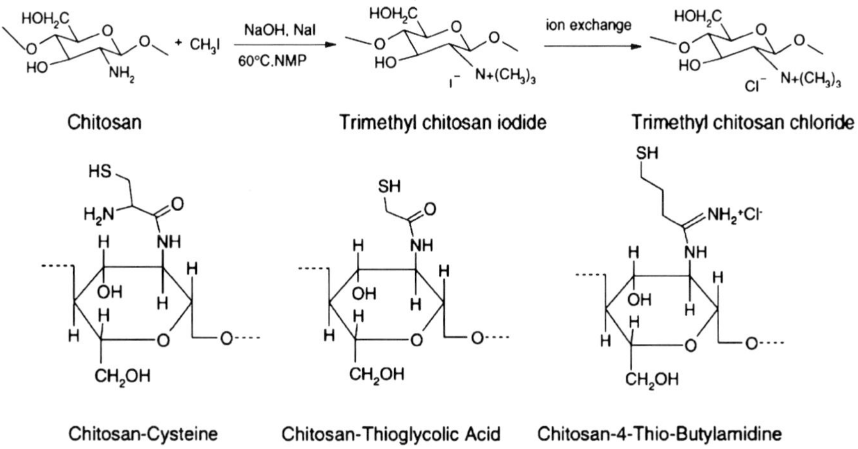

Fig. 2 Synthesis of N,N,N-trimethyl chitosan and substructure of thiolated chitosan derivatives [28, 29]

TMC and its derivatives have also been reported as promising gene vectors. Our group synthesized TMC with high Mw and studied the role of DQ in terms of gene transfection efficiency and cytotoxicity [32]. It was found that the TMC showed some toxicity under a long-term cell culture. When the DQ is larger than 12%, a further increase of the DQ lowers the gene transfection efficiency. To further improve the gene delivery efficiency and biocompatibility of TMC, thermosensitive poly(N-isopropylacrylamide) (PNIPAAm) was grafted to the TMC molecule [33]. The TMC-g-PNIPAAm/DNA can form compact particles above the lower critical solution temperature (LCST) of PNIPAAm as a result of collapse of the PNIPAAm chains. After cellular uptake of the particles, the culture was maintained below the LCST for a period of time to facilitate the unpacking of DNA from the complexes. By this strategy, the gene transfection efficiency was significantly improved while the overall good cytocompatibility was maintained. Other studies have also been performed to enhance the colloidal stability and cellular uptake of the TMC/gene particles by modifying TMC with PEG and folate [34, 35].

2.1.3 Thiolated Chitosan

Thiolated chitosan is generally formed through the reaction between primary amino groups on the chitosan molecule and thiol-bearing reagents such as cysteine, thioglycolic acid (TGA) and 4-thio-butylamidine (TBA) (Fig. 2) [29]. Thiolated chitosan shows enhanced mucoadhesiveness owing to formation of disulfide bonds between the thiol groups on chitosan and mucus glycoproteins. Moreover, the thiolated chitosan can form inter- and intramolecular disulfide bonds within a pH range of 5–6.8, endowing the molecule with in situ gelling properties, which is quite important for preparation of a delivery system.

Chitosan–TBA microparticles have been prepared by an emulsification solvent evaporation technique, along with insulin and the permeation mediator reduced glutathione for nasal administration [36]. Because of the improved mucoadhesive properties and enhanced permeation properties, the bioavailability of the chitosan–TBA/glutathione microparticles is 3.5 times of that of the systems based on unmodified chitosan. Attempts have also been made to combine the mucoadhesion of thiolated chitosan and the permeation-enhancing effects of TMC. TMC–cysteine (TMC-Cys) conjugate has been prepared and allowed to form nanoparticles with insulin through electrostatic interactions (Fig. 3) [37]. Partly attributed to the formation of disulfide bonds between TMC-Cys and mucin, the TMC-Cys/insulin nanoparticles display higher mucoadhesion and insulin transport properties. Thiolated chitosan-based gene delivery systems have been constructed as well. Through the disulfide crosslinkage under the oxidation treatment, an enhanced protection effect and sustained release of plasmid DNA are achieved, resulting in higher gene transfection efficiency [38]. TMC-Cys can enhance the positive charge and solubility of TMC and the reversible crosslinking features of thiolated chitosan, and has recently been evaluated as a gene vector (Fig. 4) [39]. Thiolated chitosan can also be used to build a porous scaffold for tissue-repairing applications. In the study carried out by Li et al. [40], composite chitosan/chitosan–TGA scaffolds with different component ratios were fabricated by a freeze-drying method. The maximum tensile strength of the scaffold is obtained with a chitosan to chitosan–TGA ratio of 3:7 and at a freezing temperature of $-20°C$. Fibroblasts exhibit preferential growth on this scaffold.

2.2 Modification by Specific Ligands

In order to endow the biomaterials with desirable interactions with cells and mediate specific cell responses and behavior, it is crucial to introduce cell-specific ligands or signaling molecules into the materials. For this purpose, many attempts

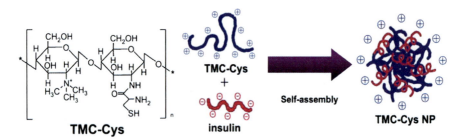

Fig. 3 Chemical structure of TMC-Cys and schematic representation of formation of self-assembled TMC-Cys/insulin nanoparticles (*TMC-Cys NP*) [37]

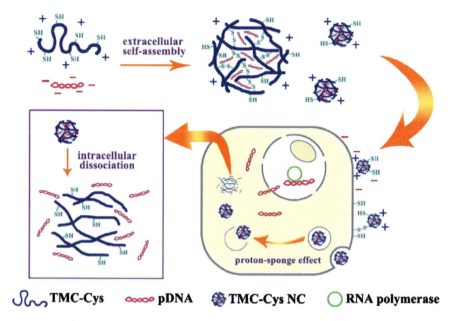

Fig. 4 Transfection process of TMC-Cys nanocomplexes (*NC*) including cell binding through electrostatic affinity and disulfide bonding, uptake via endocytosis, endosomal escape, intracellular plasmid DNA release, and nuclear transport of plasmid DNA [39]

have been made to functionalize chitosan with specific ligands. From the viewpoint of biomimetics, combination with ECM proteins like collagen, fibronectin, and laminin is an attractive strategy for chitosan modification. However, direct modification by proteins has several limitations due to the possible immunogenicity, low cell-binding efficiency, and easy denaturation. By using small peptide sequences derived from these ECMs, however, the drawbacks are overcome while the main biofunctions are retained, since the short peptides are more stable against sterilization, heat treatment, and variation in pH. In addition, implication of sugar moieties in cell signaling mechanisms and in recognition processes indicates them as another key component for chitosan modification.

2.2.1 Peptides

The arginine–glycine–aspartate (RGD) sequence or RGD-containing short peptides are by far the most widely distributed and extensively used ECM-derived biomolecules for stimulating cell attachment by specific recognition with integrins on the cell surface [41]. Various approaches have been developed to immobilize the RGD-containing peptides on chitosan. Karakecili et al. [42] grafted RGDS peptide on the surface of chitosan film by photochemical techniques based on phenyl-azido chemistry (Fig. 5). In another strategy, chitosan reacted with 2-iminothiolane to

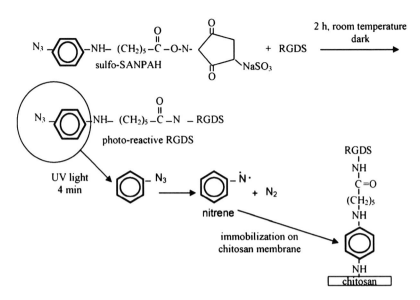

Fig. 5 Production of nitrene groups in phenyl-azido derivatized RGDS by UV irradiation and immobilization on chitosan surface [42]

generate a SH-chitosan derivative and, subsequently, RGDSGGC was introduced by disulfide bond linkage with the aid of dimethyl sulfoxide [43]. This chitosan–RGDSGGC conjugate shows excellent adhesion and proliferation for chondrocytes and fibroblasts.

A99a (ALRGDN) and AG73 (RKRLQVQLSIRT) are laminin-derived peptides with cell-specific activity. A99a is an $\alpha v\beta 3$ integrin-binding peptide, while AG73 is a syndecan-binding peptide. Two kinds of peptide-conjugated chitosan membranes were prepared by binding A99a and AG73 to maleimidobenzoyloxy–chitosan [44]. Both bioactive membranes promoted cell attachment according to the cell-type specificity, with different mechanisms: A99a–chitosan membrane recognizes an integrin receptor whereas the AG73–chitosan membrane interacts with proteoglycan. Further investigation found that the membrane structure partially influenced the cell attachment activity of A99a, but had no effect on that of AG73. Optimization of the peptide amount on the membrane was conducted to obtain the strongest cell adhesion, cell spreading, and neurite outgrowth [45]. As an example of the potential application in tissue engineering, the AG73–chitosan was reported to enable the delivery of keratinocytes to the wound bed [46].

YIGSR is another laminin-derived peptide and has been regarded as capable of enhancing neural outgrowth [47]. When YIGSR-modified chitosan/hydroxyapatite tubes were implanted as bridge grafts into the sciatic nerve of Sprague-Dawley rats, the nerve regeneration and sprouting from the proximal nerve stump were enhanced [48]. To further enhance the bioactivity of the YIGSR sequence, glycine spacers were introduced to yield the CGGYIGSR peptide [49].

The EPDIM sequence is derived from an ECM protein, βig-h3. Bae et al. [50] reported that EPDIM promoted keratinocyte adhesion, proliferation, and migration by integrin-mediated interactions. Compared to those unmodified materials, the EPDIM-immobilized chitosan porous beads significantly enhanced the growth rate of NIH3T3 fibroblasts and HaCaT keratinocytes, which is promising for the wound healing of injured tissue such as skin.

2.2.2 Sugars

Galactose is one of the most popular ligands to the asialoglycoprotein (ASGPR) receptors on the surface of hepatocytes and has been used to modify biomaterials to enhance hepatocyte adhesion as well as liver-specific functions [51]. Galactosylated chitosan (GC) is synthesized from chitosan and lactobionic acid bearing galactose ligands by using 1-ethyl-3-(3-dimethylaminopropyl) carbodiimide (EDC) as an active ester intermediate [52]. Other methods have also been developed using etherization of chitosan and galactose in THF using $BF_3.OEt_2$ as catalyst [53]. GC has been used as scaffolding material and shows good hepatocyte attachment and functions for live tissue engineering. Feng et al. [54] utilized an electrospinning technique to fabricate a GC-based nanofibrous scaffold, in which rat primary hepatocytes formed 3D flat aggregates with high mechanical stability and excellent bioactivity. The nanofibrous scaffold was further applied to develop a multilayer radial-flow bioreactor [55]. This new bioreactor showed exciting properties and might afford short-term support of patients with hepatic failure. As a gene vector, GC or its copolymers (such as GC-*g*-PEG or GC-*g*-dextran) can form complexes with DNA and exhibit hepatocyte-targeted transfection [52, 56, 57].

Lactose is a disaccharide consisting of galactose and glucose. Donati et al. [58] conjugated lactose to a highly deacetylated chitosan via a reductive N-alkylation. The resulting lactose–chitosan could induce chondrocyte aggregation, formation of nodules of high dimensions, and synthesis of aggrecans and type II collagen. The author attributed this chondro-specificity to the presence of galactose residues, implying the existence of specific interactions between galactose and chondrocyte [59]. Tan et al. [60] blended the lactose–chitosan with heparin for chondrocyte culture, resulting in better cell adhesion, proliferation, and GAG secretion.

Mannose can interact specifically with macrophages and dendritic cells via surface mannose receptors involved in endocytosis and phagocytosis [61]. A mannose moiety can be introduced onto chitosan or chitosan-*g*-polyethyleneimine (PEI) molecules by a thiourea reaction between the isothiocyanate group and the amine groups (Fig. 6) [62, 63]. The mannose-bearing polymers show enhanced macrophage-specific bioactivity both as a vaccine and as a gene delivery system.

Sugar–lectin specific interaction is an important cellular phenomenon. Li et al. [64] linked L-fucose to chitosan, which can act as a somatic agglutinin to induce bacteria aggregation. The enhanced antimicrobial activity of chitosan–L-fucose is attributed to the specific recognition and binding of the L-fucose moiety with PA-ΠP lectin on *Pseudomonas aeruginosa* surface.

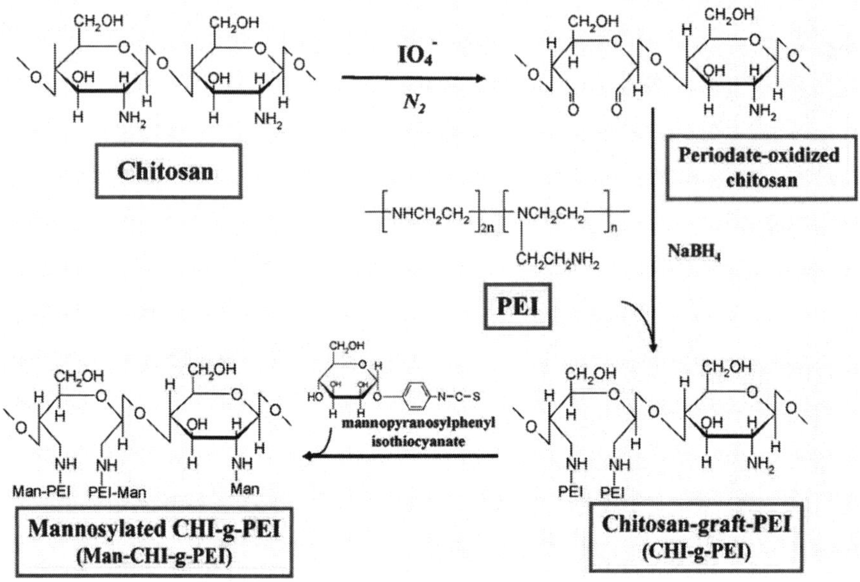

Fig. 6 Proposed reaction scheme for synthesis of mannosylated chitosan-g-PEI [62]

2.3 Modification by Macromolecules

2.3.1 Natural Macromolecules

Due to the inherent advantages like biocompatibility and biodegradability of natural macromolecules, especially ECM-derived biomacromolecules, they have been extensively used to modify chitosan to improve its biological performance as a tissue-repairing material. As the most abundant ECM component, collagen exhibits excellent cytocompatibility owing to the specific cell-binding sites such as the RGD peptide sequence [65]. However, the use of collagen is greatly limited due to its poor mechanical properties, fast biodegradation rate, and contraction during cell culture. Ma et al. [66] designed a chitosan-based dermis substitute that was more stable in terms of pore size and microstructure when cultured with cells. Our group prepared a porous scaffold consisted of collagen and chitosan by freeze-drying [18]. The chitosan molecules function as a crosslinking bridge under glutaraldehyde (GA) treatment, and thereby improve the stability of the composite against biodegradation. Moreover, the composite scaffold exhibits good cytocompatibility both in vitro and in vivo.

Gelatin is a partially hydrolyzed product of collagen [67]. Pulieri et al. [68] prepared dehydro-thermally crosslinked chitosan/gelatin blend films, in which the gelatin amount affected the physicochemical properties significantly. The blends with 80% gelatin displayed the best affinity for neuroblastoma cell attachment and proliferation. In another study, He et al. [69] developed a chitosan/gelatin hybrid scaffold with well-organized microstructures, which facilitated hepatocyte growth in vitro. Chitosan/gelatin nanofibers fabricated by electrospinning show remarkably higher tensile strength (37.91 ± 4.42 MPa) than the pure gelatin fibers (7.23 ± 1.15 MPa), which is of great significance for potential skin tissue engineering applications [70].

Chondroitin sulfate (CS) is a heparin-like GAG abundantly existing in cartilage, cornea, skin, and arterial walls. It consists of a repeating disaccharide unit of differently sulfated residues of β-D-glucuronic acid and α-D-acetylgalactosamine [71]. Thanks to the heparin-like structure, it has the ability to bind with growth factors and thereby stabilize the active conformations. Mi et al. [72] prepared a crosslinked chitosan/CS porous scaffold in which the basic fibroblast growth factor (bFGF) retained its bioactivity after release. CS is also expected to improve cytocompatibility. Chondroitin-6-sulfate is immobilized onto chitosan nonwoven fabric by glutaraldehyde [73]. Besides the increase of cell-seeding efficiency, the proliferation of fibroblasts is improved to about 45 times of that of the original chitosan scaffold.

Hyaluronic acid is composed of repeating disaccharide units of N-acetyl-D-glucosamine and D-glucuronic acid [74]. It functions as the backbone of GAG complexes in the ECM and can bind with some cell-specific receptors such as CD44 [75]. Wang et al. [76] immobilized hyaluronic acid onto the surface of chitosan film, improving the hydrophilicity and cytocompatibility. Xu et al. [77] used the chitosan/hyaluronic acid hybrid films as wound dressing, and found that with the increase of hyaluronic acid amount the water-uptake ratio and water retention capacity were enhanced while protein adsorption and fibroblast adhesion were weakened. Galactosylated hyaluronic acid is utilized to combine with chitosan to prepare a porous sponge. Fan et al. [78] concluded that in the presence of galactosylated hyaluronic acid, the mechanical strength of the sponge was improved and hepatocyte functions were promoted.

Alginate is a kind of naturally derived polysaccharide comprising 1,4-linked β-D-mamnuronic and α-L-guluronic residues. Compared to the chitosan counterpart, the chitosan/alginate hybrid scaffolds display significantly improved mechanical properties due to the ionic interaction between chitosan and alginate [79]. Li et al. [80] specially emphasized the biological effect of the alginate constituent. They found that the chitosan/alginate composites exhibited superior ability over pure chitosan scaffold in terms of HTB-94 cell proliferation and phenotype maintenance.

2.3.2 Synthetic Macromolecules

Broadly speaking, biomaterials used as supporting matrix for tissue repair applications must meet two requirements: mechanical and structural similarity to the target tissues, and appropriate interactions with cells [5]. Synthetic biopolymers have attracted much attention because they display mechanical properties and degradation behaviors more suitable for some applications than their natural counterparts mentioned above. However, the synthetic biopolymers have disadvantages such as hydrophobicity and poor cell affinity as well as lack of biological responses [81]. It is a simple but effective strategy to combine synthetic biopolymers with natural biopolymers such as chitosan by blending or coating, to generate biomaterials with a balance between the physicochemical and biological properties. The most widely used synthetic biodegradable polymers are PCL, PLA, PGA, and PLGA.

Considering the decomposition of chitosan before melt flow, it is crucial to use a common solvent for the solution blending of chitosan and synthetic biopolymers. Wan et al. [82] used hexafluoro-2-propanol as the common solvent and sodium chloride as the porogen to fabricate a chitosan/PCL scaffold, which possessed well-defined compressive properties and dimension stability in wet state. The incorporated chitosan is capable of buffering the acidic hydrolysis products of PCL during degradation and minimizing the possible side effects in vivo as well. Malheiro et al. [83] utilized a formic acid/acetone mixture (70:30 vol%) as a common solvent to obtain a fibrous chitosan/PCL hybrid scaffold by a simple wet spinning method. By optimizing the processing parameters, it is possible to tune the mechanical and biological properties. Cruze et al. [84] synthesized semi-interpenetrating polymer networks (semi-IPNs) by simultaneous precipitation of chitosan/PCL blend, followed by physical crosslinking of chitosan, and finally melt processing and leaching out to prepare porous scaffold. The resulting semi-IPNs scaffold exhibited high porosity and good mechanical properties. Xu et al. [85] prepared chitosan/PLA blend micro-/nanofibers from a trifluoroacetic acid mixture solution by electrospinning. Along with the increase of PLA content, the fiber diameter was enlarged, with a fine morphology.

2.4 Crosslinking Modification

Crosslinking is another effective approach for modulating a broad spectrum of characteristics of chitosan-based biomaterials for tissue repair. Typically, in the case of chitosan porous scaffolds, the mechanical strength and biostability can be enhanced by the crosslinking treatment. With chitosan-based hydrogel systems, the releasing profiles of drugs or bioactive factors (e.g., growth factors, cytokines, and genes) can also be regulated by the crosslinking.

Two types of crosslinking are used for the chitosan porous scaffolds: ionic crosslinking by polyanions such as triphosphate, hyaluronic acid, CS, and alginate; and covalent crosslinking by glutaraldehyde and genipin. In an effort to fabricate alginate-crosslinked chitosan scaffold incorporated with pentoxifylline (PTX), the extensive effects of various crosslinking degrees have been studied [86]. In comparison with the non-crosslinked chitosan scaffolds, the crosslinked scaffolds are of higher mechanical strength and resistance to enzymatic degradation. In addition, the crosslinking is favorable for sustained release of PTX from the scaffolds, which may be significant in reducing inflammation around wound sites.

However, ionic crosslinking is based on physical interaction and in many cases cannot provide enough stability and controllability. Therefore, the covalent crosslinking of chitosan scaffolds is performed by making use of the chemical reactions between amino and/or hydroxyl groups of chitosan and crosslinkers. Di- or polyaldehydes such as glutaraldehyde [87, 88], oxidized starch [89], and oxidized cyclodextrin [90] are the most commonly used crosslinkers for chitosan. Hoffmann et al. [91] compared the effect of glutaraldehyde and oxidized dextran, which varied in "bridge lengths" and number of aldehyde groups. Although both crosslinkers can alter the pore structure and improve the mechanical properties, glutaraldehyde favors formation of a stiffer network due to its length being smaller than that of the oxidized dextran. Due to the potential toxicity of aldehydes to cells and tissues [92, 93], a kind of diimidoester crosslinker, dimethyl-3,3′-dithio-bis-propionimidate (DTBP), is used to treat the chitosan scaffolds. DTBP has proved to be effective, because the crosslinked scaffolds exhibit greater tensile strength and a lower enzymatic degradation rate than the non-crosslinked ones [94]. Moreover, the resulting scaffolds are of lower cytotoxicity compared to those crosslinked by glutaraldehyde.

As mentioned above, it is a common strategy to combine chitosan with other polymers to generate hybrid scaffolds. Crosslinking of the chitosan-based composite materials is also important with respect to the physical and biological properties. For instance, an amide-type crosslinker 1-ethyl-3-(3-dimethylaminopropyl) carbodiimide/N-hydroxysuccinimide (EDC/NHS) is usually utilized to crosslink the systems containing amino and carboxylic groups such as collagen/chitosan composites. However, owing to the limited length of the crosslinkages [95], the carboxylic and amino groups located on adjacent collagen microfibrils are too far apart to be linked. Rafat et al. [96] cooperatively used EDC/NHS and a long-range bifunctional crosslinker PEG dibutyraldehyde (PEG-DBA). As shown in Fig. 7, EDC/NHS enables

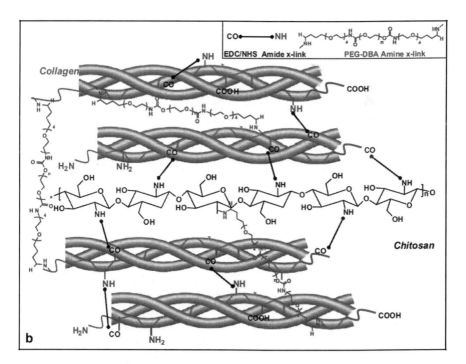

Fig. 7 Molecular and structural schematics of hybrid polymer network scaffold comprised of chitosan-embedded collagen scaffold crosslinked by PEG-DBA and EDC/NHS [96]

short-range intramolecular and intermolecular crosslinking and thereby contributes to the strength enhancement, while PEG-DBA provides long-range intermolecular and interfibrilar linkages to increase robustness and elasticity. This hybrid crosslinking approach results in well-balanced physical characteristics for the collagen/chitosan composites, which are promising candidates for tissue engineering corneal tissue. Our group [97] developed an EDC/NHS-based crosslinking method under the assistance of an amino acid (glycine, glutamic acid, or lysine) to prepare collagen scaffolds. It is demonstrated that the ratio of amino groups to carboxyl groups in the crosslinking system is the dominant factor influencing the microstructure as well as the biostability of the scaffolds. It is feasible that the amino-acid-assisted approach can be further exploited for the crosslinking of collagen/chitosan composite scaffolds.

3 Structures and Functions of Major Importance

3.1 Porous Scaffolds

As one of crucial components in tissue engineering and regenerative medicine, porous scaffolds serve as an ECM analog to support cell attachment, proliferation, differentiation, and delivery of bioactive molecules. The scaffold should have suitable pore size for cell penetration and enough interconnectivity for transport of nutrients and waste [17]. Other factors such as porosity and pore morphology influence cellular colonization rate and organization and, additionally, angiogenesis required for certain applications [98]. Freeze-drying is the most commonly used technique to fabricate chitosan-based porous scaffolds. Briefly, chitosan solution is frozen, and then the formed ice crystals are removed through sublimation during a lyophilization process to generate porosity. The above-mentioned pore parameters can be regulated by controlling solution concentration, freezing temperature [7, 99], and crosslinking treatment.

Some newly developed techniques have also been applied. Supercritical carbon dioxide (sc.CO_2) has been reported to be a promising processing medium for fabrication of porous scaffolds by the supercritical drying technique [100–102]. In a typical preparation process [103, 104], chitosan is dissolved in acetic acid and supplemented with a crosslinker such as formaldehyde, and then is stirred continuously to form a viscous hydrogel. After solvent exchange by acetone to remove any water from the system, the chitosan gel is put into a sealed chamber of sc.CO_2 extractor to react for 2 h at 40°C and 200 bar. Subsequently, a flow of CO_2 is applied through the gel to replace acetone. Finally, the temperature is increased to 20°C and the pressure is released slowly to the atmosphere, resulting in a solid scaffold with a porous structure. As CO_2 is nontoxic, inexpensive, and readily available [105], the sc.CO_2-based technique is regarded as a "green" approach. In comparison with the chitosan scaffolds prepared by the conventional freeze-drying technique, this scaffold exhibits a larger pore size and surface area, better thermal stability, and is expected to support cell growth better [103].

The replica-assisted technique is attractive for preparation of porous scaffolds because it allows good control of the micro- or nanoscale structures. In an example of replica molding, the chitosan scaffolds are formed from a network of random unbound fibers (Fig. 8) [106, 107]. After the chitosan solution is filled into the microchannels (with depths and widths ranging from 1 to 50 μm) of the polydimethylsiloxane mold, another aqueous solution is used to induce pH-dependent coagulation of the molded chitosan. Finally, the chitosan fibers are released and collected from solution, generating the desired scaffold. A remarkable advantage of this approach is that the dimension and shape of the fibers can be controlled according to the mold. In addition, the macroscopic shape of the scaffold is easily manipulated by rearrangement of the chitosan network since the fibers never leave the aqueous phase and experience no unbalanced forces. Another example of a replica-assisted fabrication process was reported by He et al. [69]. This study involved the combination of rapid phototyping, microreplication, and freeze-drying techniques to fabricate a chitosan/gelatin hybrid scaffold with a porous structure, well-organized fluid

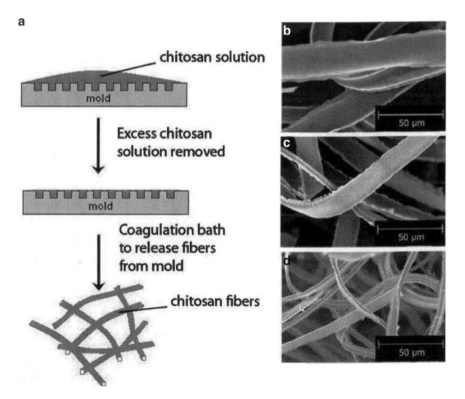

Fig. 8 Fabrication of novel random fibrous chitosan scaffolds. (**a**) Illustration of the micromolding process. (**b–d**) SEM images of chitosan scaffolds composed of fibers measuring 22 μm (**b**), 13 μm (**c**), and 4 μm (**d**) in width [106]

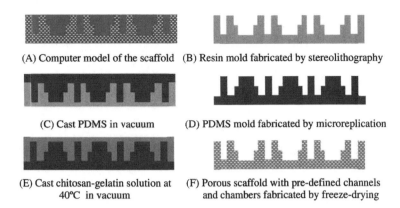

Fig. 9 Fabrication process for porous chitosan/gelatin scaffold with well-organized channels and chambers [69]

channels and hepatic chambers (Fig. 9). The resultant scaffold mimics the architecture of natural liver lobule and is promising for hepatic tissue engineering.

Fabrication of the chitosan porous scaffolds based on microsphere or particle aggregation has drawn much attention due to the combined advantages of good mechanical properties and high interconnectivity. The bonding of adjacent particles is enabled due to the bioadhesive property of chitosan, assuring the mechanical integrity of the scaffolds. Jiang et al. [108, 109] developed chitosan/PLGA hybrid scaffolds by a microsphere-based method. The chitosan/PLGA composite microspheres with diameters ranging from 500 to 710 µm were prepared by a solvent evaporation technique [110], and were then packed into a stainless steel mold. The scaffolds were formed when the adjacent microspheres were sintered together by heating the mold above the glass transition temperature of PLGA. By controlling the sintering temperature and sintering time, scaffolds with defined pore structures and mechanical properties were obtained. Malafaya et al. [111, 112] proposed another approach for construction of the chitosan particle-agglomerated scaffolds. Typically, regular particles were produced by extruding chitosan acetic acid solution through a syringe into a NaOH precipitation bath. After these prefabricated particles were pressed into molds, they were dried in an oven at 50°C for 3 days to obtain a particle-agglomerated scaffold. Recently, the bonding of chitosan microspheres has also been implemented using an acidic solvent [113].

3.2 Hydrogels

Hydrogels are highly hydrated 3D physically or chemically crosslinked polymer networks. Smart hydrogels can respond to environmental stimuli such as light, temperature, electric or magnetic fields, pH, ions, and chemical or biochemical molecules. Here, the responses may include gelation, reversible adsorption on a surface, and alteration between hydrophilic and hydrophobic states [114, 115], leading to changes in properties such as rheology, mechanical strength, cell-binding affinity, and drug-loading efficiency. In tissue repair applications, these hydrogels have attracted increasing attention because of their similarity to the ECM environment and their injectable capability. In comparison with preshaped scaffolds, the injectable hydrogel can fit any shape of the target defects and entrap cells or other biological molecules easily. In addition, minimal invasive procedures are required when using the hydrogels as tissue-repairing biomaterials, which is of great advantage for in vivo applications.

Our group has modified chitosan by sequential grafting of methacrylic acid and lactic acid to obtain a kind of crosslinkable and water-soluble chitosan derivative, chitosan–methacrylic acid–lactic acid (CML), which underwent a gelation transition under the initiation of a redox system, i.e., ammonium persulfate (APS)/N,N,N',N'-tetramethylethylenediamine (TEMED) or photoinitiator (Fig. 10) [116, 117]. In vitro culture of chondrocytes and in vivo tests demonstrated that the CML hydrogel exhibited considerable cytocompatibility and histocompatibility [116]. CML could also be combined with collagen-coated PLA microspheres, as microcarriers for cells, to form a composite hydrogel [118]. As expected, incorporation of the microcarriers substantially enhanced the mechanical strength of the hydrogel

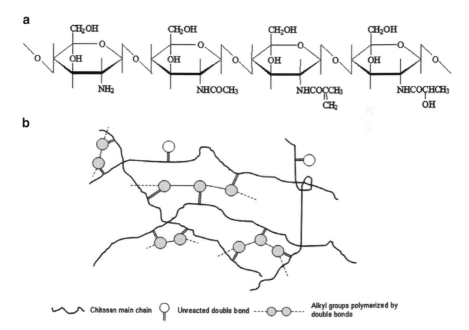

Fig. 10 (a) Molecular structure of a water-soluble and crosslinkable chitosan derivative (CML) obtained by grafting methacrylic acid and lactic acid onto the pendant amine groups of chitosan. The structure does not represent the real ratio between each monomer unit. (b) Illustration of the chitosan hydrogel network linked by alkyl chains, which are formed via C=C polymerization [116]

system. It was found that the chondrocytes were able to attach and proliferate on the surface of the microcarriers to form confluent cell layers, demonstrating the feasibility of the strategy. However, the potential cytotoxicity of the redox system APS/TEMED remains a problem. To overcome this drawback, another photoinitiator, Irgacure2959, was used to make the CML hydrogel, which showed no cytotoxicity at lower initiator concentration and is thereby more suitable for tissue repair applications [119]. In a better-designed system, a composite photoinitiated CML hydrogel was prepared by blending with PLGA particles modified by methacrylic acid-*graft*-gelatin [120]. Improved mechanical properties and cytocompatibility were achieved owing to the addition of the particles, indicating a great opportunity of this composite material to be applied in chondrogenesis.

Temperature- and/or pH-responsive chitosan hydrogels have been extensively studied because these two stimulii are applicable in vivo. Mixing chitosan with glycerol phosphate (GP) disodium salt has been proved to be a feasible approach for constructing temperature-responsive hydrogels [121]. The gelation at higher temperatures is partly attributed to the electrostatic interaction between chitosan and GP, and partly due to the salt-induced reduction of electrostatic repulsion between chitosan molecules, resulting in an increased hydrogen bonding [121]. Further in vivo experiments demonstrate that co-injection of the chitosan/GP hydrogel with embryonic stem cells improves myocardial performance in infracted rat hearts [122, 123]. A pH-responsive PVA–chitosan–poly(acrylic acid)–IPN hydrogel was prepared by Zhang et al. [124]. This hydrogel shows a swelling change in response to the pH of the medium, indicating potential application in modulating material systems for tissue repair. Ding et al. [125] reported the preparation of dually responsive injectable hydrogel by in situ crosslinking of glycol chitosan and benzaldehyde-capped poly(ethylene oxide)-*b*-poly(propylene glycol)-*b*-poly(ethylene oxide) (PEO-PPO-PEO). The hydrogels were formed in situ. The release of both the loaded hydrophobic and hydrophilic drugs could be manipulated by pH and temperature. The benzoic–imine bonds and PEO-PPO-PEO segments serve as pH-labile covalent linkers and thermosensitive moieties, respectively.

3.3 Rods

Chitosan rods are of great importance as they are promising biomaterials for bone fixation applications. However, processing chitosan into a rod is not an easy job due to its low decomposition temperature. So far, many efforts have been made to obtain chitosan rods with high-enough mechanical strength for bone repair and regeneration.

Hu and coworkers [126, 127] firstly developed an in situ precipitation approach to fabrication of 3D ordered chitosan rods with a structure of concentric circles through the formation process illustrated in Fig. 11. Briefly, the chitosan/acetic acid solution is filled into a bag made of chitosan membrane, and then immersed into 5% NaOH aqueous solution. When OH$^-$ ions from the outside solution permeate into

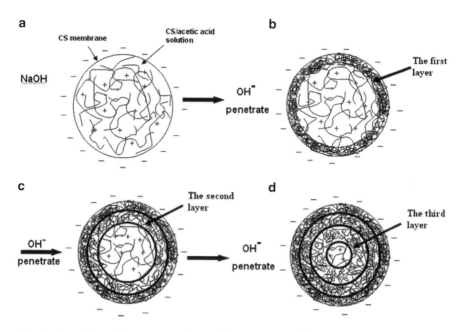

Fig. 11 Formation of chitosan gel with a multilayer structure [127]

the inner chitosan solution, the first layer of the gel is formed by precipitation due to neutralization of the protonated amino groups on chitosan. With continuous diffusion of the OH$^-$ ions, all the chitosan solution turns into gel eventually, resulting in a rod formed of concentric circles after drying. Due to the inductive effect of the OH$^-$ concentration gradient, a spoke-like oriented structure can be obtained. The chitosan rods with this special structure exhibits very good mechanical properties, with a bending strength of 92.4 MPa, bending modulus of 4.1 GPa, and shear strength of 36.5 MPa, showing a great potential to be used as a bone fixation biomaterial.

It has been widely accepted that introduction of hydroxyapatite (HA) can improve the bioactivity of bone-repairing materials and induce neo-bone formation. By using the in situ precipitation approach, a homogenous and high-strength chitosan/HA composite rod has been prepared [128]. The matrix chitosan and filler HA are simultaneously synthesized, solving the problem of aggregation of nano-sized HA when dispersed in the chitosan matrix. The bending strength and modulus of the composite rods reached 86 MPa and 3.4 GPa, respectively, which are two or three times stronger than rods of PMMA and bone cement. These chitosan/HA composite rods can be further reinforced by crosslinking with glutaraldehyde, resulting in an increment of bending strength and modulus by 107% and 52.9%, respectively. Using the in situ precipitation method, different organic or inorganic components such as cellulose fibers, CaCO$_3$, and magnetite can be combined with chitosan to generate hybrid rod materials for other specific applications [129–131].

3.4 Delivery Systems

Bioactive signals such as growth factors, hormones and functional genes play crucial roles in tissue repair and regeneration processes by mediating communication between cells and their microenvironment, and thereby modulating cellular adhesion, proliferation, migration, differentiation, and gene expression. Exogenous delivery of these bioactive biomolecules in combination with tissue-repairing biomaterials has emerged as an important approach for construction of bioactive materials that can stimulate desirable cell response and neo-tissue formation.

3.4.1 Delivery of Growth Factors

Cell growth factors such as basic or acidic fibroblast growth factor (bFGF or aFGF), transforming growth factor-beta (TGF-β), hepatocyte grow factor (HGF), vascular endothelial growth factor (VEGF), and platelet-derived growth factor (PDGF) are extensively applied in tissue repair and regeneration [132]. Due to the short half-lives, relatively large size, slow tissue penetration, and potential toxicity, many efforts have been made to develop well-designed micro-/nanovectors for delivery of these proteins.

Chitosan can be directly used to physically entrap or chemically conjugate to growth factors in various material forms such as films, fibers, porous scaffolds, and hydrogels. In a study reported by Park [133], a chitosan sponge fabricated by freeze-drying and adsorbed with PDGF-BB solution exhibited good cytocompatibility and marked increase in new bone formation. By using a simple approach, an EGF-containing chitosan gel was developed and proved favorable to promote epithelialization in burn healing [134]. Obara et al. [135] incorporated FGF-2 into a chitosan hydrogel by photocrosslinking to generate a carrier material that significantly accelerated wound closure due to its ability to retain the bioactivity of FGF-2 as well as to release it in a controlled manner. Covalent immobilization of EGF onto chitosan membranes is also achieved through photochemical reactions, leading to a bioactive material for stimulating fibroblast growth [136].

The chitosan-based microcarriers including particles, micro-/nanospheres, and microgranules have also been applied to encapsulate and deliver growth factors. Moreover, they are also easily combined with the scaffolding biomaterials to generate tissue-repairing materials with improved bioactivity. For example, TGF-β1-loaded chitosan microspheres are fabricated by an emulsion method, leading to a sustained release of TGF-β1 [137]. The porous scaffold loaded with chitosan/TGF-β1 microspheres can augment cell proliferation and production of ECM. A similar approach for providing prolonged delivery of growth factors was proposed by Liu et al. [138], in which a chitosan/gelatin hybrid scaffold containing bFGF-loaded chitosan/gelatin microspheres was used to improve skin regeneration. Recently, better designed chitosan-based nanoparticles have been reported for protection and release of bFGF. Typically, thiol-modified chitosan sulfate forms self-assembled polyelectrolyte complexes with chitosan and simultaneously incorporates bFGF, providing a novel method for specific delivery of growth factors [139].

Heparin can specifically bind and store growth factors, thus biomaterials combined with heparin are able to bind and release heparin-binding growth factors. A kind of non-anticoagulant heparin is synthesized and used to form hydrogel with water-soluble chitosan through ionic interactions, with the enhancement of the stability and bioactivity of the loaded FGF-2 [140]. Our group constructed a gelatin/chitosan/hyaluronan ternary complex scaffold and further modified the scaffold by covalent immobilization of heparin using carbodiimide [141]. The bFGF was subsequently bound onto the scaffold by a bioaffinity force. Ho et al. [142] also used a chemical method to modify chitosan/alginate scaffolds by heparin, and confirmed that the bFGF-binding efficiency of the modified scaffolds could be increased up to 15 times. Moreover, the heparin-functionalized scaffold displayed controllable release of bFGF and could prevent the growth factors from inactivation.

Inspired by the above research, some biomacromolecules with a similar structure to heparin were also used to construct tissue-repairing materials. For instance, chondroitin sulfate (CS), a heparin-like GAG with the ability to enhance the binding affinity of growth factors, is utilized to prepare a CS/chitosan sponge. The release rate of PDGF-BB from this sponge can be modulated by varying the content of CS [143]. Mi et al. [72] also demonstrated the effect of CS in a CS/chitosan composite on retaining the biological activity of bFGF, and thus enhancing vascularization of the composite. Fucoidans are fucose-containing polysaccharides that are known to bind heparin-binding growth factors and enhance their activity. It is suggested that a chitosan/fucoidan microhydrogel has high affinity for EGF-2 and can protect it from inactivation [144].

3.4.2 Delivery of DNAs and siRNAs

Another strategy for modulating the bioactivity signals for tissue repair and regeneration is to exploit plasmid DNAs or small interfering RNAs (siRNAs). Plasmid DNAs are expected to transfect cells and express the required growth factors in situ. In contrast, the application of siRNAs is used to silence targeted genes and downregulate the corresponding protein levels [145]. In this type of application, vectors are necessary to enhance the transfection efficiency of DNAs or siRNAs to target cells. Although many types of vectors have been developed so far, our focus will only be on chitosan-based delivery systems in the form of micro- or nanosized vectors, films, 3D scaffolds, gels, and their composites.

The chitosan-based nonviral vectors for systematic delivery of plasmid DNAs or siRNAs have gained increasing interest recently. Due to its cationic property at acidic pH below the pK_a, chitosan is able to bind negatively charged DNAs or siRNAs via electrostatic interaction, typically resulting in spontaneous formation of the nanosized complexes in aqueous condition. The well-defined complexes are believed to protect DNAs or siRNAs from degradation or clearance and to facilitate their cellular uptake. Many researchers have reported that the delivery efficiency of chitosan/DNA and chitosan/siRNA complexes is influenced by several formulation parameters, such as the Mw and DD of chitosan, charge ratio, ionic strength and pH of the medium, serum concentration, and cell type [146]. It is crucial to carefully optimize these parameters when designing such a delivery carrier. In addition, encapsulation and adsorption mechanisms have been exploited to construct nanosized chitosan-based nonviral vectors (Fig. 12).

Along with the progress in nanovectors for DNA or siRNA, chitosan-based gene-activated matrices or scaffolds have emerged for tissue repair and regeneration. In a gene-activated system, naked functional plasmid DNA or vector/DNA complexes are combined with the repairing materials and, subsequently, used to in situ transfect cells to express the required factors. In one typical example [147], a chitosan/PAA nanofibrous scaffold with addition of plasmid DNA exhibited significant transgenic expression in the culture of human dermal fibroblasts. Another example reported the formation of nanosized chitosan/DNA complexes and subsequent loading of the nanoparticles onto a coral scaffold [148]. Compared to the pure coral scaffolds, the gene-activated scaffolds supported the proliferation of human periodontal ligament cells and facilitated the expression of PDGFB and type I collagen both in vitro and in vivo. Several researchers [149–151] have made efforts to construct a chitosan/collagen hybrid scaffold containing functional DNAs, which has been proved to be a good substrate candidate in periodontal tissue engineering.

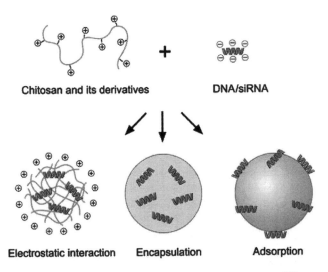

Fig. 12 Preparation of chitosan-based DNA or siRNA nanoparticles by different mechanisms [146]

4 Modulation on Stem Cells

Stem cells, whether derived from embryos, fetuses, or adults, can be simply defined as progeny of cells that are capable of differentiating into different lineages [152]. Embryonic stem cells (ESCs) are isolated from the inner cell mass of blastocysts and have the ability to be cultured and maintained in an undifferentiated and pluripotent state, and directed to differentiate into all specific cell types [153, 154]. A variety of adult stem cells (often referred as progenitor or multipotent cells), including bone marrow-derived mesenchymal stem cells (MSCs), hematopoietic stem cells (HSCs), adipose-derived stem cells (ADSCs), and neutral stem cells (NSCs), have been found more committed but less pluripotent than ESCs.

In a traditional tissue engineering approach, the matrix/cell constructs are cultured in vitro and subsequently transplanted to repair and regenerate damaged organs or tissues [2]. The shortage of cell sources remains a problem that limits the clinical application of tissue engineering. With their pluripotent and self-renewal capacity, stem cells have been regarded as an ideal choice for cell-based tissue engineering therapy, especially for the construction of complicated organs with multiple cell types. For the concept of regenerative medicine, a supporting matrix without cells is utilized to repair tissues in vivo based on the recruitment of native cells, including stem cells [3]. As a result, the stem cells play increasingly prominent roles in tissue repair and regeneration, and the interactions between stem cells and biomaterials are becoming one of the most important issues. Recently, a variety of studies have focused on the influence of chitosan and its derivatives on modulating the attachment, proliferation, and differentiation of stem cells, and thereby the properties of tissue repair and regeneration. In addition, chitosan-based composites and bioactive systems are of great significance in this regard.

4.1 Two-Dimensional Environments

The Mw is a crucial factor in determining the physical and biological properties of chitosan, and therefore might have influence on stem cell behavior. Ratanavaraporn et al. [155] investigated the influences of chito-oligosaccharide (COS) with both low and high Mw chitosan on the behavior of ADSCs and MSCs. Both types of stem cell attached and proliferated better on the COS film than on the chitosan film. In addition, under osteogenic induction, the stem cells cultured on the COS film were more favorable to osteogenic differentiation. The DD of chitosan affects the stem cell responses as well. Several reports indicate that chitosan films with a higher DD show better cell affinity to Schwann cells, fibroblasts, and chondrocytes. Zheng et al. [156] prepared eight kinds of chitosan films, with chitosan Mw ranging from 5×10^4 Da to 1×10^6 Da, and DD of either 85% or 95%. The results confirmed that the survival and proliferation of BMSCs were significantly promoted on the film of chitosan having Mw 1×10^6 Da and DD 95%.

Some researchers compared the behavior of stem cells on chitosan and other polymer substrates. It was found that the proliferation and differentiation of NSCs were inhibited on both chitosan and poly(vinylidenefluoride) (PVDF) membranes at a single-cell level [157]. However, in the form of neurospheres, the migration of NSCs was better promoted on the chitosan membranes in a serum-free environment. Similarly, in a study dealing with the effect of chitosan and collagen membranes on NSCs, the cellular responses were dependent on the presence or absence of serum in the culture medium [158]. Moreover, the chitosan/collagen hybrid membrane exhibited better ability to facilitate NSC migration from neurospheres and differentiation into neurons.

Modification with bioactive factors alters the surface characteristics of chitosan substrates and thereby their behavior in mediating stem cell responses. Two cell-binding peptides, i.e., F36(PDGRVD) and F77(KEDGRLL), were stably immobilized onto chitosan membranes, leading to a promotion of MSC adhesion and differentiation into osteoblastic cells, as demonstrated by alkaline phosphate (ALP) expression and mineralization [159]. Growth factors such as bone morphogenetic protein 2 (BMP-2) were also used to modify a titanium–chitosan substrate [160]. Although immobilization of BMP-2 results in a relatively low level of initial attachment and proliferation of BMSCs, osteogenic differentiation was remarkably promoted.

4.2 Three-Dimensional Environments

The behavior of stem cells in a 3D environment is well worth studying, since most practical applications of tissue repair and regeneration are accomplished by materials with a 3D structure, such as scaffolds, hydrogels, fibrous meshes, and microspheres.

4.2.1 Modulating Stem Cells with Chitosan Scaffolds

Similar to the situation with 2D membranes, the basic molecular characteristics of chitosan such as DD also show great influence on the ability of chitosan scaffolds to modulate stem cell behavior. The chitosan scaffolds with a high DD can maintain the viability and pluripotency of buffalo embryonic stem-like (ES-like) cells [15]. However, the cell behavior on 2D and 3D environments are quite different. Comparison of MSC behavior in both 2D plates and chitosan/gelatin/chondroitin scaffolds demonstrates that the 3D microenvironment can enhance osteogenesis and maintain the viability of cells [161]. The research by Altman et al. [162] found that the apparent elastic modulus and cytoskeleton F-actin fiber density were higher for ADSCs seeded in 3D silk fibroin/chitosan scaffolds than on 2D glass plates (Fig. 13).

Combination of chitosan with other materials to generate hybrid scaffolds is an effective approach for tailoring biomaterials with desired interactions with

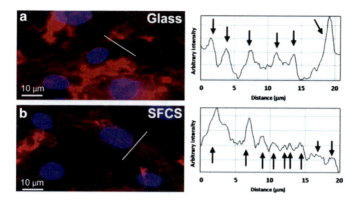

Fig. 13 Fluorescent images and the corresponding line profiles of the F-actin fibers (*red*) of ADSCs seeded on (**a**) glass surface and (**b**) silk fibroin/chitosan (*SFCS*) scaffold. F-actin fiber density of ADSCs was quantified and confirmed by line-profile analysis of the fibers using ImageJ software. The x-axis is the distance in microns, and the peaks correspond to the intensity of the rhodamine–phalloidin stain (*red*), whose peak maximum occurs at the location of the fibers along the line. Nuclei were stained with DAPI (*blue*) [162]

stem cells. Blending of gelatin into chitosan improves the spreading and proliferation of buffalo ES cells [163]. Due to the enhanced protein and calcium ion adsorption of HA, the initial adhesion, long-term growth and osteogenic differentiation of human MSCs (hMscs) are promoted by introducing HA into chitosan/gelatin composites [164]. In the research on cultivation of MSCs on coralline/chitosan scaffolds, an increase of the coralline content resulted in scaffolds exhibiting better performance in cell number, ALP activity, and osteocalcin expression, indicating the positive effect of coralline on promoting MSC proliferation and osteogenic differentiation [165].

4.2.2 Modulating Stem Cells with Chitosan Hydrogels

Chitosan-based hydrogels for stem cell cultivation and their in vivo applications will be summarized in this section. Recently, several studies have exploited the application of a kind of injectable material, i.e., chitosan/GP hydrogel, for stem cell-based therapy. The in-situ-formed chitosan gel is a good substrate for the attachment and proliferation of rat BMSCs and MDSCs. Moreover, after osteogenic factors are incorporated into the hydrogel, the rat MDSCs can be induced to differentiate into the osteogenic lineage and bone formation is stimulated [114, 166]. In another report, the chitosan/GP hydrogel is combined with ESCs in the treatment of myocardial infarction, exhibiting good delivery efficiency of stem cells and improved cardiac functions [123].

Dang et al. [167] developed a thermosensitive hydroxybutyl chitosan (HBC) and evaluated its compatibility with hMSCs. The HBC can well support hMSCs in terms of metabolic activity and ECM production. Another thermosensitive hydrogel made of chitosan-*g*-PNIPAAm is utilized for MSC culture and cartilage formation [168]. The polymer gel exhibits good cytocompatibility and can induce chondrogenic differentiation from MSCs both in vitro and in vivo. In another research, a chitosan/alginate gel was prepared to support MSCs, and was shown to be promising as an injectable material for generating new bone [169].

4.2.3 Modulating Stem Cells with Chitosan Microspheres

Biodegradable microspheres have been widely used as substrates for cell cultivation and expansion. In particular, these microspheres have potential applications in tissue engineering as injectable microcarriers for various cell types, including stem cells.

Porous chitosan microbeads are prepared by electrospraying chitosan solution into liquid nitrogen and subsequently thawing and refreezing [170]. The resulting microbeads possess controllable diameter, pore size, and porosity depending on the initial chitosan concentration. By optimizing the processing parameters, microbeads with suitable pore structures for hMSC culture are obtained, on which hMSCs can successfully attach and proliferate to form 3D aggregates by connecting the nearby microbeads. These microcarrier/cells constructs have great potential for tissue formation.

Chitosan microspheres are also combined with porous scaffold for the delivery of stem cells with high efficiency [171]. ADSCs are not only able to attach and infiltrate into the pores of the microspheres, but can also maintain multipotency after being released from the microspheres and into a collagen gel scaffold. This investigation provides a new approach for incorporation of stem-cell-loaded microspheres into suitable scaffolding architecture and for construction of tissue-engineered composite biomaterials.

It is commonly accepted that the behavior of stem cells is influenced by various signaling biomolecules. Recently, chitosan microspheres have been utilized to incorporate and release signaling biomolecules, and thus mediate the proliferation and differentiation of stem cells [172, 173]. Neurotrophin-3 (NT-3) was added to the chitosan carriers, which were further co-cultured with neural stem cells and showed good viability and increased ability to differentiate into neurons. Moreover, the amount of NT-3 for stimulating the desired cell responses was reduced, possibly due to the effect of chitosan carriers on prolonging the half-life and activity of NT-3.

5 Chitosan-Based Biomaterials for Tissue Repair Applications

5.1 Skin

Skin loss or function failure caused by trauma, burns, and chronic diseases has become a critical problem in clinical practice. To repair the skin loss and reconstruct the functions, skin substitutes such as wound dressings, xenografts, allografts, and autografts have to be employed. However, because these treatments are limited by antigenicity and donor sites, skin substitutes based on the principles of tissue engineering and regenerative medicine have become a promising alternative [174, 175]. Particularly, skin substitute made of chitosan or its derivatives have attracted much attention due to the outstanding characteristics of chitosan, such as biocompatibility, hemostatic activity, antibacterial property, and ability to accelerate the wound-healing process.

5.1.1 Membranes

Chen et al. [176] reported the preparation of an asymmetric chitosan membrane containing nanoscale type I collagen particles, which were thought to be able to facilitate the adhesion of fibroblasts. The layer towards the air allows the drainage of wound exudates, while the lower layer absorbs wound exudates and accelerates wound repair. In vivo studies indicated that the membrane could be exploited as a wound dressing and promoted the epithelialization and reconstruction of the wound. In another research, chitosan was combined with fucoidan to fabricate a wound dressing for burn healing, which significantly accelerated the wound closure and healing process [177]. The fucoidan may serve as a heparin analog and increase the binding affinity to both fibroblasts and growth factors or cytokines. Composite nano-titanium oxide–chitosan membranes are also used as artificial skin, resulting in better and faster recovery of wounds in an animal model [178]. The immune-enhancing effect of chitosan and the bactericidal effect of nano-TiO_2 are believed to contribute to this positive result.

Chitosan derivatives have also been studied for possible utilization in wound dressings. For example, three kinds of chitosan derivative (oligochitosan, N,O-carboxymethyl-chitosan, and N-carboxymethyl-chitosan) are used to form sheets and pastes, all of which exhibit appropriate cytocompatibility to the fibroblasts isolated from normal human dermis and hypertrophic scars [179].

5.1.2 Composite Scaffolds

As a scaffolding material, chitosan has disadvantages of low mechanical integrity and rapid degradation especially in acidic conditions or in the presence of lysozyme. The extensively applied approaches to overcome these drawbacks are crosslinking treatment or incorporation with other components. Adekogbe et al. [94] crosslinked a chitosan scaffold using DTBP to improve its tensile strength. Suitable water vapor transmission rate and pore structures are obtained for skin tissue engineering applications. Mao et al. [180] prepared an asymmetric scaffold composed of chitosan and gelatin by a freeze-drying technique, in which keratinocytes and fibroblasts were co-cultured to construct a bilayer skin substitute in vitro. The gelatin can improve the hydrophilicity of the scaffolds, and the composite artificial skin has suitable mechanical properties and shows no contraction. Chitosan is also used in combination with sodium alginate to form complexes, which are further fabricated into porous sponges [181]. In addition, curcumin can be incorporated into the sponge and serves as an anti-inflammatory antioxidant and can induce detoxification enzymes, ultimately improving the wound healing. By controlling the crosslinking degree, release of curcumin from the sponge can be modulated. In vivo results in Sprague-Dawley rats showed that the composite sponge had a better wound-healing effect than the traditional gauze.

We previously fabricated a porous scaffold for skin tissue engineering from a mixture of collagen and chitosan by freeze-drying [18]. Biostability of the collagen/chitosan composite scaffolds is enhanced by glutaraldehyde (GA) crosslinking. In vitro results revealed that human dermal fibroblasts could proliferate well in the scaffolds, and in vivo embedded tests further revealed that the scaffolds had the ability to support and accelerate fibroblasts infiltration from the surrounding tissues. The collagen/chitosan scaffolds were subsequently covered with a silicone membrane, which served as a temporary epidermal layer, to construct a bilayer dermal equivalent (BDE) (Fig. 14) [182]. Application on full-thickness skin defects in Bama miniature pigs demonstrated that the BDEs could induce angiogenesis and regeneration of the dermis, and finally complete healing of full-thickness skin after ultrathin skin grafting [183].

5.1.3 Hydrogels

Boucard et al. [184] prepared bilayered physical hydrogels for the treatment of full-thickness burn injuries in a pig model. The upper rigid protective layer is generated from a solution of chitosan hydrochloride in hydroalcoholic medium and is designed to provide suitable mechanical properties and ensure gas exchange. The lower layer is soft and flexible, which can fill the shape of the wound and ensure

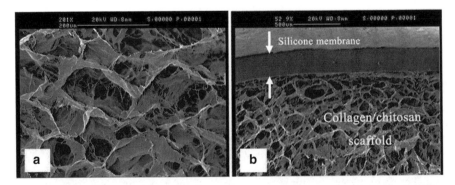

Fig. 14 SEM images showing the microstructure of (**a**) glutaraldehyde-crosslinked scaffold and (**b**) the bilayer dermal equivalent [182]

a good superficial contact. The in vivo results showed that the chitosan gels could induce inflammatory cell migration, angiogenesis, formation of the dermal–epidermal junction, and ultimately promote skin regeneration. The newly formed tissues display good flexibility, which is encouraging from the esthetic point of view. A photocrosslinkable chitosan containing azide groups and lactose moieties (Az-CH-LA) has also been utilized to form hydrogels as wound-healing materials [185]. Serum-free culture medium can be further added into the hydrogels to stimulate infiltration of neutrophils. When applied to deep burn wounds, the medium-Az-CH-LA gels not only induce formation of thicker granulation tissue than collagen sponge, but also mediate earlier degradation and angiogenic activities.

5.1.4 Gene-Activated Matrices

Angiogenesis of the dermal equivalent is one of the most crucial issues for the repair and regeneration of full-thickness skin defects. Our group used TMC as a gene vector to deliver functional genes [32]. Later, the complexes of TMC/plasmid DNA encoding VEGF (pDNA-VEGF) were incorporated into a collagen scaffold to construct a gene-activated matrix [186]. Implantation of the gene-activated matrix into Sprague-Dawley mice demonstrated that the TMC/DNA complexes remarkably promoted the in vivo expression of VEGF and thus the angiogenesis of the scaffolds. Recently, we prepared a gene-activated BDE and evaluated its biological performance for treatment of the full-thickness incisional wounds in terms of histology, immunohistochemistry, immunofluorescence, real-time quantitative PCR, and western blotting analysis in a porcine model [187]. The TMC/pDNA-VEGF group showed highest VEGF expression at both mRNA and protein levels, leading to the highest densities of newly formed and mature vessels (Fig. 15). After 112 days of ultrathin skin graft transplantation, the healing skin had a similar

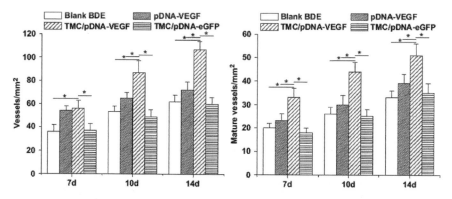

Fig. 15 Number of newly formed and mature vessels in wounds after treatment with blank BDE, and BDEs loaded with pDNA-VEGF, TMC/pDNA-VEGF, and TMC/pDNA-eGFP after 7, 10 and 14 days ($n = 6$). Asterisk denotes statistically significant difference, $P < 0.05$ [187]

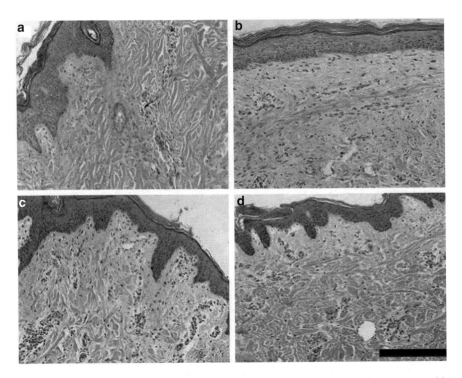

Fig. 16 H&E staining of (**a**) normal skin tissue and (**b–d**) sections of wounds after treatment with BDEs loaded with TMC/pDNA-VEGF for 10 days, followed by transplantation of ultrathin autografts for 21 days (**b**), 70 days (**c**) and 112 days (**d**). *Scale bar*: 200 μm [187]

structure and ~80% tensile strength of the normal skin (Fig. 16). Exploitation of the gene-activated BDE for the healing of full-thickness burns was also performed, showing very positive results similar to those for incisional wounds [188].

5.2 Cartilage

Due to the absence of blood vessels and lymphatic systems, injured articular cartilage has poor capacity for spontaneous self-repair [189, 190]. Surgical approaches such as abrasion, drilling, microfracture, osteochondral grafting, and autologous chondrocyte implantation have been utilized to treat and restore cartilage defects in the past decades [191]. Tissue engineering and regenerative medicine provide new opportunities for cartilage repair. Chitosan and its derivatives are among the attractive candidate materials for cartilage repair, owing to their structural similarity with GAGs and the positive effects of their degradation products on biosynthesis of articular matrix [192].

5.2.1 Pure Chitosan

Chitosan scaffolds are prepared by freeze-drying, and the effect of pore size on the behavior of cultured chondrocytes within the scaffolds has been determined [193]. More chondrocytes, collagen type II, and GAG have been measured in scaffolds with pores of 70–120 μm in diameter than those with pores of ≤10 μm. In addition, larger pore sizes can better improve the proliferation and metabolic activity of chondrocytes. Montembault et al. [194] found that in pure chitosan hydrogels, the chondrocytes could bind tightly to the surface of the fragments. The neo-formed cartilage-like ECM accumulated and was widely distributed within the construct. The optimal chitosan hydrogels are formed at a DD of 60–70% and chitosan concentration of 1.5% (w/w), which can maintain the phenotype of chondrocytes for as long as 45 days in primary culture. This research indicates that the chitosan hydrogels can act as a decoy for cartilage ECM components, leading to a biological response termed "reverse encapsulation" by the authors. Chitosan nonwoven scaffolds composed of fibers with varied width have been prepared and are expected to simulate the structure of cartilage ECM [106]. In comparison with PGA mesh, the chitosan fibrous scaffolds result in a higher matrix production per chondrocyte.

5.2.2 Chitosan Composites

In order to combine the advantages of natural biomacromolecules and synthetic polymers, chitosan/poly(butylene succinate) (CPBS) has been blended and processed into scaffolds by compression molding with salt leaching [195]. Mouse bone marrow-derived mesenchymal progenitor cells (BMC9) can grow and colonize in the scaffolds, and express collagen type II at 3 weeks, indicating that the cells are undergoing a chondrogenic differentiation. A bovine articular chondrocyte model has also been applied to establish primary cultures in CPBS scaffolds with different pore size and geometry. Large pores and random geometry promote the production of collagen type II and proteoglycans, while the production of GAG is influenced oppositely. By using the freeze-drying technique, alginate/chitosan scaffolds with semi-interpenetrating network were prepared and used to culture the ATDC5 chondrogenic cell line [196]. The hybrid scaffolds can support chondrocyte proliferation and maintain cell phenotype. In particular, the alginate/chitosan scaffolds (50:50, v/v) are proved to be promising candidates for cartilage tissue engineering.

PEO can provide advantages such as enhanced hydrophilicity for cell affinity, elasticity for cartilage analogy, and permeability for mass transport, therefore PEO/chitosan composite scaffolds have also been generated and further modified by fibronectin [197]. The growth and functions of bovine knee chondrocyte are favored under higher content of PEO and human fibronectin, revealing that the biomedical properties of solid chitosan scaffolds have been remarkably improved. Yamane et al. [198] developed a chitosan/hyaluronic acid fibrous scaffold by a wet spinning method. It was found that the scaffold with a pore size of 400 μm induced higher production of GAG and higher mRNA ratio of collagen II to collagen I

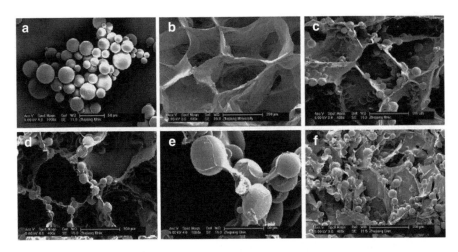

Fig. 17 SEM images of (**a**) PLGA microspheres and (**b**) the gelatin/chitosan/hyaluronan ternary complex scaffold. (**c–f**) SEM images of the ternary complex scaffold containing 30% (**c**), 50% (**d**) and 70% (**f**) PLGA microspheres. (**e**) Magnified image of (**d**) [199]

compared with those scaffolds having pore sizes of 100 or 200 µm. We [199] have fabricated a hybrid system containing gelatin/chitosan/hyaluronan scaffolds containing PLGA microspheres for cartilage tissue engineering (Fig. 17). Generally, a higher content of PLGA microspheres leads to a smaller porosity but a larger apparent density and compressive modulus. An optimized PLGA content of 50% can provide appropriate mechanical properties and also maintain the biocompatibility of the original gelatin/chitosan/hyaluronan matrix with chondrocytes.

Our group designed and fabricated a chitosan-based composite hydrogel by mixing collagen-coated PLA microcarriers into a crosslinkable chitosan hydrogel (CML) [200]. The hydrogel acts as a delivery system of microcarriers, and the microcarriers can substantially improve the mechanical strength of the hydrogel. In vitro culture revealed that the chondrocytes are able to attach and grow on the surface of microcarriers to generate cell layers, indicating the great potential of the composite system for cartilage tissue engineering. In another study, chitosan was derived by conjugation of glycolic acid (GA) and phloretic acid (PA) to obtain a water-soluble polymer (chitosan–GA/PA), which can be processed into a hydrogel by enzymatic crosslinking with horseradish peroxidase (HRP) and H_2O_2 [201]. Encapsulation and culture of chondrocytes in the hydrogels suggest that the material has an ability to support proliferation of cells and retain their round shape in vitro. Tan et al. [202] synthesized *N*-succinyl-chitosan and aldehyde hyaluronic acid for the fabrication of injectable hydrogels based on the gelation reaction between amino and aldehyde groups. Higher content of *N*-succinyl-chitosan results in a slower degradation rate and improved compressive modulus of the hydrogels. Biological studies indicate that the composite hydrogels promote survival rate and retain the spherical morphology of chondrocytes (Fig. 18). Silva et al. [203] prepared chitosan/silk sponges from blends of chitosan and *Bombyx mori* silk

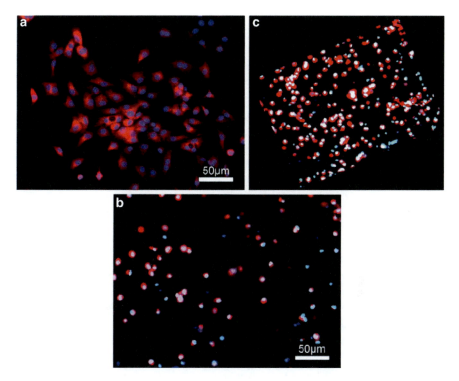

Fig. 18 (a) CLSM image showing bovine chondrocytes on the surface of a 5/5 (v/v) *N*-succinyl-chitosan/aldehyde hyaluronic acid composite hydrogel after 24-h culture. Cell-seeding density was 50,000 per well (24-well cell culture plate). (b) CLSM image showing bovine chondrocytes encapsulated in a 5/5 (v/v) *N*-succinyl-chitosan/aldehyde hyaluronic acid composite hydrogel after 24-h culture. Cell-seeding density was 5×10^6/mL. (c) 3D image of (b). Live cells were stained with Cell Tracker Orange CMRA (*red*) and all cell nuclei were stained with Hoechst 33342 (*blue*) [202]

fibroin by crosslinking with genipin. Attributed to the silk protein conformation changes, the structures of the sponges are stable and ordered. These sponges were expected to mimic the natural cartilage environment and proved to favor the adhesion, proliferation, and matrix production of chondrocyte-like cells. A chitosan–Pluronic (CP) conjugate was obtained by grafting Pluronic onto chitosan molecules and was subsequently generated into thermosensitive hydrogels as injectable cell carriers for cartilage regeneration [204]. The sol–gel transition of CP above the LCST around 25°C is thought to be based on the hydrophobic interactions between PPO moieties. The CP gels exhibit good performance in supporting chondrocyte growth and promoting ECM production. Hao et al. [205] prepared another kind of temperature-responsive hydrogel by combining chitosan, β-sodium glycerophosphate, and hydroxyethyl cellulose for cartilage tissue engineering. After transplantation of the construct cultured for 1 day to a sheep in vivo, the articular cartilage defects could be completely repaired within 24 weeks.

5.2.3 Bioactive Chitosan Composites

Bioactive agents such as peptides, growth factors, cytokines, and functional genes have been combined with the chitosan-based matrix for cartilage repair and regeneration. By coupling the carboxyl group in the RGD peptide with the amine groups in CP molecules, a RGD-conjugated CP is synthesized and fabricated into thermosensitive hydrogels [206]. The introduction of RGD enhances cell viability and GAGs expression remarkably. In order to mimic the composition of natural cartilage matrix, our group immobilized heparin onto the gelatin/chitosan/hyaluronan (82.6/16.5/0.1, w/w/w) porous scaffolds, through which bFGF was subsequently bound [141]. The chondrocytes cultured in the bFGF-immobilized scaffold displayed significantly higher viability. Quite recently, we combined stem cells and functional genes into a hydrogel/scaffold composite as a novel scaffold for in vivo restoration of full-thickness cartilage defects (Fig. 19) [207]. Here, the TMC is exploited to condense and encapsulate plasmid DNA encoding TGF-β1 to improve the transfection efficiency. The composite construct composed of BMSCs, TMC/pDNA-TGF-β1 complexes, fibrin gel, and PLGA scaffold was implanted into the full-thickness cartilage defects in New Zealand white rabbits. After 12 weeks, the cartilage was successfully repaired, as confirmed by immunohistochemical and GAGs staining, and gene expression (Fig. 20). An overall score of 2.83 was obtained based on Wakitani's standard, indicating that the composite construct is effective in restoring cartilage defects and possibly has great potential for practical applications in the near future.

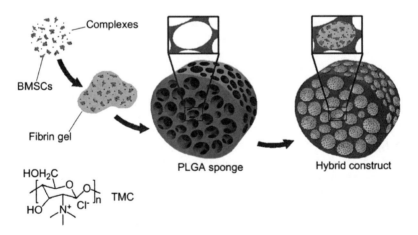

Fig. 19 Fabricating procedure of the composite construct by filling BMSCs, TMC/DNA complexes, and fibrin gel into a PLGA sponge. *Bottom left*: Chemical structure of TMC. pDNA-TGF-β1 was used in the in vivo experiment [207]

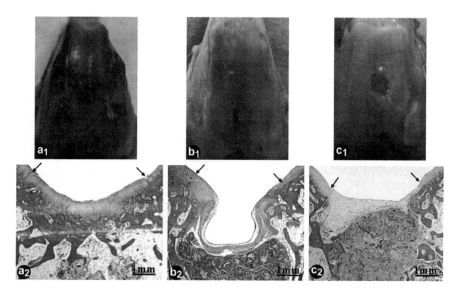

Fig. 20 (**a1–c1**) Gross view and (**a2–c2**) histological images of the neo-cartilage after transplantation for 12 weeks in rabbit knees. (**a1, a2**) PLGA/fibrin gel/BMSCs/(TMC/pDNA-TGF-β1 complexes), (**b1, b2**) PLGA/fibrin gel/BMSCs, and (**c1, c2**) PLGA/fibrin gel/(TMC/pDNA-TGF-β1 complexes). The *arrows* in (**a2–c2**) indicate the boundaries between the grafts and the host tissues [207]

5.3 Bone

Recently, in order to overcome the limitations of autologous bone graft such as availability of suitable bone, painful procedure, cosmetic disability, nerve damage, and large and unconfined cartilage defects, bone tissue engineering has been developed as an alternative to autologous bone graft treatment for the reconstruction of mass bone defect [208]. Due to its ability to promote proliferation and mineral deposition by osteoblasts, chitosan has been extensively used for bone tissue engineering [209]. In particular, because the bone ECM is composed of organic phase and HA-containing inorganic phase [210], composite materials of chitosan and inorganic bioceramics are paid considerable attention.

5.3.1 Composite Scaffolds

In order to improve the mechanical strength and biological performance of chitosan and make it more suitable for bone repair and regeneration, it has been a widely accepted approach to incorporate other biopolymers or inorganic materials into chitosan scaffolds. Furthermore, from the viewpoint of biomimetics, bone is a nanocomposite of minerals and proteins. Therefore, attempts have been made recently to develop nanocomposites for bone tissue engineering, among which the utilization of nanohydroxyapatite (nHA) has drawn increasing attention. Thain et al. [211] reported a comparative assessment of the structures, physicochemical properties, and biological performances of chitosan/nHA composites and pure chitosan scaffolds. The nHA particles exhibit a uniform dispersion in chitosan matrix and interact with chitosan via chemical affinity. Increased content of nHA leads to a decreased water-uptake ability as well as a lower degradation rate of the scaffolds. The attachment and proliferation of pre-osteoblasts are enhanced on the composites compared to those on the control. Jiang et al. [212] prepared a composite scaffold consisting of nHA, chitosan, and CMC. Biological evaluation by culture of MG63 cells and MSCs in vitro and implantation study in vivo confirmed that the composite material was both cytocompatible and histocompatible. In another study, HA was synthesized in situ and incorporated into the collagen/chitosan matrix to obtain a collagen/chitosan/HA nanocomposite [213]. Plenty of organic fibers exist and protrude out from the dense matrix containing inorganic aggregates less than 30 nm in size, suggesting improved flexibility. The collagen/chitosan/HA nanocomposite exhibits high compatibility with Ran Ros 17/2.8 osteoblasts, providing a practical approach for bone grafting nanocomposites. Sol–gel-derived bioactive glass ceramic nanoparticles (nBGC), which possessed osteoconductivity and biodegradability, have been blended with chitosan and gelatin to generate a composite scaffold [214]. The addition of nBGC results in an increase of protein adsorption and a higher amount of mineral deposits on the composite scaffolds.

5.3.2 Fibers, Membranes, and Microspheres

Nonwoven polyester fibers can be coated by chitin/chitosan with a density of 0.08 mg/cm^2 to generate a biological fixation to bone [215]. The chitin/chitosan coating acts as a bone formation accelerator, which significantly enhances the fixation strength and the area of neo-formed bone tissue. By using a sol–gel process, a silica xerogel with bone bioactivity was hybridized with chitosan to form a guiding membrane for bone regeneration (Fig. 21) [216]. In vitro bone activity of the membranes was confirmed by the findings of rapid induction of calcium phosphate minerals in simulated body fluid and higher ALP activity of osteoblastic cells. Moreover, in a rat calvarial model, the hybrid membranes exhibit the ability to promote bone regeneration. By fusing chitosan microspheres of 500–900 μm in diameter, a co-precipitated composite chitosan/nanocrystalline calcium phosphate scaffold has been prepared (Fig. 22) [217]. Compared with the pure chitosan scaffold, the composite scaffolds are much rougher and possess 20-fold bigger surface area per unit mass, which promote the adsorption of fibronectin and the attachment of cells. In addition, the proliferation of osteoblasts is significantly increased after 1 week of culture, as confirmed by dsDNA levels. Jiang et al. [109] constructed another microsphere-based system from sintered hybrid chitosan/PLGA microspheres, further functionalized by immobilization of heparin. MC3T3-E1 cells show the best activity of proliferation and differentiation in the scaffolds with low heparin loading (1.7 μg/scaffold).

Chitosan-Based Biomaterials for Tissue Repair and Regeneration 119

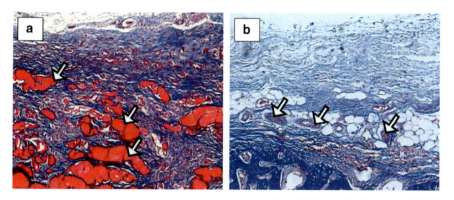

Fig. 21 Bone tissue and membranes 3 weeks after implantation of (**a**) pure chitosan membrane and (**b**) chitosan/silica xerogel hybrid membrane. For the histomorphometric analysis, the defect sites were observed at high magnification. The pure chitosan membrane was partially degraded and the remaining part (*arrows*) was surrounded by collagen fibers (*blue*), bone marrow, and osteocyte cells (*red*), as shown in (**a**). However, the hybrid membrane was almost completely degraded and the defect site (*arrows*) was replaced by a large number of collagen fibers and fresh new bone (*blue*), as shown in (**b**) [216]

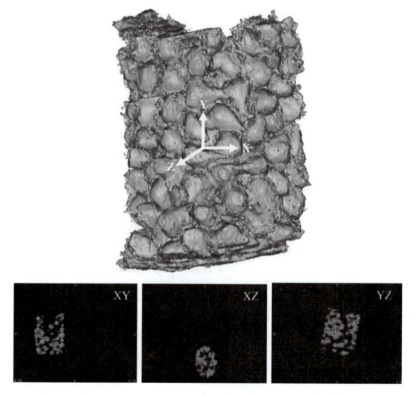

Fig. 22 Representative micro-computed tomography images of composite scaffolds in axial (*XY*), coronal (*XZ*), and sagittal (*YZ*) directions [217]

5.3.3 Systems Containing Growth Factors

Bone morphogenetic proteins (BMPs) are members of the TGF-β family and are well known for the capability of inducing bone formation. Akman et al. [218] incorporated BMP-6 into chitosan scaffolds by an embedding technique. When cultured with MC3T3-E1 cells, the BMP-6-loaded scaffolds significantly accelerated ECM production, had higher levels of ALP and osteocalcin, and showed higher mineralized tissue-forming activity than the blank scaffolds or chitosan scaffolds supplemented with same amount of BMP-6 in the culture medium. These results suggest that combination of BMP-6 with the chitosan scaffold provides an appealing approach for inducing osteoblastic differentiation and thereby bone regeneration. A sequential delivery of growth factors is achieved by incorporating BMP-2-loaded PLGA nanocapsules and BMP-7-loaded poly(3-hydroxybutyrate-co-3-hydroxyvalerate) (PHBV) nanocapsules into the chitosan-based scaffolds, into which MSCs are then seeded [219]. The early release of BMP-2 and longer term release of BMP-7 is expected, which results in a high ALP activity per cell but suppresses proliferation. These findings indicate the synergistic effect of BMP-2 and BMP-7 on bone repair. VEGF has also been applied to enhance neovascularization of the implant in bone healing. By loading VEGF-encapsulated alginate microspheres into chitosan-based scaffolds, controlled release and localization of VEGF at the desired site of defect can be achieved [220]. As a key factor in bone regeneration, PDGF can also promote angiogenesis. In a strategy proposed by Riva et al., both VEGF and PDGF were incorporated into brushite–chitosan systems [221]. In rabbit femur models, PDGF was released from the system more rapidly than VEGF, although both of them remained around the implantation sites (Fig. 23). According to the results of histological and histomorphometrical evaluation, it was concluded that bone formation was remarkably stimulated by the scaffolds loaded with PDGF andVEGF.

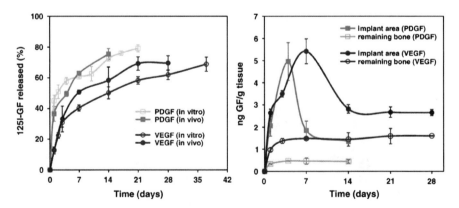

Fig. 23 *Left*: In vitro and in vivo release profiles of ^{125}I-VEGF and ^{125}I-PDGF incorporated into brushite–chitosan scaffolds. *Right*: ^{125}I-VEGF and ^{125}I-PDGF concentrations achieved in the different areas of rabbit femurs after brushite–chitosan implantation [221]

6 Conclusion

In summary, chitosan has been extensively utilized in biomaterials for tissue repair and regeneration. Physical and chemical modifications are carried out to derive chitosans with the desired structures, properties, and functions. Porous scaffolds and smart hydrogels are the most important applicable material forms, while the chitosan-based delivery systems for growth factors, DNAs, and siRNAs are also of great significance in constructing bioactive biomaterials. In particular, as stem cells play an increasingly prominent role in the field of tissue repair and regeneration, the combination and interaction between stem cells and chitosan-based materials have been specifically emphasized and discussed. Successful exploitation of chitosan-based biomaterials in different tissues and organs such as skin, cartilage, and bone suggests their promising future for repair and regeneration applications.

Acknowledgments We acknowledge financial support by the Natural Science Foundation of China (20934003), the Science Technology Program of Zhejiang Province (2009C14003, 2009C13020), and the Major State Basic Research Program of China (2011CB606203).

References

1. Tabata Y (2009) J R Soc Interface 6:S311
2. Langer R, Vacanti JP (1993) Science 260:920
3. Stevens MM, Marini RP, Schaefer D, Aronson J, Langer R, Shastri VP (2005) Proc Natl Acad Sci USA 102:11450
4. Trung TS, Thein-Han WW, Qui NT, Ng CH, Stevens WF (2006) Bioresour Technol 97:659
5. Place ES, George JH, Williams CK, Stevens MM (2009) Chem Soc Rev 38:1139
6. Suh JKF, Matthew HWT (2000) Biomaterials 21:2589
7. Madihally SV, Matthew HWT (1999) Biomaterials 20:1133
8. Eisenbarth E (2007) Adv Eng Mater 9:1051
9. Khor E, Lim LY (2003) Biomaterials 24:2339
10. Hirano S, Tsuchida H, Nagao N (1989) Biomaterials 10:574
11. Dornish M, Kaplan D, Skaugrud O (2001) Bioartificial organs III: tissue sourcing, immunoisolation, and clinical trials. Ann NY Acad Sci 944:388
12. VandeVord PJ, Matthew HWT, DeSilva SP, Mayton L, Wu B, Wooley PH (2002) J Biomed Mater Res 59:585
13. Chandy T, Sharma CP (1990) Biomater Artif Cells Artif Organs 18:1
14. Ge ZG, Baguenard S, Lim LY, Wee A, Khor E (2004) Biomaterials 25:1049
15. Muzzarelli RAA (1988) Carbohyd Polym 8:1
16. Muzzarelli RAA, Muzzarelli C (1998) Native and modified chitins in the biosphere. In: Stankiewicz BA, van Bergen PF (eds) Nitrogen-containing macromolecules in the bio- and geosphere. ACS Symposium Series 707:148
17. Thein-Han WW, Kitiyanant Y (2007) J Biomed Mater Res B 80B:92
18. Ma L, Gao CY, Mao ZW, Zhou J, Shen JC, Hu XQ, Han CM (2003) Biomaterials 24:4833
19. Desai UR (2004) Med Res Rev 24:151
20. Nagasawa K, Tohira Y, Inoue Y, Tanoura N (1971) Carbohydr Res 18:95
21. Nudga LA, Plisko EA, Danilov SN (1974) Zh Prikl Khim 47:872
22. Muzzarelli RAA (1992) Carbohyd Polym 19:231

23. Li QL, Huang N, Chen JL, Wan GJ, Zhao AS, Chen JY, Wang J, Yang P, Leng YX (2009) J Biomed Mater Res A 89A:575
24. Vikhoreva G, Bannikova G, Stolbushkina P, Panov A, Drozd N, Makarov V, Varlamov V, Gal'braikh L (2005) Carbohyd Polym 62:327
25. Qu GW, Yao Z, Zhang C, Wu XL, Ping QE (2009) Eur J Pharm Sci 37:98
26. Huang AB, Guo R, Xu SJ, Ma L, Gao CY (2009) Acta Polymerica Sin 2:7
27. Lehr CM, Bouwstra JA, Schacht EH, Junginger HE (1992) Int J Pharm 78:43
28. Mourya VK, Inamdar NN (2009) J Mater Sci Mater M 20:1057
29. Bernkop-Schnurch A, Hornof M, Guggi D (2004) Eur J Pharm Biopharm 57:9
30. Amidi M, Romeijn SG, Borchard G, Junginger HE, Hennink WE, Jiskoot W (2006) J Control Release 111:107
31. Chen F, Zhang ZR, Huang Y (2007) Int J Pharm 336:166
32. Mao ZW, Ma L, Jiang Y, Yan M, Gao CY, Shen JC (2007) Macromol Biosci 7:855
33. Mao ZW, Ma L, Yan J, Yan M, Gao CY, Shen JC (2007) Biomaterials 28:4488
34. Germershaus O, Mao SR, Sitterberg J, Bakowsky U, Kissel T (2008) J Control Release 125:145
35. Zheng Y, Cai Z, Song XR, Yu B, Bi YQ, Chen QH, Zhao D, Xu JP, Hou SX (2009) Int J Pharm 382:262
36. Krauland AH, Guggi D, Bernkop-Schnurch A (2006) Int J Pharm 307:270
37. Yin LC, Ding JY, He CB, Cui LM, Tang C, Yin CH (2009) Biomaterials 30:5691
38. Lee D, Zhang W, Shirley SA, Kong X, Hellermann GR, Lockey RF, Mohapatra SS (2007) Pharm Res 24:157
39. Zhao X, Yin LC, Ding JY, Tang C, Gu SH, Yin CH, Mao YM (2010) J Control Release 144:46
40. Li Z, Cen L, Zhao L, Cui L, Liu W, Cao YL (2010) J Biomed Mater Res A 92A:973
41. Hersel U, Dahmen C, Kessler H (2003) Biomaterials 24:4385
42. Karakecili AG, Gumusderelioglu M (2008) Colloid Surf B 61:216
43. Masuko T, Iwasaki N, Yamane S, Funakoshi T, Majima T, Minami A, Ohsuga N, Ohta T, Nishimura SI (2005) Biomaterials 26:5339
44. Mochizuki M, Kadoya Y, Wakabayashi Y, Kato K, Okazaki I, Yamada M, Sato T, Sakairi N, Nishi N, Nomizu M (2003) FASEB J 17:875
45. Hozumi K, Otagiri D, Yamada Y, Sasaki A, Fujimori C, Wakai Y, Uchida T, Katagiri F, Kikkawa Y, Nomizu M (2010) Biomaterials 31:3237
46. Ikemoto S, Mochizuki M, Yamada M, Takeda A, Uchinuma E, Yamashina S, Nomizu M, Kadoya Y (2006) J Biomed Mater Res A 79A:716
47. Itoh S, Takakuda K, Samejima H, Ohta T, Shinomiya K, Ichinose S (1999) J Mater Sci Mater M 10:129
48. Itoh S, Matsuda A, Kobayashi H, Ichinose S, Shinomiya K, Tanaka J (2005) J Biomed Mater Res B 73B:375
49. Wang W, Itoh S, Matsuda A, Aizawa T, Demura M, Ichinose S, Shinomiya K, Tanaka J (2008) J Biomed Mater Res A 85A:919
50. Bae JS, Lee SH, Kim JE, Choi JY, Park RW, Park JY, Park HS, Sohn YS, Lee DS, Lee EB, Kim IS (2002) Biochem Biophys Res Commun 294:940
51. Chung T-W, Lu Y-F, Wang S-S, Lin Y-S, Chu S-H (2002) Biomaterials 23:4803
52. Kim TH, Park IK, Nah JW, Choi YJ, Cho CS (2004) Biomaterials 25:3783
53. Song BF, Zhang W, Peng R, Huang J, Me T, Li Y, Jiang Q, Gao R (2009) Colloid Surf B 70:181
54. Feng ZQ, Chu XH, Huang NP, Wang T, Wang YC, Shi XL, Ding YT, Gu ZZ (2009) Biomaterials 30:2753
55. Chu XH, Shi XL, Feng ZQ, Gu JY, Xu HY, Zhang Y, Gu ZZ, Ding YT (2009) Biomaterials 30:4533
56. Park IK, Kim TH, Park YH, Shin BA, Choi ES, Chowdhury EH, Akaike T, Cho CS (2001) J Control Release 76:349

57. Park YK, Park YH, Shin BA, Choi ES, Park YR, Akaike T, Cho CS (2000) J Control Release 69:97
58. Donati I, Stredanska S, Silvestrini G, Vetere A, Marcon P, Marsich E, Mozetic P, Gamini A, Paoletti S, Vittur F (2005) Biomaterials 26:987
59. Colnot C, Sidhu SS, Poirier F, Balmain N (1999) Cell Mol Biol 45:1191
60. Tan HP, Lao LH, Wu JD, Gong YH, Gao CY (2008) Polym Adv Technol 19:15
61. Taylor ME, Conary JT, Lennartz MR, Stahl PD, Drickamer K (1990) J Biol Chem 265:12156
62. Jiang HL, Kim YK, Arote R, Jere D, Quan JS, Yu JH, Choi YJ, Nah JW, Cho MH, Cho CS (2009) Int J Pharm 375:133
63. Jiang HL, Kang ML, Quan JS, Kang SG, Akaike T, Yoo HS, Cho CS (2008) Biomaterials 29:1931
64. Li XB, Tushima Y, Morimoto M, Saimoto H, Okamoto Y, Minami S, Shigemasa Y (2000) Polym Adv Technol 11:176
65. Sun LP, Wang S, Zhang ZW, Wang XY, Zhang QQ (2009) Biomed Mater 4:055008
66. Ma JB, Wang HJ, He BL, Chen JT (2001) Biomaterials 22:331
67. Young BR, Pitt WG, Cooper SL (1988) J Colloid Interface Sci 124:28
68. Pulieri E, Chiono V, Ciardelli G, Vozzi G, Ahluwalia A, Domenici C, Vozzi F, Giusti P (2008) J Biomed Mater Res A 86A:311
69. He JK, Li DC, Liu YX, Yao B, Zhan HX, Lian Q, Lu BH, Lv Y (2009) Acta Biomater 5:453
70. Dhandayuthapani B, Krishnan UM, Sethuraman S (2010) J Biomed Mater Res B 94B:264
71. Bryant SJ, Davis-Arehart KA, Luo N, Shoemaker RK, Arthur JA, Anseth KS (2004) Macromolecules 37:6726
72. Mi FL, Shyu SS, Peng CK, Wu YB, Sung HW, Wang PS, Huang CC (2006) J Biomed Mater Res A 76A:1
73. Jou CH, Chen WC, Yang MC, Hwang MC, Chou WL, Lin SM, Hsu CY (2008) Polym Adv Technol 19:377
74. Kakehi K, Kinoshita M, Yasueda S (2003) J Chromatogr B 797:347
75. Aruffo A, Stamenkovic I, Melnick M, Underhill CB, Seed B (1990) Cell 61:1303
76. Wang YJ, Guo L, Ren L, Yin SH, Ge J, Gao QY, Luxbacher T, Luo SJ (2009) Biomed Mater 4:035009
77. Xu HT, Ma L, Shi HF, Gao CY, Han CM (2007) Polym Adv Technol 18:869
78. Fan JY, Shang Y, Yuan YJ, Yang J (2010) J Mater Sci Mater M 21:319
79. Li ZS, Ramay HR, Hauch KD, Xiao DM, Zhang MQ (2005) Biomaterials 26:3919
80. Li ZS, Zhang MQ (2005) J Biomed Mater Res A 75A:485
81. Ratner BR, Hoffman AS, Schoen FJ, Lemons JE (1996) Biomaterials science, 2nd edn. Academic, New York
82. Wan Y, Wu H, Cao XY, Dalai S (2008) Polym Degrad Stabil 93:1736
83. Malheiro VN, Caridade SG, Alves NM, Mano JF (2010) Acta Biomater 6:418
84. Cruz DMG, Coutinho DF, Mano JF, Ribelles JLG, Sanchez MS (2009) Polymer 50:2058
85. Xu J, Zhang JH, Gao WQ, Liang HW, Wang HY, Li JF (2009) Mater Lett 63:658
86. Lin HY, Yeh CT (2010) J Mater Sci Mater M 21:1611
87. Gupta KC, Jabrail FH (2007) Carbohydr Res 342:2244
88. Nayak UY, Gopal S, Mutalik S, Ranjith AK, Reddy MS, Gupta P, Udupa N (2009) J Microencapsul 26:214
89. Baran ET, Mano JF, Reis RL (2004) J Mater Sci Mater M 15:759
90. Paradossi G, Cavalieri F, Crescenzi V (1997) Carbohydr Res 300:77
91. Hoffmann B, Seitz D, Mencke A, Kokott A, Ziegler G (2009) J Mater Sci Mater M 20:1495
92. Mi FL, Tan YC, Liang HF, Sung HW (2002) Biomaterials 23:181
93. Lee CR, Grodzinsky AJ, Spector M (2001) Biomaterials 22:3145
94. Adekogbe I, Ghanem A (2005) Biomaterials 26:7241
95. Zeeman R, Dijkstra PJ, van Wachem PB, van Luyn MJA, Hendriks M, Cahalan PT, Feijen J (1999) Biomaterials 20:921

96. Rafat M, Li FF, Fagerholm P, Lagali NS, Watsky MA, Munger R, Matsuura T, Griffith M (2008) Biomaterials 29:3960
97. Ma L, Gao CY, Mao ZW, Zhou J, Shen JC (2004) Biomaterials 25:2997
98. Madihally SV, Flake AW, Matthew HWT (1999) Stem Cells 17:295
99. Mao JS, Zhao LG, Yin YJ, Yao KD (2003) Biomaterials 24:1067
100. Arora KA, Lesser AJ, McCarthy TJ (1999) Macromolecules 32:2562
101. Mooney DJ, Baldwin DF, Suh NP, Vacanti LP, Langer R (1996) Biomaterials 17:1417
102. Shi C, Huang Z, Kilic S, Xu J, Enick RM, Beckman EJ, Carr AJ, Melendez RE, Hamilton AD (1999) Science 286:1540
103. Rinki K, Dutta PK (2010) J Macromol Sci A 47:429
104. Rinki K, Dutta PK (2010) Int J Biol Macromol 46:261
105. Temtem M, Casimiro T, Mano JF, Aguiar-Ricardo A (2007) Green Chem 9:75
106. Ragetly GR, Slavik GJ, Cunningham BT, Schaeffer DJ, Griffon DJ (2010) J Biomed Mater Res A 93A:46
107. Slavik GJ, Ragetly G, Ganesh N, Griffon DJ, Cunningham BT (2007) J Mater Chem 17:4095
108. Jiang T, Abdel-Fattah WI, Laurencin CT (2006) Biomaterials 27:4894
109. Jiang T, Khan Y, Nair LS, Abdel-Fattah WI, Laurencin CT (2010) J Biomed Mater Res A 93A:1193
110. Borden M, Attawia M, Khan Y, Laurencin CT (2002) Biomaterials 23:551
111. Malafaya PB, Pedro AJ, Peterbauer A, Gabriel C, Redl H, Reis RL (2005) J Mater Sci Mater M 16:1077
112. Malafaya PB, Santos TC, van Griensven M, Reis RL (2008) Biomaterials 29:3914
113. Kucharska M, Walenko K, Butruk B, Brynk T, Heljak M, Ciach T (2010) Mater Lett 64:1059
114. Cho MH, Kim KS, Ahn HH, Kim MS, Kim SH, Khang G, Lee B, Lee HB (2008) Tissue Eng Part A 14:1099
115. Crescenzi V, Cornelio L, Di Meo C, Nardecchia S, Lamanna R (2007) Biomacromolecules 8:1844
116. Hong Y, Song HQ, Gong YH, Mao ZW, Gao CY, Shen JC (2007) Acta Biomater 3:23
117. Hong Y, Mao ZW, Wang HL, Gao CY, Shen JC (2006) J Biomed Mater Res A 79:913
118. Hong Y, Gong YH, Gao CY, Shen JC (2007) J Biomed Mater Res A 85:628
119. Hu XH, Gao CY (2008) J Appl Polym Sci 110:1059
120. Hu XH, Zhou J, Zhang N, Tan HP, Gao CY (2008) J Mech Behav Biomed Mater 1:352
121. Chenite A, Buschmann M, Wang D, Chaput C, Kandani N (2001) Carbohyd Polym 46:39
122. Lu SH, Wang HB, Lu WN, Liu S, Lin QX, Li DX, Duan C, Hao T, Zhou J, Wang YM, Gao SR, Wang CY (2010) Tissue Eng Part A 16:1303
123. Lu WN, Lu SH, Wang HB, Li DX, Duan CM, Liu ZQ, Hao T, He WJ, Xu B, Fu Q, Song YC, Xie XH, Wang CY (2009) Tissue Eng Part A 15:1437
124. Zhang J, Yuan K, Wang YP, Zhang ST, Zhang J (2007) J Bioact Compat Pol 22:207
125. Ding CX, Zhao LL, Liu FY, Cheng J, Gu JX, Dan S, Liu CY, Qu XZ, Yang ZZ (2010) Biomacromolecules 11:1043
126. Hu QL, Qian XZ, Li BQ, Shen JC (2003) Chem J Chin Univ 24:528
127. Li YZ, Wang YX, Wu D, Zhang K, Hu QL (2010) Carbohyd Polym 80:408
128. Hu QL, Li BQ, Wang M, Shen JC (2004) Biomaterials 25:779
129. Wang ZK, Hu QL, Dai XG, Wu H, Wang YX, Shen JC (2009) Polym Compos 30:1517
130. Cui W, Hu QL, Wu JD, Li BQ, Shen JC (2008) J Appl Polym Sci 109:2081
131. Hu QL, Chen ZK, Chen L, Shen JC (2006) Chem J Chin Univ 27:575
132. Chen FM, Zhang M, Wu ZF (2010) Biomaterials 31:6279
133. Park YJ, Lee YM, Park SN, Sheen SY, Chung CP, Lee SJ (2000) Biomaterials 21:153
134. Alemdaroglu C, Degim Z, Celebi N, Zor F, Ozturk S, Erdogan D (2006) Burns 32:319
135. Obara K, Ishihara M, Ishizuka T, Fujita M, Ozeki Y, Maehara T, Saito Y, Yura H, Matsui T, Hattori H, Kikuchi M, Kurita A (2003) Biomaterials 24:3437
136. Karakecli AG, Satriano C, Gumusderelioglu M, Marletta G (2008) Acta Biomater 4:989

137. Kim SE, Park JH, Cho YW, Chung H, Jeong SY, Lee EB, Kwon IC (2003) J Control Release 91:365
138. Liu HF, Fan HB, Cui YL, Chen YP, Yao KD, Goh JCH (2007) Biomacromolecules 8:1446
139. Ho YC, Wu SJ, Mi FL, Chiu YL, Yu SH, Panda N, Sung HW (2010) Bioconjug Chem 21:28
140. Fujita M, Ishihara M, Simizu M, Obara K, Ishizuka T, Saito Y, Yura H, Morimoto Y, Takase B, Matsui T, Kikuchi M, Maehara T (2004) Biomaterials 25:699
141. Tan HP, Gong YH, Lao LH, Mao ZW, Gao CY (2007) J Mater Sci Mater M 18:1961
142. Ho YC, Mi FL, Sung HW, Kuo PL (2009) Int J Pharm 376:69
143. Park YJ, Lee YM, Lee JY, Seol YJ, Chung CP, Lee SJ (2000) J Control Release 67:385
144. Nakamura S, Nambu M, Ishizuka T, Hattori H, Kanatani Y, Takase B, Kishimoto S, Amano Y, Aoki H, Kiyosawa T, Ishihara M, Maehara T (2008) J Biomed Mater Res A 85A:619
145. Grimm D (2009) Adv Drug Deliver Rev 61:672
146. Mao SR, Sun W, Kissel T (2010) Adv Drug Deliver Rev 62:12
147. Wang JW, Chen CY, Kuo YM (2010) J Appl Polym Sci 115:1769
148. Zhang YF, Wang YN, Shi B, Cheng XR (2007) Biomaterials 28:1515
149. Peng L, Cheng XR, Zhuo RX, Lan J, Wang YN, Shi B, Li SQ (2009) J Biomed Mater Res A 90A:564
150. Zhang YF, Cheng XR, Wang JW, Wang YN, Shi B, Huang C, Yang XC, Liu TJ (2006) Biochem Biophys Res Commun 344:362
151. Zhang YF, Shi B, Li CZ, Wang YN, Chen Y, Zhang W, Luo T, Cheng XR (2009) J Control Release 136:172
152. Dawson E, Mapili G, Erickson K, Taqvi S, Roy K (2008) Adv Drug Deliver Rev 60:215
153. Evans ND, Gentleman E, Polak JM (2006) Mater Today 9:26
154. Mitjavila-Garcia MT, Simonin C, Peschanski M (2005) Adv Drug Deliver Rev 57:1935
155. Ratanavaraporn J, Kanokpanont S, Tabata Y, Damrongsakkul S (2009) Carbohyd Polym 78:873
156. Zheng L, Cui HF (2010) J Mater Sci Mater M 21:1713
157. Hung CH, Lin YL, Young TH (2006) Biomaterials 27:4461
158. Yang ZY, Mo LH, Duan HM, Li XG (2010) Sci China Life Sci 53:215
159. Lee JY, Choo JE, Choi YS, Shim IK, Lee SJ, Seol YJ, Chung CP, Park YJ (2009) Biotechnol Appl Biochem 52:69
160. Lim TY, Wang W, Shi ZL, Poh CK, Neoh KG (2009) J Mater Sci Mater M 20:1
161. Machado CB, Ventura JMG, Lemos AF, Ferreira JMF, Leite MF, Goes AM (2007) Biomed Mater 2:124
162. Altman AM, Gupta V, Rios CN, Alt EU, Mathur AB (2010) Acta Biomater 6:1388
163. Thein-Han WW, Saikhun J, Pholpramoo C, Misra RDK, Kitiyanant Y (2009) Acta Biomater 5:3453
164. Zhao F, Grayson WL, Ma T, Bunnell B, Lu WW (2006) Biomaterials 27:1859
165. Gravel M, Gross T, Vago R, Tabrizian M (2006) Biomaterials 27:1899
166. Kim KS, Lee JH, Ahn HH, Lee JY, Khang G, Lee B, Lee HB, Kim MS (2008) Biomaterials 29:4420
167. Dang JM, Sun DDN, Shin-Ya Y, Sieber AN, Kostuik JP, Leong KW (2006) Biomaterials 27:406
168. Cho JH, Kim SH, Park KD, Jung MC, Yang WI, Han SW, Noh JY, Lee JW (2004) Biomaterials 25:5743
169. Park DJ, Choi BH, Zhu SJ, Huh JY, Kim BY, Lee SH (2005) J Cranio Maxillo Surg 33:50
170. Maeng YJ, Choi SW, Kim HO, Kim JH (2010) J Biomed Mater Res A 92A:869
171. Natesan S, Baer DG, Walters TJ, Babu M, Christy RJ (2010) Tissue Eng Part A 16:1369
172. Yang ZY, Duan HM, Mo LH, Qiao H, Li XG (2010) Biomaterials 31:4846
173. Li XG, Yang ZY, Zhang AF (2009) Biomaterials 30:4978
174. Yannas IV (1985) Abstr Pap Am Chem Soc 190:38
175. Yannas IV (1995) Adv Polym Sci 122:219

176. Chen KY, Liao WJ, Kuo SM, Tsai FJ, Chen YS, Huang CY, Yao CH (2009) Biomacromolecules 10:1642
177. Sezer AD, Hatipoglu F, Cevher E, Ogurtan Z, Bas AL, Akbuga J (2007) AAPS PharmSciTech 8:E1–E8
178. Peng CC, Yang MH, Chiu WT, Chiu CH, Yang CS, Chen YW, Chen KC, Peng RY (2008) Macromol Biosci 8:316
179. Rasad MSBA, Halim AS, Hashim K, Rashid AHA, Yusof N, Shamsuddin S (2010) Carbohyd Polym 79:1094
180. Mao JS, Zhao LG, de Yao K, Shang QX, Yang GH, Cao YL (2003) J Biomed Mater Res A 64A:301
181. Dai M, Zheng XL, Xu X, Kong XY, Li XY, Guo G, Luo F, Zhao X, Wei YQ, Qian ZY (2009) J Biomed Biotechnol 2009:595126
182. Shi YC, Ma L, Zhou J, Mao ZW, Gao CY (2005) Polym Adv Technol 16:789
183. Ma L, Shi YC, Chen YX, Zhao HH, Gao CY, Han CM (2007) J Mater Sci Mater M 18:2185
184. Boucard N, Viton C, Agay D, Mari E, Roger T, Chancerelle Y, Domard A (2007) Biomaterials 28:3478
185. Kiyozumi T, Kanatani Y, Ishihara M, Saitoh D, Shimizu J, Yura H, Suzuki S, Okada Y, Kikuchi M (2007) Burns 33:642
186. Mao ZW, Shi HF, Guo R, Ma L, Gao CY, Han CM, Shen JC (2009) Acta Biomater 5:2983
187. Guo R, Xu SJ, Ma L, Huang AB, Gao CY (2010) Biomaterials 31:7308
188. Guo R, Xu SJ, Ma L, Huang AB, Gao CY (2010) Biomaterials 32:1019
189. Temenoff JS, Mikos AG (2000) Biomaterials 21:431
190. Cucchiarini M, Thurn T, Weimer A, Kohn D, Terwilliger EF, Madry H (2007) Arthritis Rheum 56:158
191. Evans CH, Gouze E, Gouze JN, Robbins PD, Ghivizzani SC (2006) Adv Drug Deliver Rev 58:243
192. Kim IY, Seo SJ, Moon HS, Yoo MK, Park IY, Kim BC, Cho CS (2008) Biotechnol Adv 26:1
193. Griffon DJ, Sedighi MR, Schaeffer DV, Eurell JA, Johnson AL (2006) Acta Biomater 2:313
194. Montembault A, Tahiri K, Korwin-Zmijowska C, Chevalier X, Corvol MT, Domard A (2006) Biochimie 88:551
195. Oliveira JT, Correlo VM, Sol PC, Costa-Pinto AR, Malafaya PB, Salgado AJ, Bhattacharya M, Charbord P, Neves NM, Reis RL (2008) Tissue Eng Part A 14:1651
196. Tigli RS, Gumusderelioglu M (2009) J Mater Sci Mater M 20:699
197. Kuo YC, Hsu YR (2009) J Biomed Mater Res A 91A:277
198. Yamane S, Iwasaki N, Kasahara Y, Harada K, Majima T, Monde K, Nishimura SI, Minami A (2007) J Biomed Mater Res A 81A:586
199. Tan HP, Wu JD, Lao LH, Gao CY (2009) Acta Biomater 5:328
200. Hong Y, Gong YH, Gao CY, Shen JC (2008) J Biomed Mater Res A 85A:628
201. Jin R, Teixeira LSM, Dijkstra PJ, Karperien M, van Blitterswijk CA, Zhong ZY, Feijen J (2009) Biomaterials 30:2544
202. Tan HP, Chu CR, Payne KA, Marra KG (2009) Biomaterials 30:2499
203. Silva SS, Motta A, Rodrigues MT, Pinheiro AFM, Gomes ME, Mano JF, Reis RL, Migliaresi C (2008) Biomacromolecules 9:2764
204. Park KM, Lee SY, Joung YK, Na JS, Lee MC, Park KD (2009) Acta Biomater 5:1956
205. Hao T, Wen N, Cao JK, Wang HB, Lu SH, Liu T, Lin QX, Duan CM, Wang CY (2010) Osteoarthr Cartilage 18:257
206. Park KM, Joung YK, Park KD, Lee SY, Lee MC (2008) Macromol Res 16:517
207. Wang W, Li B, Li YL, Jiang YZ, Ouyang HW, Gao CY (2010) Biomaterials 31:5953
208. Damien CJ, Parsons JR (1991) J Appl Biomater 2:187
209. Di Martino A, Sittinger M, Risbud MV (2005) Biomaterials 26:5983
210. Thein-Han WW, Kitiyanant Y, Misra RDK (2008) Mater Sci Tech Lond 24:1062
211. Thein-Han WW, Misra RDK (2009) Acta Biomater 5:1182
212. Jiang LY, Li YB, Xiong CD (2009) J Biomed Sci 16:65

213. Wang XL, Wang XM, Tan YF, Zhang B, Gu ZW, Li XD (2009) J Biomed Mater Res A 89A:1079
214. Peter M, Binulal NS, Nair SV, Selvamurugan N, Tamura H, Jayakumar R (2010) Chem Eng J 158:353
215. Kawai T, Yamada T, Yasukawa A, Koyama Y, Muneta T, Takakuda K (2009) J Biomed Mater Res B 88B:264
216. Lee EJ, Shin DS, Kim HE, Kim HW, Koh YH, Jang JH (2009) Biomaterials 30:743
217. Chesnutt BM, Viano AM, Yuan YL, Yang YZ, Guda T, Appleford MR, Ong JL, Haggard WO, Burngardner JD (2009) J Biomed Mater Res A 88A:491
218. Akman AC, Tigli RS, Gumusderelioglu M, Nohutcu RM (2010) Artif Organs 34:65
219. Yilgor P, Tuzlakoglu K, Reis RL, Hasirci N, Hasirci V (2009) Biomaterials 30:3551
220. De la Riva B, Nowak C, Sanchez E, Hernandez A, Schulz-Siegmund M, Pec MK, Delgado A, Evora C (2009) Eur J Pharm Biopharm 73:50
221. De la Riva B, Sanchez E, Hernandez A, Reyes R, Tamimi F, Lopez-Cabarcos E, Delgado A, Evora C (2010) J Control Release 143:45

Use of Chitosan as a Bioactive Implant Coating for Bone-Implant Applications

Megan R. Leedy, Holly J. Martin, P. Andrew Norowski, J. Amber Jennings, Warren O. Haggard, and Joel D. Bumgardner

Abstract Chitosan is the deacetylated derivative of the natural polysaccharide, chitin. Chitosan has been shown to be biocompatible, biodegradable, osteoconductive, and to accelerate wound healing. These characteristics are largely due to its structural and chemical homology to hyaluronic acid and other proteoglycans found in extracellular matrices. Because of these properties, chitosan has been investigated as a coating for implant materials to promote osseointegration, and as a potential vehicle to deliver therapeutic agents to the local implant–tissue interface. The coating of chitosan onto implant alloy surfaces has been achieved via chemical reactions and electrodeposition mechanisms as well as by other methods such as dip coating and layer-by-layer assembly. This work examines the different mechanisms and bond strengths of chitosan coatings for implant alloys, coating composition and physiochemical properties, degradation, delivery of therapeutic agents, such as growth factors and antibiotics, and in vitro and in vivo compatibilities.

Keywords Biocompatibility · Chitosan coatings · Dental/craniofacial implants · Electrodeposition · Local controlled drug delivery · Orthopedic implants · Physical characteristics · Silane deposition and bonding

Contents

1 Introduction	130
2 Chitosan Bound to Titanium by Alkyloxysilane Deposition	133
2.1 Solution Casting of Chitosan	133

2.2 Silane Compounds 133
2.3 Ethanol/Water and Alkyloxysilanes 135
2.4 Toluene and Alkyloxysilanes 143
2.5 Physical Adsorption of Chitosan on Implant Surfaces 145
2.6 Summary of Chemical and Physical Bonding Methods for Chitosan Coatings to Implant Alloy Surfaces 147
3 Electrodeposition 147
3.1 Basics of the Electrodeposition Method 147
3.2 Electrodeposition of Chitosan with Calcium Phosphate Materials 149
3.3 Electrodeposition of Chitosan–CaP Composite Coatings 150
3.4 Summary of Electrodeposited Chitosan–CaP Coatings 156
4 Overview of Other Chitosan-Based Coatings 156
5 Summary 157
References 158

1 Introduction

Procedures using titanium and titanium-based alloy implants are highly successful and established therapies for restoring bone and joint function in orthopedics and for replacing missing bone and teeth in dental/craniofacial applications. In 2004, over a million total joint replacement procedures were performed [1]. In 2006, the number of dental implants placed in the USA was over five million, with an estimated market of one billion dollars [2]. The success of these implant therapies is due in part to the ability of titanium and its alloys to osseointegrate or to become well integrated into the surrounding bone. Studies have demonstrated that these devices have predictable long-term clinical success of 72–92% at 10 years for total joint devices, and 81–91% for dental implants at up to 15 years [3–9]. The osseointegration properties of titanium and its alloys and their clinical success have led to an expansion of their use for younger patient populations and for patients with diseased or altered bone physiology. Given the younger patient population and increased life expectancies, as well as use in patients with diseased or altered bone, the demand for longer functional lifetime service of these implant devices is increasing.

To meet these demands, implant designers and engineers have focused on improving osseointegration of implants through surface modifications and coatings (see Fig. 1), and many reviews are available [10–16]. In general, microsurface roughness and metal bead coatings increase mechanical interlocking between surrounding bone and implant but do not result in direct bone–implant bonding [11, 15]. Calcium phosphate and bioglass-based coatings are reported to develop direct bone–implant bonding but the coatings are brittle and subject to coating–substrate interfacial fracture [10, 14, 16–18]. Nanostructured surfaces show promise for promoting osteoblast attachment, growth, and differentiation in vitro but there are conflicting reports on the benefits in vivo, due in part to differences in surface topographical characteristics and/or chemical compositions [14, 15, 19–22]. Chitosan, a biocompatible biopolymer, has received attention as a potential coating

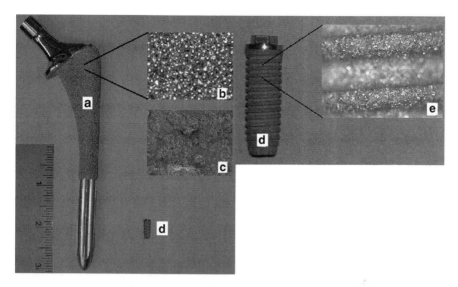

Fig. 1 Photograph of (**a**) femoral hip stem with (**b**) inset of the microbeaded surface. (**c**) Photomicrograph of a plasma-deposited calcium phosphate coating on a hip stem (image kindly provided by Smith & Nephew, Memphis, TN, USA). (**d**) Dental implant with (**e**) inset showing a titanium plasma-sprayed surface coating

material for orthopedic and dental/craniofacial implants due to its osteogenic and biodegradable/drug delivery properties, ability to accelerate wound healing, and flexibility in processing and modification [23–29].

Chitosan (1-4, 2-amino-2-deoxy-β-D-glucan) is the deacetylated derivative of chitin (1-4, 2-acetoamido-2-deoxy-β-D-glucan), a linear polysaccharide found in the exoskeletons of arthropods and in cell walls of some fungi and plankton. Chitin is obtained largely from the seafood processing industry by crushing and washing shells from lobsters, crabs, and shrimp, then removing calcium minerals with strong acid and removing proteinaceous material with alkali. Additional treatment with strong alkali removes acetyl [–C(=O)–CH3] side groups. When more than 50% of the acetyl groups are removed, the polymer is called chitosan [23]. The fraction of acetyl side groups removed from polymer chain is termed the degree of deacetylation (DDA) and ranges from 50–100%. A major advantage of deacetylating chitin is that chitosan is soluble in dilute acids at pH < 6 due to protonation of amino groups. This makes chitosan highly versatile and flexible for chemical and physical modifications, whereas chitin is generally insoluble in aqueous solutions making processing more difficult [23, 25].

Biocompatibility of chitosan is largely attributed to its similarity to hyaluronic acid and glycosaminoglycan extracellular matrix molecules (Fig. 2) [23, 30–32]. This similarity is reported to result in the organization of physiologically functioning collagen fibers in reconstructed tissues [31–34]. The cationic nature of chitosan attracts negatively charged cytokines and growth factors and is believed to help

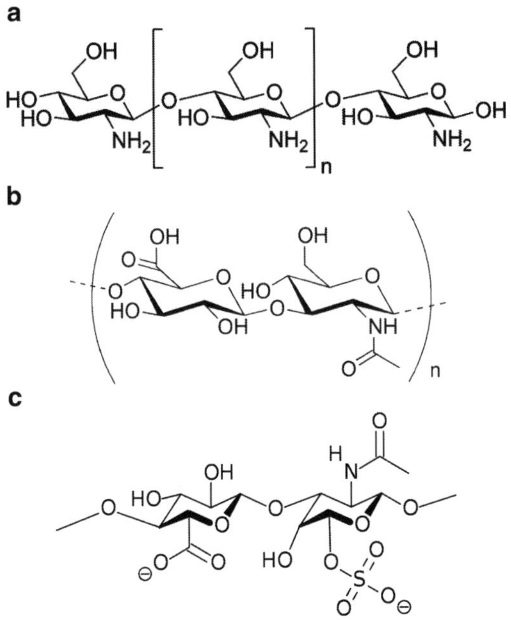

Fig. 2 Repeat units of (**a**) chitosan, (**b**) hyaluronan, and (**c**) chondroitin sulfate

protect and concentrate cytokines and growth factors secreted by cells at local sites for accelerated healing [31, 33, 35–40]. Increasing the DDA increases the net positive charge of chitosan, which is correlated with increased cell attachment [38–45]. In vitro studies have reported that chitosan films enhance the differentiation of osteoprogenitor cells and elaboration of extracellular matrix, and inhibit fibroblast proliferation [38, 46–51]. Degradation is primarily by lysozyme action and hydrolysis [23, 30, 52–55]. Degradation products, including saccharides and glucosamines, are part of normal metabolism and may be incorporated into glycoproteins or excreted as carbon dioxide during respiration [23, 30, 56]. In addition, chitosan degradation products are reported to stimulate an increase in the expression of osteogenic genes such as bone morphogenetic protein and alkaline phosphatase in bone cultures and in vivo models [30, 33, 49, 57, 58]. Degradation of chitosan is inversely proportional to DDA since high DDA polymer structure also allows for tighter chain packing and increased crystallinity, thereby limiting enzyme access to polymer chains, as compared to low DDA polymers [23, 30, 40, 53, 54, 59–61]. Thus, DDA provides a mechanism for control of polymer degradation and release of therapeutic agents [23, 28–30]. Many studies have documented the osteoconductive and osteoinductive properties of chitosan and modified chitosans in animal models [24, 25, 31–34, 60, 62–64]. Indeed, a methyl-pyrrolidinone-modified chitosan promoted osteoconduction and formation of new mechanically functional bone in ten human patients with surgical wounds from wisdom tooth avulsions [65]. Extensive reviews on properties and advantages of chitosan materials for biomedical applications are available [23–29, 66]. Collectively, these studies highlight the potential for chitosan to enhance osseointegration of orthopedic and dental/craniofacial implants and as a vehicle to deliver therapeutic agents to the local implant–tissue interface.

Because of the desirable osteoconductive and controllable biodegradation/drug release characteristics of chitosan, it is been investigated as a coating for implant devices. The coating of chitosan onto implant alloy surfaces has been achieved via physical adsorption, chemical reaction, and electrodeposition mechanisms as well as other methods. This work examines the different mechanisms and bond strengths of chitosan coatings for implant alloys, coating compositions and physicochemical properties, degradation, delivery of therapeutic agents, and in vitro and in vivo compatibilities.

2 Chitosan Bound to Titanium by Alkyloxysilane Deposition

2.1 Solution Casting of Chitosan

Using chitosan as an implant coating for bone implants, such as joint replacements or dental/craniofacial applications, requires that chitosan is firmly bound to the implant surface in order to withstand the mechanical forces associated with implant placement and to secure the implant in place during osseointegration. Therefore, efforts to bond chitosan to metal implant surfaces have been made, starting with simple solution casting, whereby chitosan is poured over the metal surface and allowed to dry [46]. However, chitosan does not bond strongly to implant alloy surfaces due to a lack of surface reactivity, passivation, and the large size of the chitosan molecule. The weak bonding produced, on the order of 0.50 MPa, is not likely to be able to withstand the stress of implantation into bone [46]. In an effort to improve the adhesion strength of chitosan to a metal implant surface, silane chemical reactions have been explored.

2.2 Silane Compounds

Silanes are often used to modify metal oxide surfaces, especially those rich in hydroxyl groups, to enable a broad range of functionalities such as hydrophilicity, immobilization of therapeutic agents, polymers, and cells, and the creation of model surfaces [67–72]. The easiest methods of deposition of silane compounds involve dipping or solution casting techniques. Other methods for depositing silanes include microwave and vapor deposition techniques [70, 71, 73].

Silane compounds contain silicon with one to four additional groups. The simplest silane compound, commonly referred to as "silane", is silicon tetrahydride, which contains silicon and four hydrogen molecules [74]. Typically, silicon tetrahydride (silane) is not used for attaching molecules to material surfaces. However, silane molecules can be modified to produce a silicon "anchor" with two to four different sites or active groups. The addition of active groups provides the mechanism by which a silane can be used as a linker molecule to attach another molecule or a coating material to the surface of a substrate material via covalent bonds [71, 75, 76].

One compound typically added to the silicon is oxygen with an alkane attachment, such as methoxy- or ethoxy-. One to four of these units can be attached, although for most coating purposes, one to three of these units are attached (as shown in Fig. 3) to form a network on the material surface. The fourth group is then used to form a bond with molecules to be coated or attached to the material surface. When only a single oxygen with an alkane is bound to the silicon, this group is referred to as -oxy- with the proper chain length alkane name (e.g., -methoxysilane), and the remaining groups are identified as di- (e.g., -dimethyl-methoxysilane) (Fig. 3a). The attachment of two -oxy- groups is identified as di- (e.g.,-dimethoxysilane), while the remaining group is referred to without a preceding suffix (e.g., -methyl-dimethoxysilane) (Fig. 3b). Finally, in compounds with three alkane-oxygen groups, the groups are referred to as tri- (e.g., -trimethoxysilane) (Fig. 3c) [77]. The final group is typically an alkane with a reactive end group, such as nitrogen, alcohol, allyl, aldehyde, or acetone. A portion of the name of the silane molecule is based on the length of the alkane, with the rest of the silane name being comprised of the terminal end of this portion of the molecule [77]. For example, acetoxyethyl-triethoxysilane contains an acetoxy group connected to an ethyl group connected to the silicon, which also has three ethoxy groups attached (Fig. 3d).

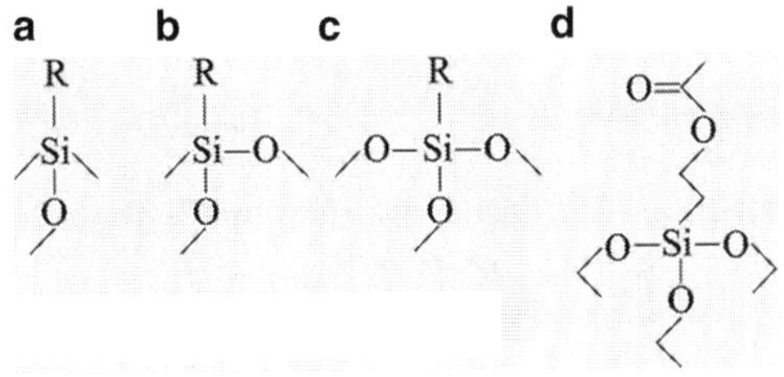

Fig. 3 Nomenclature for silanes based on pendant groups attached to silicon: (**a**) R-dimethylmethoxysilane, (**b**) R-methyldimethoxysilane, (**c**) R-trimethoxysilane, (**d**) acetoxyethyl-triethoxysilane

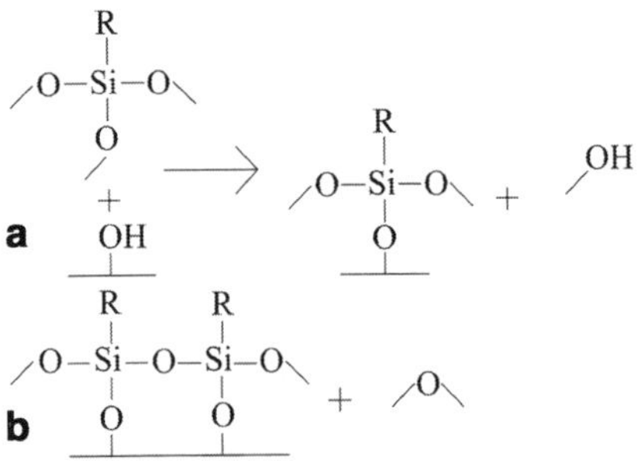

Fig. 4 Two different reactions on implant surfaces, where (**a**) is the reaction between the surface water and the silane molecule and (**b**) is the polysiloxane reaction between neighboring R-trimethoxysilanes

Fig. 5 Two silane molecules showing different reactive ends: (**a**) aminopropyltriethoxysilane and (**b**) triethoxsilylbutyraldehyde

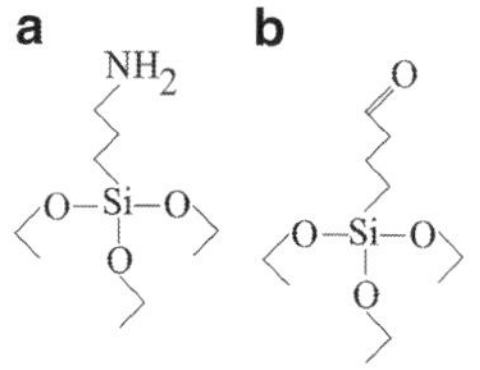

The -oxy- ending groups typically react with absorbed surface water or hydroxylated surface groups and release an alcohol or water group (Fig. 4a) [70, 71, 75]. Trialkylsilanes also will react with neighboring silanes, to create a self-assembled monolayer network (Fig. 4b) [70, 71, 75]. These reactions result in a linker molecule strongly bound to the substrate material surface. By choosing a silane molecule with the desired reactive end group, one can form a bond between molecules or compounds of the coating and the surface-bound silane, thereby creating a strong covalent bond between coating molecules and material surface. Careful control of the silane deposition conditions is needed to prevent thick, multilayer silane networks or silane self-polymerization reactions from occurring, which can result in reduced and inhomogeneous silane bonding [70, 71, 75, 78].

Silane compounds are used in the modification of biomedical implant surfaces because titanium, stainless steel, and cobalt–chromium alloys readily form oxide surfaces that are naturally rich in hydroxyl groups. An amine-ending silane, aminopropyltriethoxysilane (APTES), has been investigated as a way to attach many different compounds, including enzymes, proteins, and chitosan to medical implant alloys [46, 67–72, 79–82]. An advantage of the amino-silane is that its reactive amine end can be used "as is" or modified with additional linker molecules to produce the desired functional end group. In the case of chitosan polymer, which is also rich in amino groups, the amino end of the APTES (Fig. 5a) was modified with a second linker molecule, glutaraldehyde, to produce a reactive aldehyde group (Fig. 5b) for bonding to the amino groups in the chitosan polymer (Fig. 6a, b) [46]. There is no need for a second linker molecule when using a silane with an aldehyde end, such as triethoxsilylbutyraldehyde (TESBA) (Fig. 5b) [84].

2.3 Ethanol/Water and Alkyloxysilanes

Initial efforts to bond chitosan coatings to metal implant surfaces used ethanol/water solutions, ranging from 95% ethanol and 5% water to 70% ethanol and 30% water, to deposit APTES onto the surface of titanium substrates [39, 46, 75, 78]. Ethanol and water have been used to deposit the silane because they are safe and easy to use. The use of ethanol/water to deposit APTES significantly increased the bond strength of chitosan on titanium from a mean 0.5 MPa for chitosan simply absorbed to the titanium to 1.5 MPa (Table 1) [46]. Using an isocyantopropyltriethoxysilane (ICPTES), mechanical bond strengths were increased to between

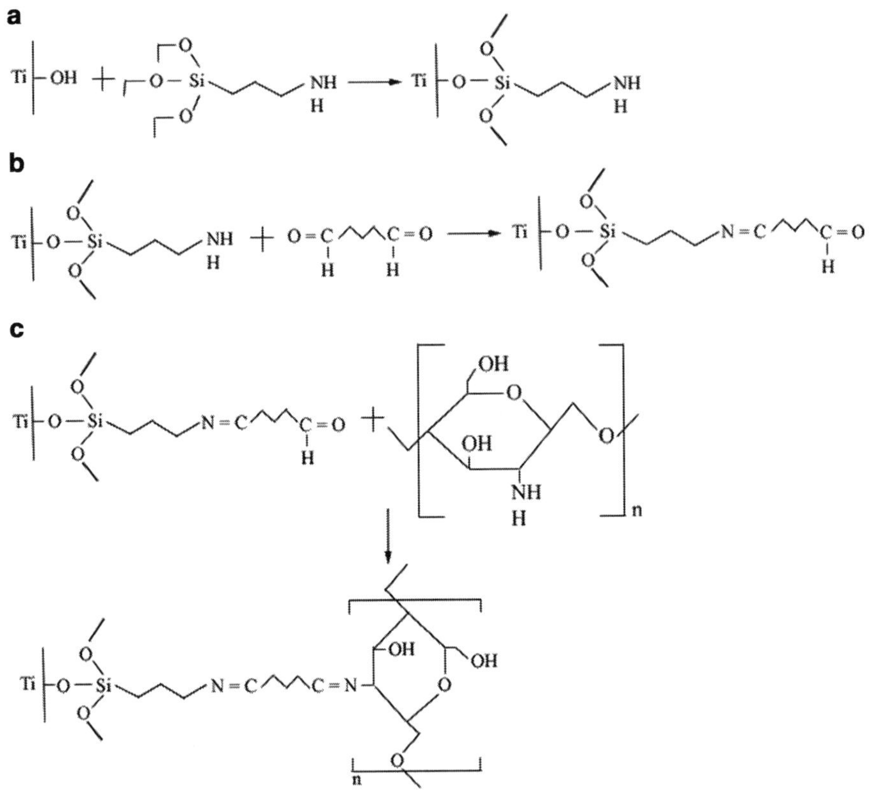

Fig. 6 Aminopropyltriethoxysilane reaction series with a titanium surface, where (a) is the reaction between the titanium surface and APTES, (b) is the reaction between the terminal amine end of APTES and glutaraldehyde, and (c) is the reaction between the aldehyde end of glutaraldehyde and chitosan. Reprinted with kind permission from Martin et al. [83], American Chemical Society, © 2007

Table 1 Adhesion strength of chitosan coatings bound to titanium via alkyloxysilane deposition

Chitosan bonding method	DDA (%)	MW (KDa)	Adhesion strength (MPa)	Reference
Loctite glue; no chitosan	–	–	5.92 ± 0.20	[85]
Solution cast chitosan; no bonding	91.2	200	0.51 ± 0.15	[46]
APTES in ethanol/water	91.2	200	1.55 ± 0.11	[46]
APTES in ethanol/water with sterilization	91.2	200	1.75 ± 0.25	[46]
ICPTES in ethanol/water	80.6	220	3.80 ± 1.20	[86]
ICPTES in ethanol/water	81.7	315	2.20 ± 1.30	[86]
ICPTES in ethanol/water	92.3	137	2.75 ± 1.25	[86]
APTES in toluene	86.4	–	20.41 ± 3.65	[85]
APTES in toluene with sterilization	86.4	–	22.72 ± 3.71	[87]
TESBA in toluene	86.4	–	19.11 ± 5.43	[85]
TESBA in toluene with sterilization	86.4	–	14.99 ± 0.01	[87]

APTES aminopropyltriethoxysilane, *ICPTES* isocyantopropyltriethoxysilane, *TESBA* triethoxsilylbutyraldehyde

Use of Chitosan as a Bioactive Implant Coating for Bone-Implant Applications

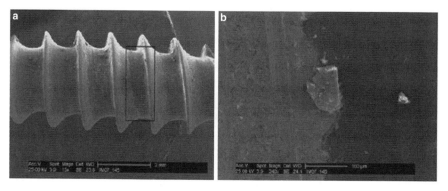

Fig. 7 SEM images of a gas sterilized chitosan-coated stainless steel screw following functional bone simulation testing where (**a**) shows the section of the screw where the chitosan coating was removed and (**b**) is a higher magnification showing where the chitosan coating separated from the surface of the stainless steel screw. Reprinted with kind permission from Greene et al. [88], Springer Science+Business Media, © 2008

2.2 and 3.8 MPa (Table 1) [86]. Greene et al. [88] used the APTES–glutaraldehyde linking chemistry to coat chitosan onto a 316L stainless steel screw via a dip-coating process. They screwed chitosan-coated screws into solid rigid polyurethane foam simulating the density of bone and showed that approximately 90% of the chitosan coating was retained even in hydrated conditions, based on change in mass (Fig. 7) [88]. This observation suggests that the silane bonding mechanism may provide sufficient coating bond strength to resist forces associated with implantation into bone. The studies by Bumgardner et al., Yuan et al., and Greene et al. [46, 86, 88] also showed that neither ethylene oxide gas sterilization, DDA of the chitosan, nor the inclusion of up to 2 wt% gentamicin in the chitosan solution used to make the coating had any significant effect on coating bond strengths to titanium or stainless steel surfaces (Table 1 and Fig. 7). Furthermore, in vitro studies for up to 8 weeks showed that the coatings exhibited little dissolution in physiological solutions with or without lysozyme, indicating potential for the coatings to be retained on implant surfaces in vivo [46, 86]. It was noted by Yuan et al. that the molecular weight (MW) of the chitosan coatings retained on the titanium surface decreased by 69–85% over 5 weeks, with the higher DDA chitosan coatings exhibiting less percentage change in MW than the lower DDA materials. This decrease in MW may actually be of benefit since low MW chitosans are reported to enhance bone cell differentiation and healing [30, 33, 49, 57, 58].

Although the studies cited above demonstrate the potential for chemically bonding chitosan to an implant surface, the mechanical bond strengths measured are still lower than the 6.7–26 MPa bond strengths reported for plasma-sprayed hydroxyapatite coatings [16, 46]. In the initial studies by Bumgardner et al., Yuan et al. and Greene et al. [46, 86, 88], the surfaces of the titanium and stainless steel screw were roughened with 80 grit silicon carbide paper or grit blasting with 220 grit silica beads, respectively, in an attempt to maximize the surface area of silane deposition. However, it is likely that multilayer silane networks and/or silane self-

Table 2 Elastic modulus and hardness of chitosan coatings determined from nano-indentation methods

Chitosan coating bonding method	DDA (%)	MW (KDa)	Hardness (GPa)	Elastic modulus (GPa)	Reference
Chitosan with no treatment	82.5	92.7	0.176 ± 0.004	4.39 ± 0.06	[89]
APTES in ethanol/water on glass	76.1	3,200	0.130 ± 0.003	3.58 ± 0.06	[90]
APTES in ethanol/water on glass	92.3	7,520	0.120 ± 0.001	3.54 ± 0.03	[90]
APTES in ethanol/water on glass	95.6	2,430	0.120 ± 0.005	3.85 ± 0.07	[90]
APTES in toluene	86.4	–	0.234 ± 0.011	3.49 ± 0.35	[85]
APTES in toluene with sterilization	86.4	–	0.186 ± 0.026	2.99 ± 0.97	[87]
TESBA in toluene	86.4	–	0.209 ± 0.024	4.08 ± 0.65	[85]
TESBA in toluene with sterilization	86.4	–	0.148 ± 0.019	2.23 ± 0.78	[87]

polymerization reactions occurred due to excess water in roughened surface crevices and thereby limited bonding of the coating to the substrate alloy [78, 80].

To further explore the characteristics of silane-deposited chitosan coatings, nano-indentation methods have been used to investigate the mechanical properties of chitosan films and coatings. These properties were investigated in part because chitosan materials are semicrystalline and their nanoscale mechanical properties are likely to be different to the macroscale properties and to be important to protein–cell interactions. The nanohardness and nanomodulus of chitosan coatings, bonded via ethanol/water-deposited APTES or ICPTES to titanium or glass surfaces, were not remarkably different from simple chitosan films (Table 2) [84, 89, 90]. These results suggest that the silane bonding process does not have a significant effect on chitosan nanomechanical properties. This, however, could be because the chitosan coatings evaluated were considered thick (~350 μm) relative to the penetration depth of in the nano-indentation tests (<10% of thickness) and as such reflect chitosan film properties rather than any effect of the silane–glutaraldehyde bonding process.

Majd et al. did identify small but statistically significant differences in modulus of the coatings based on DDA and MW of the chitosan, but also noted that brief heat treatments during the coating process had no effect [90]. The presence of needle-like, sheet-like, and small spherulite crystals identified in atomic force microscopy imaging and changes in crystallinity index values as determined in X-ray diffraction were also observed to vary with the DDA and MW of the chitosan material [90]. These observations suggest an interaction between DDA and MW effects on chitosan nanomechanical properties but the study was not able to clearly separate out the effects [90]. Additional studies are needed to better delineate the role of these factors on nanomechanical properties and their importance to interactions between chitosan coatings and host cells or tissues.

In vitro studies by Bumgardner et al. showed that, after only 15 min, the number of cells from a human osteoprogenitor cell line on chitosan-coated titanium was eightfold higher than on the control titanium surface [39]. This increase in cell attachment was attributed in part to the increased attachment or adsorption of

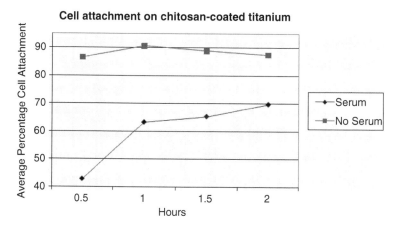

Fig. 8 Attachment of human osteoprogenitor cells to chitosan films (77–92% DDA) in DMEM balanced salt solution as compared to DMEM balanced salt solution supplemented with 10% fetal bovine serum

proteins by the chitosan material (~1.3-fold increase in albumin and fibronectin) and to electrostatic charge attraction between the cationic chitosan polymer and the cells. High levels of protein and cell attachment to chitosan substrates have been reported by others [38, 41, 44]. In an unreported follow-up study by Bumgardner and coworkers, the attachment of the same human osteoprogenitor cells over the 0.5–2 h time frame was increased 15–40% on chitosan films ranging from 76 to 92% DDA in serum-free medium as compared to serum-supplemented medium, but there was no correlation to DDA (Fig. 8). These data suggest that the initial high level of cell attachment observed by Bumgardner et al. [39] and others is due primarily to electrostatic charge interactions. Longer term interactions between chitosan substrates and cells may be more dependent on DDA, since it has been noted that low DDA chitosans tend to support less cell growth due to increased degradation, as compared to high DDA chitosans which have reduced degradation rates [38, 40, 91, 92].

In vitro cell growth using a rat osteosarcoma cell line was tested on titanium surfaces that were either passivated (control) or coated via water/ethanol APTES deposition with three different DDA chitosans [86]. The cells appeared to grow as well on the chitosan-coated samples as on the uncoated titanium controls. Interestingly, there was little difference in cell growth on the three different DDA chitosan coatings. The lack of differences in the growth of cells between the three chitosan coatings may have been due to a combination of several factors. First, all three chitosans had relatively high DDAs (81–92%), which are known to support cell growth. Second, the cells were seeded at a high density (10^5 cells/cm^2), which would have limited overall total growth. Third, the chitosan coating may have interfered with the method of measuring DNA as an estimator of cell growth since chitosan is known to strongly bind to DNA molecules [93]. This latter issue could

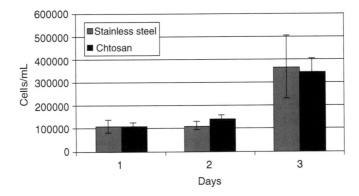

Fig. 9 Growth of an osteoblastic precursor cell line is similar on both chitosan-coated stainless steel coupons and uncoated stainless steel coupons. Adapted from Greene et al. [88], Springer Science+Business Media, © 2008

be why there was a high variation in values for DNA measured for cells on the test chitosan coatings and may actually result in an underestimation of the number of cells. Also, as noted by Yuan et al. [86] there may be issues related to the manufacturer of the chitosans because previous reports have shown that cell responses can be variable between sources (e.g., crab, shrimp, squid pen, fungi) and between production lots [47, 94, 95]. Hence, although the results of Yuan et al. [86] do support the general hypothesis that chitosan coatings are able to support the growth of osteoblasts, they also highlight the importance of developing high quality and consistent chitosan materials for predictable and repeatable biological performance characteristics.

To avoid possible interference of chitosan in estimating cell growth via DNA quantification, Greene et al. employed a double trypsinization method to collect normal human fibroblasts and cells from a human osteoblastic precursor cell line from chitosan coatings bonded to stainless steel as compared to uncoated stainless steel coupons. Their results showed that both the fibroblasts and osteoprecursor cells grew equally well on the chitosan coatings as on the uncoated controls (Fig. 9) [88].

On the basis of the promising in vitro results for bonding chitosan via silane reactions to implant alloys, and for supporting bone cell attachment and growth, Bumgardner et al. evaluated the ability of chitosan-coated titanium to osseointegrate in a rabbit tibia model as compared to uncoated titanium and calcium phosphate (CaP) sputter-coated titanium [62]. In their study, a 92% DDA chitosan was bonded via the ethanol/water deposition of APTES to titanium pins. The high DDA chitosan was selected so that degradation of the coating would be slow and support a creeping substitution mechanism for osseointegration. Test chitosan-coated implants and control calcium-phosphate-coated and uncoated titanium implants were press-fitted into drilled defects and histologically evaluated at 2-, 4-, 8- and 12-week time points. During implantation, no visible loss of the chitosan or CaP coatings were noted. Undecalcified histological analyses showed

Use of Chitosan as a Bioactive Implant Coating for Bone-Implant Applications 141

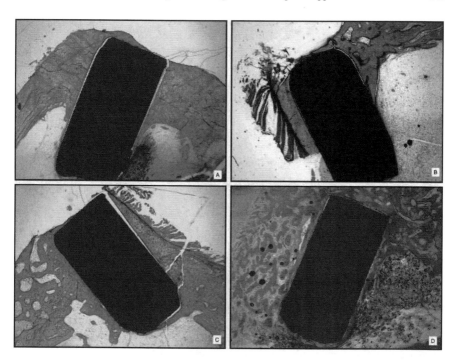

Fig. 10 Photomicrographs of paragon-stained sections of (**a**) CaP-coated, (**b**) chitosan-coated, and (**c**) uncoated titanium pins after 12 weeks in rabbit tibia. A mixture of mature lamellar and new bone was observed around all implanted pins. (**d**) Good bone formation was also observed around a chitosan-coated titanium pin that had migrated toward the rabbit tibial marrow space (original magnification 2×). Reprinted with kind permission from Bumgardner et al. [62], Wolters Kluwer Health/Lippincott Williams & Wilkins, © 2007

that the bone formation sequence of initial woven bone followed by more mature lamellar bone, was similar for all three implant types over the 12-week period (Fig. 10) [62]. In addition to the bone formation surrounding the three types of titanium pins, there was minimal inflammatory response caused by the chitosan coatings, which was similar to the CaP sputtered-coated titanium and the uncoated titanium. The study was limited in that several of the implants in all test groups migrated into the bone marrow space, which prevented additional histomorphometric analyses. However, even in the marrow space, the chitosan-coated implants were well tolerated and showed no evidence of fibrous tissue encapsulation. The study was not able detect an acceleration of the osseointegration process with the chitosan coating. This may be due in part to low degradation of the high DDA chitosan material since some critical level of degradation may be needed to stimulate the osteogenic process, as has been suggested by others [33, 49, 60]. Nevertheless, this work demonstrated that chitosan-coated implants are capable of osseointegrating [62].

Chitosan coatings, in addition to their potential for providing a favorable surface for osseointegration, have biodegradation characteristics that may provide unique opportunities for controlled delivery of therapeutic agents such as growth factors, cytokines, or antimicrobials to the implant–tissue interface. To address the problem of infection of internal fracture fixation devices in highly compromised patients, Greene et al. [88] added gentamicin at 2 wt% of chitosan to a 1 wt% chitosan (92% DDA) solution used to make coatings on stainless steel. They reported that gentamicin was released in a typical burst-release mechanism with ~1 mg/mL gentamicin released within the first hour, and then decreasing to 0.05 mg/mL at 4 days. The antibiotic-loaded coatings inhibited the growth of *Staphylococcus aureus* in zone-of-inhibition tests and were not cytotoxic to fibroblastic or mesenchymal cells [88]. To prevent early bacterial colonization on dental implants placed in at-risk patients, Norowski was able to incorporate the antibiotic tetracycline at 20 wt% or the antimicrobial chlorhexidine at 0.02 wt% of coatings made with an 81% DDA chitosan bonded to titanium [96, 97]. Coatings released 89% of the tetracycline in 7 days and 100% chlorhexidine in 2 days in vitro. Released tetracycline inhibited the growth (95–99.9%) of model anaerobic and aerobic pathogens (*Actinobacillus actinomycetemcomitans* and *Staphylococcus epidermidis*) for up to 7 days with no cytotoxicity to human fibroblastic or osteoblastic cells. The chlorhexidine released from the coatings was active against pathogens for 1–2 days (56–99.5% inhibition), but was toxic to cells on the first day of elution. Chlorhexidine was incorporated at lower levels in an attempt to minimize potential toxicity, but antimicrobial properties were also reduced [96, 97]. In a follow-up study, Norowski et al. implanted antimicrobial-loaded chitosan-coated titanium pins in the latissimus dorsi of Sprague-Dawley rats to evaluate the general tissue response and inflammation using hematoxylin and eosin (H&E) histology [97]. They showed that the tetracycline- and chlorhexidine-loaded chitosan coatings induced minor to moderate inflammation, similar or less than that produced by the degradable Vicryl sutures (polyglactin 910, Ethicon) used to seal the muscle pouch incision [97]. Leedy [98] loaded chitosan coatings bonded to titanium via adsorption with vascular endothelial growth factor as a potential mechanism to enhance osseointegration via local stimulation of angiogenesis, especially in patients on bis-phosphonate therapies for osteoporosis or myeloid cancer. The growth factor was rapidly released over 3 days from coatings with an initial peak of ~44 ng/mL/cm^2 at day 1 and 0.15 ng/mL/cm^2 at day 3. The growth-factor-loaded coatings enhanced the viability of endothelial cells and significantly stimulated the proliferation of osteoblastic cells in vitro [98].

These studies demonstrate that chitosan coatings can be bonded via silane reactions to implant alloy surfaces and that coatings retain the high biocompatibility and osteoconductive characteristics of chitosan materials in vitro and in vivo. However, the long-term stability and strength of the silane bonds requires additional study since the silane–hydroxyl group bond is subject to hydrolysis [80, 99]. Additional research is still needed to fully investigate and evaluate the effects of DDA, MW, and other processing steps (e.g., heat treatments, sterilization) on physical–mechanical and degradation properties of chitosan coatings and on cell attachment, growth, differentiation, and matrix development. This information will be needed to understand and optimize chitosan coatings for the osseointegration of implant devices and for the delivery of therapeutic agents at the implant–tissue interface.

2.4 Toluene and Alkyloxysilanes

While studies have largely focused on the deposition of silanes on implant alloys in an ethanol/water solution, a major issue of adhesion strength remains because the bond strengths are typically lower than those of more traditional CaP coatings [16, 39]. It has been noted that while the increased bond strengths for hydroxyapatite coatings were developed in part to overcome their brittle nature, it is not clear if these same high bond strengths are necessary for the more elastomeric chitosan biopolymer [46]. Nevertheless, efforts to enhance the strength of the silane-based bonds have been pursued [84, 85].

It is known that surface water and/or hydroxyl groups are needed to initiate the reaction between the implant surface and the silane molecule but the presence of excess water can also lead to reactions with the -oxy- ends and the amine ends of the silanes, resulting in the formation of polysiloxanes, alcohols, and nitrogen oxides (Fig. 11a–c) and destruction of the silane molecules [70, 71, 76, 80, 100, 101]. Although the entire concentration of silane in the ethanol/water solution typically used in deposition processes does not fully react, deleterious reactions with water does lead to a reduction in the amount of silane available for bonding and, hence, to lower bond strengths. In an effort to improve the surface coverage of the silane molecule on the titanium surface, toluene has been investigated as a solvent to deposit silanes for bonding chitosan [76, 80, 83–85].

Using toluene to deposit APTES onto titanium samples, Martin et al. was able to increase the bond strength of the chitosan coating to titanium more than tenfold as compared to the ethanol/water-deposited APTES (Table 1) [85]. This increase in bond strength was attributed to increased silane deposition with toluene solvent as

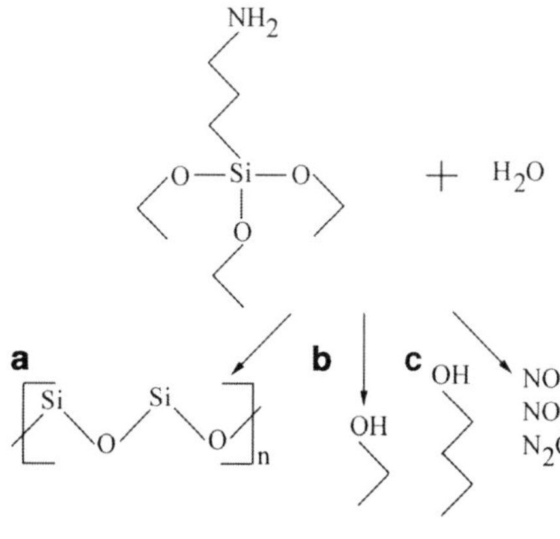

Fig. 11 Different compounds are formed when APTES or TESBA react with water: (**a**) polysiloxanes produced between silicon and oxygen bonds, (**b**) alcohols produced between water and alkyloxy- ends or alcohols produced between water and the TESBA aldehyde end, and (**c**) nitrogen oxides produced between water and the APTES amine end

compared to ethanol/water solvent, as measured by X-ray photoelectron spectroscopy [83, 84]. However, while an increase in bond strength was observed when using toluene solvent to deposit the silane, the true strength of the titanium–APTES–glutaraldehyde–chitosan bond was not able to be determined because fracture during testing occurred at the glue–pin interface instead of at the chitosan–titanium interface [85]. Nevertheless, the significance of this result was that the bond strength of the chitosan coatings made using toluene to deposit the silane could achieve values on par with those of traditional CaP coatings. Similar to the ethanol/water system, sterilization had little effect on the adhesion strength of the chitosan coating (Table 1) [102], and no differences in surface chemistry of the chitosan coatings attached to titanium using either silane solvent were noted [83]. Furthermore, there were no differences detected in bulk or nanomechanical properties of the coatings made using the two different silane solvent methods (Table 2) [85]. These studies suggest that the toluene not only increased the effectiveness of silane deposition for increased bonding, but also did not affect the overall physical-chemical aspects of the chitosan polymer coating.

To simplify the chitosan coating process, Martin et al. investigated the use of an aldehyde silane, TESBA, for bonding chitosan to implant surfaces (Fig. 5b). The advantage of the TESBA molecule is that it provides, in a single molecule, the reactive aldehyde group for bonding chitosan polymer chains, whereas the amino-silanes require a second linker molecule, glutaraldehyde, to create the reactive aldehyde group for bonding. Their results showed that the TESBA molecules were able to be deposited via both ethanol/water and toluene solvents and to bond the chitosan coatings to the titanium substrate [85]. Similar to the results with the amino-silane, deposition of the TESBA in toluene resulted in increased bond strength of the chitosan coating as compared to the deposition of the TESBA in ethanol/water (Table 1). Chemical composition, bulk, and nanomechanical properties of the chitosan coatings were also similar to coatings attached to titanium surfaces using the amino-silanes deposited by either the ethanol/water or toluene solvents (Table 2) [84, 85]. The observed decrease in the TESBA bond strength of sterilized coatings was attributed to presence of air bubbles in the glue used in the test and not necessarily to any effect of the sterilization, since fracture still occurred at the glue–pin interface and not within the coating or between the coating–titanium surface. It is noted though that although the bond strengths were reduced in this group, they were still tenfold higher than bond strengths produced using ethanol/water as the solvent (Table 1) [102]. The results of these studies indicate that aldehyde-silanes are able to effectively bond chitosan to implant alloy surfaces.

Martin et al. in a preliminary in vitro investigation evaluated the 2-h attachment and 6-day growth of human osteosarcoma bone cells on 86% DDA chitosan coatings bound via toluene-deposited APTES or TESBA solvents to titanium as compared to uncoated titanium control [87]. They observed that cell attachment increased with time, but that there were no differences between the test chitosan coatings or uncoated controls. For cell growth, increases in cell numbers were observed over the 6-day evaluation period on the test chitosan coatings and uncoated controls. There were no differences in the growth of the cells on the test chitosan coatings or controls at days 1 and 3. However, by day 6, significantly more cells were observed on the uncoated titanium controls, followed by the TESBA-bound chitosan, and the statistically lowest number of cells were seen on the APTES-bound chitosan coatings. These data, while in general agreement with the accepted compatibility of chitosan materials, are different from previously reported studies in which significantly greater osteoblastic cell attachment and 3-day growth was observed on a 91% DDA chitosan coating bonded to titanium via an ethanol/water-deposited silane than on uncoated titanium [39, 46]. Because past studies have noted no effect of the toluene silane deposition method on the chemistry and nanomechanical properties of the chitosans [83–85], and other researchers have not reported any adverse effects of toluene-deposited silanes on cells or tissues [68, 82, 103, 104], it is unlikely that there is toxicity associated with the use of the toluene solvent. Differences between the studies are probably due to differences in type (86% DDA vs. 92% DDA) and/or MW of chitosan used to make the coatings or the type of cells (human osteoblastic precursor, rat or human osteosarcoma) used to evaluate cellular responses, or a combination of these factors. Further, although Martin et al. noted there was some reduction in the growth of the osteoblastic cells by day 6 on the chitosan coatings made using the toluene solvent method as compared to the uncoated titanium controls [87], it is not clear if the reduction in growth was a result of a shift in cells to a matrix elaboration versus proliferation stage since chitosan materials are widely reported to enhance bone cell differentiation and matrix production [30, 33, 49, 57, 58]. Additional studies are needed to evaluate the biocompatibility of the chitosan coatings attached to an implant surface via toluene-deposited silanes.

2.5 *Physical Adsorption of Chitosan on Implant Surfaces*

Chitosan coatings for hard tissue implant and drug delivery applications have also been investigated by simply adsorbing chitosan films onto implant surfaces via solution casting techniques or by spreading chitosan onto implant surfaces [57, 105–111]. In general, these studies have focused on the in vitro and in vivo compatibility and ability to deliver growth factors but have not focused on coating adhesion and bonding.

In a series of studies, the Lopez–Lacomba group investigated the in vitro ability of chitosan films to support osteoblastic cell growth and as a delivery vehicle for the bone morphogenetic protein (BMP), and then used simple solution casting techniques to absorb chitosan onto implant surfaces for in vivo evaluation [57, 106–108]. Their results showed that chitosan films were easily loaded with BMP by swelling, and that the films exhibited a slow degradation and release of BMP with as much as 80–85% of the BMP being retained in the films after 7 days [107]. The BMP-loaded chitosan films and the BMP released from the films both supported the growth and differentiation of a mouse osteoblastic precursor cell line [57, 106, 107]. Based on these results, the group coated titanium pins, approximately 3.7 mm in diameter, by submerging in a 1 wt% chitosan (~85% DDA, MW 5.61 kDa) in 1 wt% acetic acid solution and then drying under a laminar air flow. The coatings were neutralized in a phosphate buffer, loaded with 80–100 μg BMP per 1.96 cm^2 coating area and then implanted in rabbit tibial defects [105–107]. Their results showed increased bone formation and apposition as well as significantly increased removal torque for the chitosan-coated implants loaded with BMP as compared to uncoated titanium controls. They did report some coating fracture upon implantation but most of the coating remained [106, 107]. In a follow-up rodent muscle pouch model, they demonstrated the osteoinductivity of the BMP-loaded chitosan coatings as compared to uncoated titanium controls [57]. Hence, these studies further support the potential of chitosan coatings as a vehicle for delivery of therapeutic agents to the implant–tissue interface for promoting osseointegration. However, the lack of a strong chitosan bonding to underlying implant surface may be an issue in clinical applications such as immediate loading of dental implants, where potential shear forces during early healing processes may further damage the coating.

Composite chitosan–apatite coatings were made on Ti-6Al-4V alloy samples using a dip-coating process [109, 110]. In one study, chitosan–apatite composite material was first made via a co-precipitation reaction using chitosan dissolved in citric acid and then adding in calcium acetate and ammonium phosphate [109]. Coatings were made by extracting Ti-6Al-4V rods 12 × 1 mm through the chitosan–apatite solution at a rate of 1,000 μm/s, drying in air overnight and then neutralizing in 2 M NaOH for 2 h. By controlling the relative concentration of calcium acetate and ammonium phosphate, the amount of apatite in the coatings ranged from 42% to ~90%. The process yielded coatings ~1 μm thick and were reported to have adhesive tensile strengths greater than 15 MPa, the strength of the glue used in the tests, since fracture occurred at the pin–glue interface and not at the coating–substrate interface [109]. In a related study, calcium-deficient apatite powders were mixed at 35–80% with chitosan dissolved in citric acid and similarly dip-coated onto Ti-6Al-4V rods [110]. These coatings ranged in thickness from 1 to 4 μm depending on the number of coating repetitions, and also exhibited adhesive strengths greater than the 15 MPa of the glue–pin strength. Both types of coatings exhibited bioactivity based on the ability to support apatite deposition when immersed in simulated body fluids [109, 110]. Although these results are promising, it is unfortunate that key aspects of the coating method such as the type of chitosan (e.g., of different DDA and/or MW) and the concentration of citric acid used to make coating solutions were not provided. Further, the mechanism for obtaining the high adhesive bond strengths is not clear because the surface of the Ti-6Al-4V alloys had been polished to a relatively fine surface finish with 1 μm diamond paste. Additionally, the degradation, stability, and compatibility of coating with host cells and tissues will need to be evaluated.

In an interesting application, Kawai et al. investigated the potential of a chitosan coating on a non-woven polyester fabric for bone anchorage of ligament grafts. The investigators simply spread a commercial chitin/chitosan material (Chitipack P; Sunfive, Tottori, Japan) over the fabric to a density of 0.08 mg/cm^2 [111]. Chitin/chitosan-coated and -uncoated fabrics were implanted into holes in the distal femoral metaphyses of rats and evaluated histologically and mechanically after 1 or 2 weeks post-implantation. They reported that the chitin/chitosan-coated fabrics exhibited a significant threefold increase in tensile fixation strengths (24.3 ± 10.2 N) as compared to the uncoated fabrics (8.59 ± 9.33 N) after 2 weeks. The mean area of bone formation filling for the chitin/chitosan-coated fabric (0.532 ± 0.145 mm^2) was also significantly greater than that for the uncoated fabric (0.113 ± 0.049 mm^2). The authors concluded that spreading chitin/chitosan as a coating onto the fabric has the potential to enhance biological fixation of fibrous materials to bone for tendon and ligament repair [111].

2.6 Summary of Chemical and Physical Bonding Methods for Chitosan Coatings to Implant Alloy Surfaces

These studies demonstrate the following points:

1. Silane molecules are able to bond chitosan to implant surfaces
2. Silane-bonded coating strengths can achieve values similar to those of CaP coatings
3. Chemical bonding and physical adsorption coating processes can yield bond strengths that may be sufficient to resist forces associated with implantation into bone
4. Coating bond strengths are not affected by gas sterilization
5. Chitosan coatings are able to support bone cell attachment and growth
6. Chitosan coatings are capable of supporting and enhancing osseointegration similarly to calcium-phosphate-coated and uncoated implants
7. Coatings may double as drug delivery vehicles for the delivery of therapeutic agents to the implant–tissue interface

Further research is needed to determine what strengths and/or bonding conditions are necessary for the stability of the chitosan coatings under in vivo conditions, the quality of the osseointegration over time, and what chitosan coating characteristics (e.g., silane bonding, type of chitosan) are needed to optimize osseointegration and/or local drug delivery for osseointegration.

3 Electrodeposition

3.1 Basics of the Electrodeposition Method

Electrodeposition uses an electrical current to cause the deposition of a charged material from a conductive solution onto a target surface. In the academic and industrial sector, there is much interest in electrodeposition of materials due to the wide range of applications in processing advanced materials and coatings [112]. Advantages of electrodeposition include the following:

- Easily modified for specific application
- Short formation times
- Simple apparatus and low equipment costs
- Complex shapes and porous structures can be coated
- High level of automation
- Microstructural homogeneity of deposits
- Room temperature processing
- Suitability for co-deposition of materials
- Easy control of thickness and morphology through simple adjustments of deposition time and applied potential [112–117]

Two different electrodeposition techniques are currently in use: electrolytic and electrophoretic. Electrolytic deposition occurs at the surface of the cathode when water is reduced to produce hydrogen gas and hydroxyl ions, which results in an increased pH at the electrode surface [115, 118]. Electrophoretic deposition occurs when charged particles, dispersed or suspended in liquid medium, are attracted to and deposited onto a conductive substrate of opposite charge in the presence of an electric field [112, 113, 119].

Coatings produced from electrodeposition are dependent on factors related to the coating materials, the electrolytic medium for coating, the electrical nature of electrodes, and electrical conditions [112]. The particle charge, particle size, and viscosity of the suspension along with the applied electric field all influence the deposition rate [112, 117]. The pH of the suspension affects the particle charge distribution and ionic conductivity of the suspension, which in turn affects the electrophoretic mobility of the particles [117]. If the suspension is too conductive, the motion of particles through the electrolytic medium is low and if the conductivity of suspension is too high, the particles charge electronically and lose stability [112]. Optimum characteristics for the electrolytic suspension are low viscosity, high dielectric constant, and low conductivity [112]. Current density influences the rate of mass deposition on the cathode, with higher current densities causing faster deposition kinetics, but at the cost of surface inhomogeneity [112, 117, 120]. The current density, as well as the concentration of solution and deposition time, controls thickness of the deposited layer on the substrate [112, 117, 118, 120]. The ability to manipulate these parameters allows electrodeposition to be a highly versatile technique for many applications, including fabrication of coatings and surfaces for biomedical applications. For example, electrodeposition methods are used to create diamond [121], CaP [122–125], bioglass [126], and antimicrobial surface coatings [127, 128] to improve the wear, osteogenetic, and antibacterial properties of implants as well as to modify and/or create nanostructures on implant surfaces to improve host–implant interactions [129–132].

Because chitosan is an amino-rich polysaccharide that is positively charged under acidic conditions, it can be electrodeposited by electrolytic and

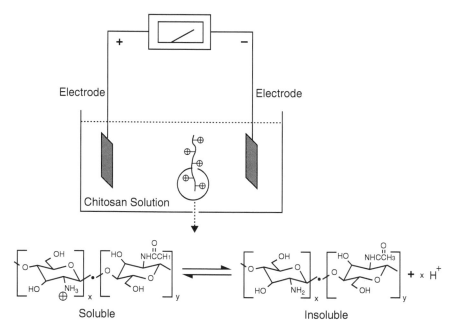

Fig. 12 Acidic chitosan solution contacting electrodes. A thin layer of insoluble chitosan is deposited at the negative electrode. Reprinted with kind permission from Wu et al. [133], American Chemical Society, © 2002

electrophoretic processes [115, 133, 134]. Figure 12 illustrates the electrodeposition of chitosan.

When dissolved in an acidic medium, chitosan becomes a polyelectrolyte solution carrying positive charges due to the presence of protonated amino groups [115, 118]. The positively charged chitosan macromolecules move toward the cathode through electrophoresis when an electric field is applied [114, 118]. Water is reduced at the cathode surface, resulting in a localized increase in pH [115, 118]. Chitosan amino groups are deprotonated when the pH is above 6.3; therefore, in the presence of the localized region of high pH, the deposited chitosan loses its charge and forms an insoluble deposit on the cathode surface [114, 115, 118, 133]. Due to the pH-dependent solubility of chitosan, the electric field is only required for the deposition of the chitosan and not to retain the chitosan layer [133]. Figure 13 shows what occurs at the surface of the cathode during this process [135].

3.2 Electrodeposition of Chitosan with Calcium Phosphate Materials

While many studies have investigated the electrodeposition of chitosan for biosensor applications [136–138] and dental and orthopedic applications, research has

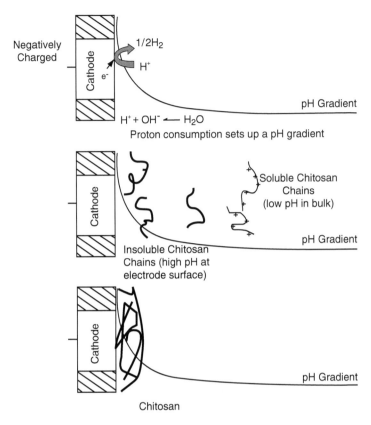

Fig. 13 Electrodeposition of chitosan showing that high localized pH is generated electrochemically at the cathode surface due to the hydrogen evolution reaction. The rate of this electrochemical reaction is proportional to the current density and can be adjusted by the applied voltage. Reprinted with kind permission from Fernandes et al. [135], American Chemical Society, © 2003

focused on the co-electrodeposition of chitosan with CaP mineral [114, 115, 117, 118, 139–142]. The rationale for the co-electrodeposition is to take advantage of the biodegradability and bioactivity of both CaP and chitosan in forming a biomimetic organic–inorganic coating for improved osseous healing while maintaining sufficient coating strength [63, 114, 115, 117, 140, 143–145].

3.3 Electrodeposition of Chitosan–CaP Composite Coatings

Redepenning et al. developed a novel electrodeposition method of composite coatings of brushite ($CaHPO_4 \cdot 2H_2O$) and chitosan on titanium to achieve an electrodeposited coating with material properties similar to bone [115]. They

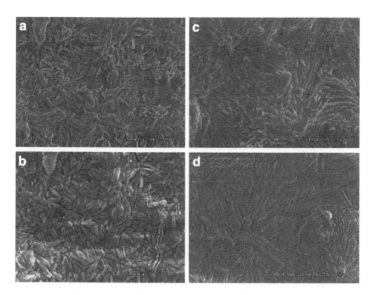

Fig. 14 Scanning electron photomicrographs of electrodeposited coatings onto titanium: (**a**) brushite; (**b**) brushite after conversion to hydroxyapatite; (**c**) brushite–chitosan composite; (**d**) brushite–chitosan composite coating after conversion to HA–chitosan. Reprinted with kind permission from Redepenning et al. [115], John Wiley & Sons, Inc., © 2003

prepared an electrolyte solution by mixing 48.5 mL stock brushite solution with 1.5 mL of 4 wt% solution of chitosan (85% DDA) containing an equimolar amount of acetic acid. The current density during the deposition was ramped from 100 to 68.5 mA/cm^2 at 0.15 mA/s/cm^2. The brushite–chitosan composites were converted to hydroxyapatite (HA)–chitosan composites by bathing samples in aqueous solutions of sodium hydroxide for 7 days at room temperature. Scanning electron microscope (SEM) images of the deposited coatings showed that chitosan appeared only as a thin film that coated the crystalline inorganic regions while partially filling the interstitial voids (Fig. 14). SEM images also showed the incorporation of chitosan into the HA coatings, resulting in highly ordered coatings. It was determined that the chitosan served as an adhesive, helping to bond the HA particles to the surface, since on highly polished surfaces the composite can be removed with a sharp razor. While Redepenning et al. demonstrated that composite coatings of HA and chitosan can be fabricated on titanium through electrodeposition, there are no data reported on the degradation of deposited coatings, on their mechanical stability, or on their ability to improve the biological performance of metallic implants [115].

Wang et al. developed a composite CaP–chitosan coating on Ti6-Al-4V plates through electrodeposition in which the CaP phase of the hybrid coating was a mixture of octacalcium phosphate (OCP) and HA [140]. The electrolyte solution was prepared by adding a 1 wt% chitosan (85% DDA) solution in 1% acetic acid into a supersaturated CaP solution to obtain final chitosan concentrations of 0.05, 0.1, and 0.2 g/L [140]. The deposition was processed at 52°C for 15 h with solution buffered to pH 6.8–6.9 and current maintained at 2.0 mA/cm^2. Coatings were uniformly deposited across the alloy surface, with chitosan-rich regions surrounding CaP globules (as observed in SEM images), suggesting that the chitosan material spread and integrated with the CaP crystals. Chitosan-rich regions increased with chitosan concentration in solution, but the coating thickness and surface roughness decreased. Scratch tests were performed on the fabricated coatings and it was reported that the addition of chitosan did not affect the first-crack forces (~6 N) or load forces for total delamination (~12 N). It was demonstrated by DNA content that the number of bone marrow stromal cells attached to the hybrid coatings with chitosan was ninefold greater after 1 day and 20-fold greater after 3 days in comparison to the electrodeposited CaP coatings without chitosan [140].

To optimize the electrodeposited coatings, Wang et al. investigated the influence of current density (1–5 mA/cm^2), acetic acid concentration, and chitosan concentration on the deposition of the composite chitosan–CaP coatings [120]. Increased current densities of 4–5 mA/cm^2 as compared to 1–2 mA/cm^2 led to an accelerated coating deposition process and more chitosan deposition. Increasing acetic acid (from 0.05 to 0.15 M) and chitosan (from 0.05 to 0.15 g/L) concentrations, however, inhibited CaP deposition.

Electrodeposited chitosan–CaP hybrid coatings were evaluated in vitro for the ability to support proliferation and differentiation of osteoblastic cells [146]. Deposited hybrid coatings were prepared using electrolyte solutions containing 0.1 and 0.2 g/L of chitosan in supersaturated CaP solution. The CaP–chitosan electrodeposited coatings demonstrated higher proliferation rates (four cell doublings vs. two cell doublings) and a higher differentiation capacity of MC3T3-E1 cells than the CaP coatings after 9 days in culture. Alkaline phosphatase activity and collagen production as indicators of differentiation, were enhanced by the incorporation of chitosan into the coatings. The chitosan concentration in solution used to make the coatings did not have a significant effect on cell responses [146]. The level of bone sialoprotein mRNA on the CaP–chitosan coatings increased 6.63- to 6.74-fold, while that of osteocalcin mRNA increased 4.68- to 5.59-fold in comparison to cells seeded on the CaP coatings. The differences in cellular response between composite and plain CaP coatings appear to be related to composition and solubility of the coating [146]. In a follow-up study, Wang et al. evaluated the electrodeposited CaP–chitosan coatings in a rabbit femoral defect and compared bone formation, bone-implant contact, and coating degradation to electrodeposited CaP coatings and uncoated Ti-6Al-4V cylinders over 52 weeks [142]. Interestingly, they reported that early bone formation and bone-implant contact values at 2, 4, and 26 weeks were greater for the non-chitosan-coated implants and that there was some fibrous tissue formation observed at 2 and 4 weeks around the CaP–chitosan-coated implants. They further reported that there was degradation for both the CaP–chitosan and CaP coatings as early as 2 weeks, with the CaP–chitosan coating exhibiting more degradation, though no inflammatory reactions were observed. Wang et al. speculated that the early fibrous tissue formation was either because the increased degradation of the CaP–chitosan coatings outpaced bone formation, or because the coating influenced early blood clot and inflammatory reactions [142]. Nevertheless, by 52 weeks, there were no differences in bone formation or bone-implant contact between the CaP–chitosan-coated, CaP-coated, and uncoated groups. Though not specifically stated, these results suggest that either changing the amount of chitosan in the electrodeposited coatings or increasing chitosan DDA may help to reduce degradation and perhaps improve bone formation.

Lu et al. fabricated CaP–chitosan composite coatings on titanium through electrodeposition in an effort to prepare pure OCP microfiber–chitosan coatings to improve surface bioactivity of orthopedic implants [114]. CaP–chitosan coatings were prepared on cathodic Ti plates in the electrolyte of an aqueous solution of 12.5 mM Ca(NO$_3$)$_2$, 5 mM NH$_4$H$_2$PO$_4$, and 4 wt% chitosan (the source of chitosan, DDA, or other chitosan characteristics were not given in the article) buffered at pH 5. The electrodeposition was conducted for 1 h for each specimen at room temperature with the current maintained at 1.0 mA/cm^2. OCP–chitosan coatings were uniformly deposited across the surface and the incorporation of chitosan led to crystalline OCP microfibers at pH 5, while large flaky OCP crystals were observed in pure OCP coatings [114]. The OCP microfibers were woven together to form porous structures, and chitosan was entrapped in the recesses and covered the fibers. The incorporation of chitosan led to a significant increase in adhesion strength from 1.31 ± 0.33 MPa (pure OCP) to 7.13 ± 1.99 MPa (composite) [114]. The authors attributed the increase in coating adhesion strength to crosslinking of the chitosan during the electrodeposition process, though the mechanism for how crosslinking of the chitosan would increase the adhesion strength of the coating is not clear [114]. The adhesion strength of electrodeposited OCP coatings is known to be low, as demonstrated by this study, but the adhesion strength was improved by incorporating chitosan into the OCP coatings [114]. The study also claimed bioactivity properties, based on SEM observations of a layer of CaP formed on both the pure OCP and OCP–chitosan electrodeposited coatings after 7 days immersion in acellular simulated body fluid [114]. However, no studies of in vitro or in vivo degradation or cellular responses were performed on these coatings.

Pang and Zhitomirsky used electrodeposition techniques to deposit composite HA–chitosan coatings onto platinum and stainless steel foils, stainless steel wires, and graphite substrates for biomedical implant applications [118, 147]. Electrodeposition was performed from suspensions of 0–8 g/L HA nanoparticles in a mixed ethanol–water solvent, containing 0–0.5 g/L chitosan (85% DDA, MW 200,000) dissolved in 1% acetic solution. Coatings were made using current densities ranging from 0.1 to 3 mA/cm^2. The deposition from aqueous solutions was accompanied by significant hydrogen gas evolution, which resulted in porous films. The porosity decreased with increasing ethanol content in the mixed ethanol/water solvent and with decreasing current density. Uniform and smooth films were obtained at low current densities of 0.1–0.2 mA/cm^2. During this investigation, no electrophoretic deposition was seen with pure HA suspensions, but the addition of chitosan in to solution resulted in the co-deposition of chitosan and HA, demonstrating that chitosan promotes the electrophoretic deposition of HA and enables the formation of adherent coatings at room temperature [118, 147]. HA content in coatings increased with HA concentration and the amount of chitosan was found to be 38.2 wt% and 8.0 wt% for the films prepared from the 0.5 g/L chitosan solutions containing 1 and 8 g/L HA, respectively. In general, the composite HA/chitosan coatings fabricated by Pang et al. contained a higher percentages of chitosan than the electrodeposited composite coatings fabricated by Redepenning et al. (1.2–16 wt% chitosan) as well as those fabricated by Wang et al. (2.3–5.1 wt% chitosan) [115, 118, 120]. Pang and Zhitomirsky further demonstrated a near-linear dependence of coating thickness on deposition time, indicating that the technique provides a constant deposition rate. SEM images showed relatively uniform deposits of different thicknesses in the range of up to 50 µm [118]. It was demonstrated that the composite coating could act as a protective layer and improve the corrosion resistance of stainless steel in the body fluid environment. This corrosion resistance was determined by the electrochemical methods of measuring impedance values and Tafel curves [118]. However, if the coating is damaged, for instance during implantation, it is unclear if this will contribute to crevice/pitting-type corrosion, especially for stainless steel alloy substrate devices, and thereby lose any protective value of the coating [148].

Silica, silver, bioactive glass, heparin, and $CaSiO_3$ have been incorporated into the electrodeposition process of chitosan and HA to try and improve performance of composite coatings for biomedical implants that interface with bone tissue [116, 119, 134, 139, 149]. While the electrodeposition methods and mechanical and adhesion strength of the coatings are commonly reported in these studies, little biological data has been gathered on the response of cells or tissues to these composite coatings.

Sharma et al. fabricated a novel bioactive porous apatite–wollastonite/chitosan composite coating on titanium through electrophoretic deposition [117]. In contrast to previous fabrication methods for composite coatings, in which the electrolyte solution consisted of a ratio of the ceramic and chitosan solutions, Sharma et al. electrodeposited the materials in alternating steps. Ceramic suspension was prepared by ultrasonically dispersing 2 g/L of apatite–wollastonite powder (formed by a modified sol–gel route) in ethanol with fixed pH of 1.6, and a 0.2% chitosan (90% DDA) solution was prepared in 2% acetic acid. To start, the titanium was coated with a thin layer of chitosan by applying a 1 mA/cm^2 fixed current density followed by three alternate coating cycles of ceramic (3 mA/cm^2 fixed current density) and chitosan to obtain a homogenous composite [117]. The pH and current densities used were optimized in the study to obtain two different coatings: a uniform, dense coating and a porous coating with ceramic particles sandwiched between polymer layers. When coatings were soaked in simulated body fluid, apatite formed on the composite coating from day 7 to day 21, which indicated favorable bioactivity [117]. Standard tape tests demonstrated an increase in mechanical strength in that 66% of the coated area was removed from ceramic coatings whereas only 21% was removed from composite coatings [117]. The bioactivity and improved mechanical strength of the composite coatings show promise for

Fig. 15 Radiographic images for (**a**) electrophoretic deposited apatite–wollastonite/chitosan coatings on titanium and (**b**) uncoated titanium implant in a rabbit tibia after 42 days. Reprinted with kind permission from Sharma et al. [141], Springer Science+Business Media, © 2009

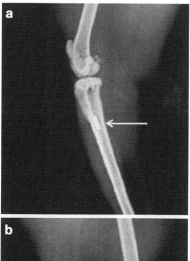
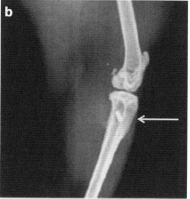

improving the performance of metallic implants. Sharma et al. subsequently evaluated the bone formation to the electrophoretic apatite–wollastonite/chitosan composite coatings in a 6-weeks rabbit tibial defect as compared to uncoated titanium [141]. On the basis of radiographic and histological analyses, they reported faster bone healing and formation to the coated implants as compared to the uncoated titanium. By 6 weeks, they noted extensive lamellar bone formation and Haversian systems with osteocytes in lacunae without intervening fibrous tissue adjacent to the coated as compared to the uncoated implants. Some radiolucent shadowing was observed at the uncoated implants, which might indicate some incomplete healing (Fig. 15). The authors concluded that their apatite–wollastonite/chitosan-coated implants enhanced early bone formation as compared to uncoated implants. However, the in vivo degradation, mechanical strength, and long-term integration of the coated implants still need to be assessed.

3.4 Summary of Electrodeposited Chitosan–CaP Coatings

Electrodeposition processes have shown promise in their ability to create coatings on implant materials and alloys using chitosan due to its cationic nature. The main focus of electrodeposition research using chitosan has focused on composite coatings of chitosan and CaP materials. The fabrication of pure chitosan coatings by electrodeposition for bone applications has not yet been fully investigated. There is wide variation in the electrolyte solutions, materials, processing temperatures, and current densities used to make the coatings during the electrodeposition process. These differences have led to composite coatings with different compositions and morphologies. Although these coatings have shown cytocompatibility in in vitro studies, in vivo data are currently mixed regarding the benefits. Additionally, the stability and degradation of the coatings have not yet been fully addressed in these studies and this will need to be determined if the coatings are to be used for enhancing osseointegration of implants devices. It has been demonstrated that incorporation of chitosan into electrodeposited CaP coatings leads to more organized coatings, higher bond strengths, and better bioactivity than electrodeposited CaP coatings alone. Ultimately, direct comparison studies of the electrodeposited chitosan–CaP coatings with current CaP, titanium plasma sprayed, or nanostructured implant coatings will need to be undertaken. Further, the opportunity to use these coatings as a local drug delivery vehicle has not been well explored and may provide additional benefit.

4 Overview of Other Chitosan-Based Coatings

The focus of this work has been on the development of adherent or bonded chitosan coatings on implant alloys for orthopedic and dental/craniofacial applications. However, there are other coating strategies that have used chitosan as part of their coating platforms, though not all have focused on coating implant alloys. For example, dip-coating processes in which substrate materials are submerged, dipped, or placed in a viscous flow of chitosan-based solutions, have been used to coat tablets to control drug delivery [150, 151] or to control the release of therapeutic agents from other drug delivery vehicles, such as calcium sulfate and chitosan [152, 153]. Peng et al. used a spin-coating technique to deposit an alginate–chitosan hydrogel onto an electrodeposited CaP coating to slow coating degradation and as a potential drug delivery mechanism. In general, these coatings showed benefit in controlling and extending the release of pharmacological agents and in decreasing degradation of calcium-based materials [154]. Thierry et al. used a chitosan–poly (ethylene oxide) polymer blend to solution-coat NiTi cardiovascular stents to reduce restenosis [155]. They showed that the coating maintained integrity during stent deployment, was hemocompatible, and could be used as a drug reservoir to decrease platelet adhesion [155]. Jun et al. used a spin-coating methodology to deposit <2-μm thick hybrid silica xerogel–chitosan gel onto titanium [156]. The coatings exhibited >60 MPa tensile bond strengths, supported rapid precipitation of HA onto the surfaces from simulated body fluids, and enhanced osteoblastic cell growth and viability in vitro [156].

Patz et al. used a novel physical vapor deposition method, matrix assisted pulsed laser evaporation (MAPLE) to coat chitosan onto a titanium wire mesh [157]. The process uses a laser to evaporate a frozen solution that contains a dilute concentration of solute coating material. The solvent material absorbs the energy of the laser, which protects the solute coating material, and is volatilized along with the coating material. The larger heavier solute molecules deposit rapidly on the substrate surface. The process provides excellent control over several film coating parameters, including thickness, roughness, and homogeneity [157]. The MAPLE chitosan coating showed high coating uniformity on the mesh (demonstrating the ability to coat complex shapes and internal surfaces) and compatibility with cultured bone cells [157].

Layer-by-layer self-assembly techniques have also been used to make polyelectrolyte films and coatings using chitosan polymers on glass, silicon wafers, and polyethylene terephthalate materials as well as on titanium, Ti-6Al-4V, NiTi, stainless steel alloys, and CaP coatings [158–167]. The technique is a relatively low cost, simple technique that can be performed with minimal equipment at room temperature, to prepare complex polymer membranes or coatings. The method takes advantage of the static or hydrogen-bond interactions between different kinds of macromolecules. The process results in very thin membranes and coatings that retain the original and desirable properties of the component polymers. Chitosan lends itself very well to this process due to its cationic characteristics when combined with anionic components such heparin, hyaluronic acid, oxy-chitin, gelatin, and bioglass particles [158–167]. These coatings have been used as possible means to control cell or bacterial adhesion and or delivery of therapeutic agents, such as growth factors and antimicrobials [158–167].

5 Summary

Chitosan has much potential for use in orthopedic and dental/craniofacial implant coatings due in part to its biocompatibility, osteoconductive properties, and biodegradabilty. The chemical and processing flexibility also provide many avenues for developing coatings on implants, including chemical bonding, electrodeposition, and physical adsorption. While many of these studies have demonstrated the osteocompatibility of chitosan coatings, the real advantage of the coatings is due to their ability to also act as mechanisms to control the local delivery of therapeutic agents, such as antimicrobials and growth factors, and even to control cell or bacterial attachments through the control of cell-mediated integrin binding. These properties and characteristics may be of particular value in improving implant integration and performance in patients that suffer from chronic disorders, such as diabetes or osteoporosis, or are otherwise predisposed to complications, such as infection. Additional research is needed to optimize chitosan characteristics, such as DDA, MW, and crystallinity, and/or in combining chitosan with other polymers and compounds, in order to promote healing and osseointegration, as well as to provide effective local delivery of therapeutic agents.

Acknowledgement Authors would like to acknowledge the Biomaterials Applications of Memphis (BAM) Research Laboratories at the University of Memphis-University of Tennessee Health Science Center for assistance in preparing work.

References

1. American Acadamy of Orthopedic Surgeons (2009) Arthritis and related conditions. AAOS Now 2009, vol 3. http://www.aaos.org/news/aaosnow/mar09/research6.asp. Accessed 28 Aug 2010
2. American Academy of Implant Dentistry (2010) Dental implants facts and figures. http://www.aaid.com/about/Press_Room/Dental_Implants_FAQ.html. Accessed Dec 2010
3. Epinette JA, Manley MT (2008) Uncemented stems in hip replacement–hydroxyapatite or plain porous: does it matter? Based on a prospective study of HA Omnifit stems at 15-years minimum follow-up. Hip Int 18(2):69–74
4. Eskelinen A et al (2006) Uncemented total hip arthroplasty for primary osteoarthritis in young patients: a mid-to long-term follow-up study from the Finnish Arthroplasty Register. Acta Orthop 77(1):57–70
5. Haddad SL et al (2007) Intermediate and long-term outcomes of total ankle arthroplasty and ankle arthrodesis. A systematic review of the literature. J Bone Joint Surg Am 89(9):1899–1905
6. Dixon MC et al (2005) Modular fixed-bearing total knee arthroplasty with retention of the posterior cruciate ligament. A study of patients followed for a minimum of fifteen years. J Bone Joint Surg Am 87(3):598–603
7. Simonis P, Dufour T, Tenenbaum H (2010) Long-term implant survival and success: a 10-16-year follow-up of non-submerged dental implants. Clin Oral Implants Res 21(7):772–777
8. Pjetursson BE et al (2007) Comparison of survival and complication rates of tooth-supported fixed dental prostheses (FDPs) and implant-supported FDPs and single crowns (SCs). Clin Oral Implants Res 18(Suppl 3):97–113
9. Lambert FE et al (2009) Descriptive analysis of implant and prosthodontic survival rates with fixed implant-supported rehabilitations in the edentulous maxilla. J Periodontol 80(8):1220–1230
10. de Jonge LT et al (2008) Organic-inorganic surface modifications for titanium implant surfaces. Pharm Res 25(10):2357–2369
11. Pilliar RM (2005) Cementless implant fixation–toward improved reliability. Orthop Clin North Am 36(1):113–119
12. Groll J et al (2009) Novel surface coatings modulating eukaryotic cell adhesion and preventing implant infection. Int J Artif Organs 32(9):655–662
13. Liu Y et al (2006) Incorporation of growth factors into medical devices via biomimetic coatings. Philos Transact A Math Phys Eng Sci 364(1838):233–248
14. Coelho PG et al (2009) Basic research methods and current trends of dental implant surfaces. J Biomed Mater Res B Appl Biomater 88(2):579–596

15. Wennerberg A, Albrektsson T (2010) On implant surfaces: a review of current knowledge and opinions. Int J Oral Maxillofac Implants 25(1):63–74
16. Yang Y, Kim KH, Ong JL (2005) A review on calcium phosphate coatings produced using a sputtering process – an alternative to plasma spraying. Biomaterials 26(3):327–337
17. Kitsugi T et al (1996) Bone-bonding behavior of plasma-sprayed coatings of Bioglass R, AW-glass ceramic, and tricalcium phosphate on titanium alloy. J Biomed Mater Res 30(2):261–269
18. Ducheyne P (1985) Bioglass coatings and bioglass composites as implant materials. J Biomed Mater Res 19(3):273–291
19. Bjursten LM et al (2010) Titanium dioxide nanotubes enhance bone bonding in vivo. J Biomed Mater Res A 92(3):1218–1224
20. Vignoletti F et al (2009) Early healing of implants placed into fresh extraction sockets: an experimental study in the beagle dog. De novo bone formation. J Clin Periodontol 36(3):265–277
21. Webster TJ, Smith TA (2005) Increased osteoblast function on PLGA composites containing nanophase titania. J Biomed Mater Res A 74(4):677–686
22. Zhao L et al (2010) The influence of hierarchical hybrid micro/nano-textured titanium surface with titania nanotubes on osteoblast functions. Biomaterials 31(19):5072–5082
23. Khor E (2001) Chitin: fulfilling a biomaterials promise. Elseveir, Amsterdam
24. Khor E, Lim LY (2003) Implantable applications of chitin and chitosan. Biomaterials 24(13):2339–2349
25. Di Martino A, Sittinger M, Risbud MV (2005) Chitosan: a versatile biopolymer for orthopaedic tissue-engineering. Biomaterials 26(30):5983–5990
26. Kim IY et al (2008) Chitosan and its derivatives for tissue engineering applications. Biotechnol Adv 26(1):1–21
27. Jayakumar R et al (2010) Novel chitin and chitosan nanofibers in biomedical applications. Biotechnol Adv 28(1):142–150
28. Sinha VR et al (2004) Chitosan microspheres as a potential carrier for drugs. Int J Pharm 274(1–2):1–33
29. Panos I, Acosta N, Heras A (2008) New drug delivery systems based on chitosan. Curr Drug Discov Technol 5(4):333–341
30. Kumar MN et al (2004) Chitosan chemistry and pharmaceutical perspectives. Chem Rev 104(12):6017–6084
31. Muzzarelli R et al (1988) Biological activity of chitosan: ultrastructural study. Biomaterials 9(3):247–252
32. Muzzarelli RA et al (1999) Biochemistry, histology and clinical uses of chitins and chitosans in wound healing. EXS 87:251–264
33. Muzzarelli RA et al (1994) Stimulatory effect on bone formation exerted by a modified chitosan. Biomaterials 15(13):1075–1081
34. Ueno H et al (1999) Accelerating effects of chitosan for healing at early phase of experimental open wound in dogs. Biomaterials 20(15):1407–1414
35. Masuoka K et al (2005) The interaction of chitosan with fibroblast growth factor-2 and its protection from inactivation. Biomaterials 26(16):3277–3284
36. Azad AK et al (2004) Chitosan membrane as a wound-healing dressing: characterization and clinical application. J Biomed Mater Res B Appl Biomater 69(2):216–222
37. Kratz G et al (1998) Immobilised heparin accelerates the healing of human wounds in vivo. Scand J Plast Reconstr Surg Hand Surg 32(4):381–385
38. Amaral IF et al (2007) Attachment, spreading and short-term proliferation of human osteoblastic cells cultured on chitosan films with different degrees of acetylation. J Biomater Sci Polym Ed 18(4):469–485
39. Bumgardner JD et al (2003) Contact angle, protein adsorption and osteoblast precursor cell attachment to chitosan coatings bonded to titanium. J Biomater Sci Polym Ed 14(12):1401–1409

40. Chang J et al (2008) Biological properties of chitosan films with different degree of deacetylation. J Mater Sci Technol 24(5):700–708
41. Mao JS et al (2004) A preliminary study on chitosan and gelatin polyelectrolyte complex cytocompatibility by cell cycle and apoptosis analysis. Biomaterials 25(18):3973–3981
42. Prasitsilp M et al (2000) Cellular responses to chitosan in vitro: the importance of deacetylation. J Mater Sci Mater Med 11(12):773–778
43. Chatelet C, Damour O, Domard A (2001) Influence of the degree of acetylation on some biological properties of chitosan films. Biomaterials 22(3):261–268
44. Hamilton V et al (2007) Bone cell attachment and growth on well-characterized chitosan films. Polym Int 56(5):241–247
45. Luna SM, Silva SS, Gomez ME, Mano JF, Reis RL (2010) Cell adhesion and proliferation onto chitosan-based membranes treated by plasma surface modification. J Biomater Appl (in press) doi: 10.1177/0885328210362924
46. Bumgardner JD et al (2003) Chitosan: potential use as a bioactive coating for orthopaedic and craniofacial/dental implants. J Biomater Sci Polym Ed 14(5):423–438
47. Chung L et al (1994) Biocompatibility of potential wound management products: fungal mycelia as a source of chitin/chitosan and their effect on the proliferation of human F1000 fibroblasts in culture. J Biomed Mater Res 28:463–469
48. Klokkevold PR et al (1996) Osteogenesis enhanced by chitosan (poly-N-acetyl glucosaminoglycan) in vitro. J Periodontol 67(11):1170–1175
49. Ohara N et al (2004) Early gene expression analyzed by cDNA microarray and RT-PCR in osteoblasts cultured with water-soluble and low molecular chitooligosaccharide. Biomaterials 25(10):1749–1754
50. Fakhry A et al (2004) Chitosan supports the initial attachment and spreading of osteoblasts preferentially over fibroblasts. Biomaterials 25(11):2075–2079
51. Lahiji A et al (2000) Chitosan supports the expression of extracellular matrix proteins in human osteoblasts and chondrocytes. J Biomed Mater Res 51(4):586–595
52. Aiba S (1991) Studies on chitosan: 3. Evidence for the presence of random and block copolymer structures in partially N-acetylated chitosans. Int J Biol Macromol 13(1):40–44
53. Tomihata K, Ikada Y (1997) In vitro and in vivo degradation of films of chitin and its deacetylated derivatives. Biomaterials 18(7):567–575
54. Kurita K et al (2000) Enzymatic degradation of β-chitin: susceptibility and the influence of deacetylation. Carbohydr Polym 42(1):19–21
55. Nguyen T et al (2008) Molecular stability of chitosan in acid solutions stored at various conditions. J Appl Polym Sci 107:2588–2593
56. Kohn P, Winzler J, Hoffman RC (1962) Metabolism of D-glucosamine and N-acetyl-D-glucosamine in the intact rat. J Biol Chem 237:304–308
57. Abarrategi A et al (2009) Gene expression profile on chitosan/rhBMP-2 films: a novel osteoinductive coating for implantable materials. Acta Biomater 5(7):2633–2646
58. Matsunaga T et al (2006) Chitosan monomer promotes tissue regeneration on dental pulp wounds. J Biomed Mater Res A 76:711–720
59. Li Q et al (1992) Applications and properties of chitosan. J Bioactive Compatible Polym 7(4):370–397
60. Hidaka Y et al (1999) Histopathological and immunohistochemical studies of membranes of deacetylated chitin derivatives implanted over rat calvaria. J Biomed Mater Res 46 (3):418–423
61. Bagheri-Khoulenjani S, Taghizadeh S, Mirzadeh H (2009) An investigation on the short-term biodegradability of chitosan with various molecular weights and degrees of deacetylation. Carbohydr Polym 78(4):773–778
62. Bumgardner JD et al (2007) The integration of chitosan-coated titanium in bone: an in vivo study in rabbits. Implant Dent 16(1):66–79
63. Chesnutt BM et al (2009) Composite chitosan/nano-hydroxyapatite scaffolds induce osteocalcin production by osteoblasts in vitro and support bone formation in vivo. Tissue Eng A 15(9):2571–2579

64. Reves B (2008) Preliminary investigation of lyophilization to improve drug delivery of chitosan-calcium phosphate bone scaffold construct. MS Thesis, Biomedical Engineering, University of Memphis
65. Muzzarelli RA et al (1993) Osteoconduction exerted by methylpyrrolidinone chitosan used in dental surgery. Biomaterials 14(1):39–43
66. Shi C et al (2006) Therapeutic potential of chitosan and its derivatives in regenerative medicine. J Surg Res 133(2):185–192
67. Gupta R, Chaudhury NK (2007) Entrapment of biomolecules in sol-gel matrix for applications in biosensors: problems and future prospects. Biosens Bioelectron 22(11): 2387–2399
68. Morra M (2006) Biochemical modification of titanium surfaces: peptides and ECM proteins. Eur Cell Mater 12:1–15
69. Puleo DA, Nanci A (1999) Understanding and controlling the bone-implant interface. Biomaterials 20(23–24):2311–2321
70. Shriver-Lake L (1998) Silane-modified surfaces for biomaterial immobilization. In: Cass AEG, Ligler FS (eds) Immobilized biomolecules in analysis: a practical approach. Oxford University Press, Oxford, p 216
71. Weetall HH (1993) Preparation of immobilized proteins covalently coupled through silane coupling agents to inorganic supports. Appl Biochem Biotechnol 41(3):157–188
72. Hanawa T (2009) An overview of biofunctionalization of metals in Japan. J R Soc Interface 6(Suppl 3):S361–S369
73. Arroyo-Hernandez M, Perez-Rigueiro J, Martinez-Duart JM (2006) Formation of amine functionalized films by chemical vapour deposition. Mater Sci Eng C Biomimetic Supramol Syst 26(5–7):938–941
74. Topchiev AV, Andrianov KA (1953) Basic nomenclature and classification of low-molecularweight organo-silicon compounds. Russ Chem Bull 2(3):439
75. Duchet J et al (1997) Influence of the deposition process on the structure of grafted alkylsilane layers. Langmuir 13(8):2271
76. Van Der Voort P, Vansant EF (1996) Silylation of the silica surface: a review. J Liq Chromatogr Related Technol 19(17):2723–2752
77. ACS (1974) Chapter 38: silicon compounds. In: Fletcher JH, Dermer OC, Fox RB (eds) Nomenclature of organic compounds: principles and practice, vol 126. American Chemical Society, Washington, pp 293–298
78. Kallury K, MacDonald P, Thompson M (1994) Effect of surface water and base catalysis on the silaniation of silica by (aminopropyl)alkoxysilanes studied by x-ray photoelectron spectroscopy and 13C cross-polarization/magic angle spinning nuclear magnetic resonance. Langmuir 10(2):492–499
79. Puleo DA (1995) Activity of enzyme immobilized on silanized Co-Cr-Mo. J Biomed Mater Res 29(8):951–957
80. Puleo DA (1997) Retention of enzymatic activity immobilized on silanized Co-Cr-Mo and Ti-6Al-4V. J Biomed Mater Res 37(2):222–228
81. Dee KC, Andersen TT, Bizios R (1998) Design and function of novel osteoblast-adhesive peptides for chemical modification of biomaterials. J Biomed Mater Res 40(3):371–377
82. Zreiqat H et al (2003) Differentiation of human bone-derived cells grown on GRGDSP-peptide bound titanium surfaces. J Biomed Mater Res A 64(1):105–113
83. Martin HJ et al (2007) XPS study on the use of 3-aminopropyltriethoxysilane to bond chitosan to a titanium surface. Langmuir 23(12):6645
84. Martin HJ et al (2008) An XPS study on the attachment of triethoxysilylbutyraldehyde to two titanium surfaces as a way to bond chitosan. Appl Surf Sci 254(15):4599
85. Martin HJ et al (2008) Enhanced bonding of chitosan to implant quality titanium via four treatment combinations. Thin Solid Films 516(18):6277

86. Yuan Y et al (2008) Mechanical property, degradation rate, and bone cell growth of chitosan coated titanium influenced by degree of deacetylation of chitosan. J Biomed Mater Res B Appl Biomater 86(1):245–252
87. Martin H, Schulz KH, Bumgardner J (2008) Comparing the attachment and growth of bone cells on chitosan bound by two silane molecules to titanium for use in joint replacements. In: American Institute of chemical engineers annual meeting, Philadelphia
88. Greene AH et al (2008) Chitosan-coated stainless steel screws for fixation in contaminated fractures. Clin Orthop Relat Res 466(7):1699–1704
89. Wang SF et al (2005) Biopolymer chitosan/montmorillonite nanocomposites: preparation and characterization. Polym Degrad Stab 90(1):123
90. Majd S et al (2009) Effects of material property and heat treatment on nanomechanical properties of chitosan films. J Biomed Mater Res B Appl Biomater 90(1):283–289
91. Freier T et al (2005) Controlling cell adhesion and degradation of chitosan films by N-acetylation. Biomaterials 26(29):5872–5878
92. Wenling C et al (2005) Effects of the degree of deacetylation on the physicochemical properties and Schwann cell affinity of chitosan films. J Biomater Appl 20(2):157–177
93. Strand SP et al (2010) Molecular design of chitosan gene delivery systems with an optimized balance between polyplex stability and polyplex unpacking. Biomaterials 31(5):975–987
94. Hamilton V et al (2006) Characterization of chitosan films and effects on fibroblast cell attachment and proliferation. J Mater Sci Mater Med 17(12):1373–1381
95. Rhazi M et al (2000) Investigation of different natural sources of chitin: influence of the source and deacetylatino process on the physicochemical characteristics of chitosan. Polym Int 49:337–344
96. Norowski P (2008) Chitosan as an antimicrobial coating for titanium implants. MS Thesis, Biomedical engineering. University of Memphis
97. Norowski PA, Courtney HS, Babu J, Haggard WO, Bumgardner JD (2011) Chitosan coatings deliver antimicrobials from titanium implants: a preliminary study. Implant Dent 20:56–67
98. Leedy M (2009) In vitro evaluation of 87.4% DDA chitosan on titanium for the local delivery of vascular endothelial growth factor. MS Thesis, Biomedical Engineering, University of Memphis
99. Wasserman S, Tao Y, Whitesides G (1989) Structure and reactivity of alkylsiloxane monolayers formed by reaction of alkyltrichlorosilanes on silicon substrates. Langmuir 5(4):1074–1087
100. Gelest (2004) Aminopropyltriethoxysilane. Material safety data sheet, Version 1. http://www.gelest.com/msds.asp?SIA0610.1. Accessed 12 Feb 2009
101. Gelest (2007) Triethoxysilylbutyraldehyde. Material safety data sheet, Version 3. http://www.gelest.com/msds.asp?SIT8185.3. Gelest, Morrisville, PA, Accessed 12 Feb 2009
102. Martin HJ, Schulz KH, Bumgardner JD (2008) Comparing the mechanical properties of chitosan films bound to titanium following deposition, neutralization, and sterilization. In: Abstracts American Institute of chemical engineers annual meeting, Philadelphia, Nov 2008. 613a. http://aiche.confex.com/aiche/2008/techprogram/P128853.HTM
103. Muller R et al (2006) Influence of surface pretreatment of titanium- and cobalt-based biomaterials on covalent immobilization of fibrillar collagen. Biomaterials 27(22):4059–4068
104. Pegg EC et al (2009) Mono-functional aminosilanes as primers for peptide functionalization. J Biomed Mater Res A 90(4):947–958
105. Martinex-Corria R et al (2011) The use of chitosan/BMP-2 complex in bone substitutes and implant surfaces. In: Gottlander R, van Steenberghe D (eds) Proceedings of the first P-I Brånemark scientific symposium, Gothenburg 2009: osseointegration and related treatment modalities: future perspectives, quality of life and treatment simplification. Quintessence Publishing, London, pp 105–122
106. López-Lacomba JL et al (2006) Use of rhBMP-2 activated chitosan films to improve osseointegration. Biomacromolecules 7(3):p792–p798

107. Abarrategi A et al (2008) Chitosan film as rhBMP2 carrier: delivery properties for bone tissue applications. Biomacromolecules 9(2):771–718
108. Abarrategi A et al (2008) Improvement of porous beta-TCP scaffolds with rhBMP-2 chitosan carrier films for bone tissue application. Tissue Eng A 14(8):1305–1319
109. Peña J et al (2006) Room temperature synthesis of chitosan/apatite powders and coatings. J Europ Ceram Soc 26:3631–3638
110. Peña J et al (2006) New method to obtain chitosan/apatite materials at room temperature. Solid State Sci 8:513–519
111. Kawai T et al (2009) Biological fixation of fibrous materials to bone using chitin/chitosan as a bone formation accelerator. J Biomed Mater Res B Appl Biomater 88(1):264–270
112. Besra L, Liu M (2007) A review on fundamentals and applications of electrophoretic deposition (EPD). Prog Mater Sci 52(1):1
113. Van der Biest OO, Vandeperre LJ (1999) Electrophoretic deposition of materials. Annu Rev Mater Sci 29(1):327–352
114. Lu X, Leng Y, Zhang Q (2008) Electrochemical deposition of octacalcium phosphate microfiber/chitosan composite coatings on titanium substrates. Surf Coat Technol 202(13):3142
115. Redepenning J et al (2003) Electrochemical preparation of chitosan/hydroxyapatite composite coatings on titanium substrates. J Biomed Mater Res A 66(2):411–416
116. Sun F, Pang X, Zhitomirsky I (2009) Electrophoretic deposition of composite hydroxyapatite-chitosan-heparin coatings. J Mater Process Technol 209(3):1597
117. Sharma S, Soni VP, Bellare JR (2009) Chitosan reinforced apatite-wollastonite coating by electrophoretic deposition on titanium implants. J Mater Sci Mater Med 20(7):1427–1436
118. Pang X, Zhitomirsky I (2005) Electrodeposition of composite hydroxyapatite-chitosan films. Mater Chem Phys 94(2–3):245
119. Pang X, Casagrande T, Zhitomirsky I (2009) Electrophoretic deposition of hydroxyapatite-CaSiO3-chitosan composite coatings. J Colloid Interface Sci 330(2):323
120. Wang J, van Apeldoorn A, de Groot K (2006) Electrolytic deposition of calcium phosphate/chitosan coating on titanium alloy: growth kinetics and influence of current density, acetic acid, and chitosan. J Biomed Mater Res A 76(3):503–511
121. Said R et al (2010) Effects of bias voltage on diamond like carbon coatings deposited using titanium isopropoxide (TIPOT) and acetylene/argon mixtures onto various substrate materials. J Nanosci Nanotechnol 10(4):2552–2557
122. Eliaz N et al (2009) The effect of surface treatment on the surface texture and contact angle of electrochemically deposited hydroxyapatite coating and on its interaction with bone-forming cells. Acta Biomater 5(8):3178–3191
123. Song Y et al (2010) Electrodeposition of Ca-P coatings on biodegradable Mg alloy: in vitro biomineralization behavior. Acta Biomater 6(5):1736–1742
124. Wang J et al (2009) Fluoridated hydroxyapatite coatings on titanium obtained by electrochemical deposition. Acta Biomater 5(5):1798–1807
125. Lopez-Heredia MA, Weiss P, Layrolle P (2007) An electrodeposition method of calcium phosphate coatings on titanium alloy. J Mater Sci Mater Med 18(2):381–390
126. Borrajo JP et al (2007) In vivo evaluation of titanium implants coated with bioactive glass by pulsed laser deposition. J Mater Sci Mater Med 18(12):2371–2376
127. Eby DM, Luckarift HR, Johnson GR (2009) Hybrid antimicrobial enzyme and silver nanoparticle coatings for medical instruments. ACS Appl Mater Interfaces 1(7):1553–1560
128. Jing H, Yu Z, Li L (2008) Antibacterial properties and corrosion resistance of Cu and Ag/Cu porous materials. J Biomed Mater Res A 87(1):33–37
129. Cunha L et al (2010) Ti-Si-C thin films produced by magnetron sputtering: correlation between physical properties, mechanical properties and tribological behavior. J Nanosci Nanotechnol 10(4):2926–2932
130. Lin C et al (2008) Electrophoretic deposition of HA/MWNTs composite coating for biomaterial applications. J Mater Sci Mater Med 19(7):2569–2574
131. Wilks SJ et al (2009) Poly(3, 4-ethylenedioxythiophene) as a micro-neural interface material for electrostimulation. Front Neuroeng 2:7

132. Yao C, Webster TJ (2006) Anodization: a promising nano-modification technique of titanium implants for orthopedic applications. J Nanosci Nanotechnol 6(9–10):2682–2692
133. Wu L-Q et al (2002) Voltage-dependent assembly of the polysaccharide chitosan onto an electrode surface. Langmuir 18(22):8620–8625
134. Zhitomirsky D et al (2009) Electrophoretic deposition of bioactive glass/polymer composite coatings with and without HA nanoparticle inclusions for biomedical applications. J Mater Process Technol 209(4):1853
135. Fernandes R et al (2003) Electrochemically induced deposition of a polysaccharide hydrogel onto a patterned surface. Langmuir 19:4058–4062
136. Kang X et al (2007) A novel glucose biosensor based on immobilization of glucose oxidase in chitosan on a glassy carbon electrode modified with gold-platinum alloy nanoparticles/multiwall carbon nanotubes. Anal Biochem 369(1):71–79
137. Zeng X et al (2009) Electrodeposition of chitosan-ionic liquid-glucose oxidase biocomposite onto nano-gold electrode for amperometric glucose sensing. Biosens Bioelectron 24(9):2898–2903
138. Zhou Q et al (2007) Electrodeposition of carbon nanotubes-chitosan-glucose oxidase biosensing composite films triggered by reduction of p-benzoquinone or H_2O_2. J Phys Chem B 111(38):11276–11284
139. Grandfield K, Zhitomirsky I (2008) Electrophoretic deposition of composite hydroxyapatite-silica-chitosan coatings. Mater Charact 59(1):61
140. Wang J, de Boer J, de Groot K (2004) Preparation and characterization of electrodeposited calcium phosphate/chitosan coating on Ti6Al4V plates. J Dent Res 83(4):296–301
141. Sharma S et al (2009) Bone healing performance of electrophoretic deposited apatite-wollastonite/chitosan coating on titanium implants in rabbit tibiae. J Tissue Eng Regen Med 3(7):501–511
142. Wang J et al (2010) Early bone appositin and 1 yr performance of electrodeposited calcium phosphate coatings: an experimental study in rabbit femora. Clin Oral Impl Res 21:951–960
143. Muzzarelli C, Muzzarelli RA (2002) Natural and artificial chitosan-inorganic composites. J Inorg Biochem 92(2):89–94
144. Xu HH et al (2002) Processing and properties of strong and non-rigid calcium phosphate cement. J Dent Res 81(3):219–224
145. Yamaguchi I et al (2001) Preparation and microstructure analysis of chitosan/hydroxyapatite nanocomposites. J Biomed Mater Res 55(1):20–27
146. Wang J, de Boer J, de Groot K (2008) Proliferation and differentiation of MC3T3-E1 cells on calcium phosphate/chitosan coatings. J Dent Res 87(7):650–654
147. Pang X, Zhitomirsky I (2007) Electrophoretic deposition of composite hydroxyapatite-chitosan coatings. Mater Charact 58(4):339
148. Singh R, Dahotre NB (2007) Corrosion degradation and prevention by surface modification of biometallic materials. J Mater Sci Mater Med 18(5):725–751
149. Pang X, Zhitomirsky I (2008) Electrodeposition of hydroxyapatite-silver-chitosan nanocomposite coatings. Surf Coat Technol 202(16):3815
150. Tavakol M et al (2009) Sulfasalazine release from alginate-N, O-carboxymethyl chitosan gel beads coated by chitosan. Carbohydr Polym 77:326–330
151. Malaekeh-Nikouei M, Tabassi SAS, Jaafari MR (2008) Preparation, characterization, and mucoadhesive properties of chitosan-coated microspheres encapsulated with cyclosporine A. Drug Dev Ind Pharm 34:492–498
152. Cui X et al (2008) Effects of chitosan-coated pressed calcium sulfate pellet combined with recombinant human bone morphogenetic protein 2 on restoration of segmental bone defect. J Craniofac Surg 19(2):459–465
153. Reves BT et al (2009) Lyophilization to improve drug delivery for chitosan-calcium phosphate bone scaffold construct: a preliminary investigation. J Biomed Mater Res B Appl Biomater 90(1):1–10

154. Peng P et al (2008) Concurrent elution of calcium phosphate and macromolecules from alginate/chitosan hydrogel coatings. Biointerphases 3(4):105–116
155. Thierry B et al (2003) Bioactive coatings of endovascular stents based on polyelectrolyte multilayers. Biomacromolecules 4:1564–1571
156. Jun S-H et al (2010) A bioactive coating of a silica xerogel/chitosan hybrid on titanium by a room temperature sol–gel process. Acta Biomater 6:302–307
157. Patz TM et al (2007) Matrix assisted pulsed laser evaporation of biomaterial thin films. Mater Sci Eng C 27:514–522
158. Couto DS, Alves NM, Mano JF (2009) Nanostructured multilayer coatings combining chitosan with bioactive glass nanoparticles. J Nanosci Nanotech 9:1741–1748
159. Dong P et al (2009) Biocompatibility of chitosan/heparin multilayer coatings on NiTi. Mater Sci Forum 610–613:1179–1182
160. Meng S et al (2009) The effect of a layer-by-layer chitosan–heparin coating on the endothelialization and coagulation properties of a coronary stent system. Biomaterials 30:2276–2283
161. Chua P-H et al (2008) Surface functionalization of titanium with hyaluronic acid/chitosan polyelectrolyte multilayers and RGD for promoting osteoblast functions and inhibiting bacterial adhesion. Biomaterials 29:1412–1421
162. Li QL et al (2007) Ultar-thin film of chitosan and sulfated chitosan on titanium oxide by layer-by-layer self assembly method. Key Engr Mater 330–332:645–648
163. Cai K et al (2005) Polysaccharide-protein surface modification of titanium via a layer-by-layer technique: characterization and cell behaviour aspects. Biomaterials 26:5960–5971
164. Richert L et al (2004) Layer by layer buildup of polysaccharide films: physical chemistry and cellular adhesion aspects. Langmuir 20:448–458
165. Ruan Q et al (2009) Investigation of layer-by-layer assembled heparin and chitosan multilayer films via electrochemical spectroscopy. J Colloid Interface Sci 333:725–733
166. Fu J et al (2006) Construction of antibacterial multilayer films containing nanosilver via layer-by-layer assembly of heparin and chitosan-silver ions complex. J Biomed Mater Res A 79A:665–674
167. Muzzeralli RAA et al (2001) Chitosan-oxychitin coatings for prosthetic materials. Carbohydr Polym 45:35–41

New Techniques for Optimization of Surface Area and Porosity in Nanochitins and Nanochitosans

Riccardo A. A. Muzzarelli

Abstract This chapter outlines the beneficial activities of chitosan and then describes the earliest observations of the expanded structure of isolated chitosans from filamentous fungi, most notably cultivated *Absidia coerulea*. Fungal chitin–glucan complexes are currently being evaluated in animal models of atherosclerosis and obesity. Impressive advances in the reactivity of chitins and chitosans of various origins have been made possible by the isolation of nanofibrils with surface area as high as 700 m^2/g by mechanically disassembling the structures occurring in vivo. These procedures lend themselves to easy scaling-up, in contrast to electrospinning that moreover often involves the use of dangerous solvents. By drying chitosan preparations with the aid of supercritical CO$_2$, aerogels with surface area of 50–750 m^2/g are obtained, and can be easily crosslinked with genipin in order to optimize the average pore size for the preparation of scaffolds of interest in orthopedics.

Keywords Electrospinning · Nanochitin · Nanochitosan · Nanofibrils

Contents

1 Introduction 168
2 Isolation of Expanded Chitin Structures from Fungi 169
3 Chitin and Chitosan Nanofibrils 173
    3.1 Mechanically Isolated Nanofibrils in the Presence of Acetic Acid 173
    3.2 Mechanically Defibrillated Nanochitosans 175
    3.3 Nanochitosan Obtained from Partially Deacetylated Chitin or from Deacetylated Nanochitin 176

R.A.A. Muzzarelli (✉)
University of Ancona, Ancona, Italy
e-mail: muzzarelli.raa@gmail.com; www.chitin.it

4	Electrospun Nanofibers	178
5	Supercritical Drying	181
6	Conclusion	184
References		184

1 Introduction

Chitosan, collagen, gelatin, and alginate have been studied because of their inherent hydrophilicity and the presence of properties similar to those of the extracellular matrix, which provides a suitable environment for cell growth. Nevertheless, scaffolds made of these biopolymers are mechanically weak, which limits their use as regenerating templates for semi-hard and hard tissues, such as cartilage and bone. There are various means of improving the mechanical properties, such as crosslinking, blending, and chemical modifications.

Proteoglycans on the other hand are major components of the extracellular matrix, and consist of glycosaminoglycans linked to proteins. Although each of them has a distinctive chemical composition, glycosaminoglycans are typically composed of repeating disaccharide units consisting of an amino sugar (GlcNAc or GalNAc) and an uronic acid (either glucuronate or iduronate), and include polymers such as heparin, heparan sulfate, chondroitin, keratin, and dermatan. Although they are a minor component of the extracellular matrix (generally $\leq$ 5% dry weight), glycosaminoglycans constitute more than 70% of the volume of the hydrated extracellular matrix.

The glycosaminoglycans also constitute a compatible interface between cells and their surrounding microenvironment. Many cell adhesion compounds as well as a number of adhesive glycoproteins, including laminin and fibronectin, have heparan sulfate-binding sites. Heparan sulfate proteoglycans, such as syndecan, consist of a core protein anchored in the plasma membrane and carrying extracellular chains of heparan sulfate. The resulting sugar-based boundary between the cell surface and the matrix can be up to 4 µm thick in chondrocytes, which is an exceptional case where hyaluronic acid (a glycosaminoglycan containing up to 50,000 monosaccharide units) constitutes a significant proportion of the surface-associated glycans [1].

When a scaffold capable of favoring cell development is desired, certain crucial characteristic properties of the material should be enhanced and optimized, in particular when the scaffold is expected to medicate living tissue losses. Hydrophilicity, biocompatibility, absence of cytotoxicity, immune-enhancing capacity, optimum porosity, high surface area and other characteristics should be possessed by the candidate scaffold. Little by little it has been realized that the use of unrefined chitins and chitosans for this kind of purpose is not advisable. Instead, there is a need for well-conceived and manufactured scaffolds with pore dimensions suitable for cell life, very large surface area for the best possible colonization, and chemical functions compatible with the expected role of the implanted material for effective wound healing and tissue regeneration. Progressively, from irregularly shaped chitin powders, investigations have moved to films, microspheres, hydrogel particles of various sizes, nanocrystals, nanofibers, and a variety of composites [2, 3].

Pharmaceutical excipients have been viewed as inert materials, but this view has changed because today's excipients have novel functions that range from stabilization of formulations to active roles in enhancing drug uptake and specific drug delivery. Chitin and chitosan are not expected to exert pharmacological activity, although their potential for use in medical devices and in wound healing has centered around biological and biochemical activity; for example, a role for chitosan in the wound healing process has been demonstrated through macrophage activation, stimulation of cell proliferation, and histo-architectural tissue organization [4, 5] with supporting evidence from induced wound models [6].

The efficacy of chitosan as a haemostatic agent is another example. In vitro studies with blood have indicated that its haemostatic mechanism is independent of the classical coagulation cascade and it is due to an interaction between the cell membrane of erythrocytes and chitosan, with clot formation in the absence of coagulation factors or platelets, according to early reports by Klokkevold et al. [7] and more recently by Scherer et al. [8]. It is thought that, because the outer membranes of erythrocytes and platelets are negatively charged, they form polyelectrolyte complexes with the cationic chitosan leading to platelet activation and thrombus formation. Such action has been utilized in medical devices such as Celox and chitosan-containing dressings for the treatment of bleeding, and have been supported by evidence of reduced bleeding and enhanced haemostasis in experimental animal models.

The purpose of this chapter is to direct attention to some chemical procedures that permit modification of the porosity and surface area of chitosan. It seems that these procedures hold the key to a more expanded development of chitin-derived biomedical items.

2 Isolation of Expanded Chitin Structures from Fungi

A four-stage procedure for the isolation of the chitin–glucan complex from the biomass of *Armillariella mellea* and the yellow morel *Morchella esculenta*, belonging to the classes Basidiomycetes and Ascomycetes, respectively, has been developed by Ivshina et al. [9]. The steps are deproteinization (2% NaOH plus 0.1% sodium stearate, 83–85 °C, 2 h), demineralization (1% HCl, 55–60 °C, 2 h), depigmentation (5% H_2O_2 in ammonia, 30–35 °C, 4 h), followed by final removal of residual protein (2% NaOH, 83–85 °C, 2 h). The content of chitin in the final products was 70% for *A. mellea* and 50% for *M. esculenta*. During the course of the isolation, the colors changed from dark brown and dark beige to light cream. The chitin content in the isolated complexes was ca. 80% and 47% respectively, the degree of acetylation was 0.80 and 0.41 respectively, while the degree of crystallinity was 61 for both. Pyrolytic gas chromatography in agreement with other analytical techniques demonstrated the identity of fungal and arthropod chitin [9].

Solid-state fermentation of *Lentinus edodes* was found to be an efficient approach to chitosan production; in fact, the chitosan yield was 6.18 g/kg and the degree of acetylation was 12.5% at 12 days after inoculation. These data are of particular significance. The solid-state fermentation gave yields 50 times higher than submerged fermentation, and the chitosan had smaller degree of acetylation than crustacean commercial chitosans, which means advantageous applicability thanks to higher charge density [10, 11].

A number of yeasts and filamentous fungi, for example, *Saccharomyces cerevisiae, Mucor rouxii, Phycomyces blakeesleanus, Choanephora cucurbitarum, Neurospora crassa, Streptomyces* spp, *Absidia* spp., and *Rhizopus* spp., contain chitin or chitosan in their cell walls and septa [12–15]. In the order Mucorales, many strains have interesting productivity of chitosan [16] in particular certain strains of *Absidia* [17]. A molecular weight (MW) as high as 700 kDa and yields of 1.0–1.3 g/L of submerged culture medium were obtained. Many authors adopted the reported protocol for isolation and purification of the chitin/chitosan–glucan complex and subsequent extraction of chitosan with the aid of dilute acetic acid. For example, the mycelia of cultured *Absidia glauca* var. *paradoaxa* were treated with hot 2% NaOH to isolate the alkali-insoluble polysaccharides, from which the extraction of chitosan was carried out with 2% acetic acid at room temperature. The chitosan extracted had degree of deacetylation of 0.86 and viscosity of 4.0 cP at 0.1% chitosan in 0.5% acetic acid, which indicates low MW [18]. The procedure followed by Niederhofer and Muller [19] with *A. coerulea* was similar but with more refinements: chitosan with average MW of 45 kDa was extracted from the raw material. Taking into account the solubility of low MW chitosan up to alkaline pH ranges, reprecipitation and washing with ethanol was adopted to avoid losses.

Wu et al. [20] found that the maximum glucosamine level in the *A. niger* mycelium was 11.10% dry weight, whereas in that of *M. rouxii* it was 20.13%. *M. rouxii* contained both chitin and chitosan, whereas *A. niger* contained only chitin. The yields of crude chitin from *A. niger* and *M. rouxii* were 24.01 and 13.25%, respectively, and the yield of chitosan from *M. rouxii* was 12.49%. Significant amounts of glucan (7.4–39.8%) were associated with chitinous compounds from both species and could not be eliminated by the extraction method used. The degrees of acetylation were determined to be 0.76 and 0.50 for chitin from *A. niger* and *M. rouxii*, respectively, and 0.19 for *M. rouxii* chitosan. According to Chatterjee et al. [21], the production yield of chitosan from *M. rouxii* can be improved with the aid of plant growth hormones, i.e., indoleacetic acid, indolebutyricacid, kinetin, and gibberellic acid. The yield of chitosan increased 34–69%, gibberellic acid being the most potent enhancer.

In consideration of the large spent biomass generated during the production of citric acid, several authors have studied the recovery of the chitin–glucan complex from *A. niger*. In the earliest report on the isolated chitosan–glucan from *A. niger*, Muzzarelli et al. [22] investigated extensively the preparative conditions under 16 sets of five parameters: the statistical evaluation indicated that a 4-h treatment with 40% NaOH aqueous solution without nitrogen blanketing at 128 °C provided satisfactory yield (44%) and chitosan content (>32%). The isolated powders where white and turned light brown upon drying at 60 °C. These products were not fully soluble in 5% acetic acid, but dispersions were obtained upon prolonged stirring. The amount of chitosan was determined in the dispersions with the aid of potassium polyvinylsulfate and sodium molybdate, which produce analytically valid polyelectrolyte complexes (as also observed with alginate). The infrared spectra taken on the fractions obtained after filtration indicated different ratios of chitosan and glucan. The collection percentages of eight transition metal ions were definitely higher than the corresponding values for animal chitosan, despite the fact that the complex contains nearly 50% chitosan by weight. Evidently, the surface area is much bigger: in fact the filamentous mycelia shapes were still visible under the microscope in rather frail films, obtained thanks to the preserved typical filmogenicity of chitosan [22]. Evidence of the covalent binding of chitin with glucans was confirmed many years later for a variety of fungi [23] and by Zamani et al. [24] among others.

The contributions by Nwe et al. [25, 26] about the production and applications of fungal chitosans dealt with a method to produce high quality and quantity of fungal chitosan from the cell wall of *Gongronella butleri* and *A. coerulea*. The α-1,4 glycosidic bond between chitosan and glucan in the chitosan–glucan complex was cleaved in part by a heat-stable α-amylase. On the other hand, pure chitosan could be obtained from the cell wall of fungus *G. butleri* USDB 0201 with the aid of the enzyme Termamyl. Nwe and coworkers further optimized the conditions for production of chitosan with high yield using solid substrate fermentation. Free chitosan (6.5 g/100 g of mycelia) and total chitosan (8–9 g/100 g of mycelia) were isolated from *A. coerulea*. Nwe et al. [26] further applied fungal chitosan in plant tissue culture.

The chitin–glucan from *A. niger* was later produced by Kitozyme (Belgium). Analysis by ^{13}C-solid state NMR showed that the poly(*N*-acetyl-D-glucosamine) and the $\beta(1,3)$-D-glucan were present in the ratio 35:65 (w/w). The material was studied in an animal model of atherosclerosis by Berecochea-Lopez et al. [27]: it strongly reduced the area of aortic fatty streak deposition by 87–97%, and cardiac production of superoxide anion by 25%. On the other hand, it enhanced liver superoxide dismutase activity by 7–45% and glutathione peroxidase activity by 38–120%. These findings support the view that long-term consumption of chitin–glucan has potential effects against atherosclerosis, the underlying mechanism being related mainly to improving the defenses against antioxidants. No undesirable or toxic effects were detected, nor evidence of other clinical signs. Thus, at low doses, chitin–glucan was deemed to be a safe nutraceutical supplement. Certain aspects of the work were confirmed by Neyrinck et al. [28], who concluded that fungal chitosan (from the same producer) counteracts some inflammatory disorders and metabolic alterations that occur in diet-induced obese mice since it decreases feed efficiency, adipocytokine secretion, fat mass, and ectopic fat deposition in the liver and muscle.

Muzzarelli et al. [29] found that the chitosan–glucan complex in *A. coerulea* grown aerobically for 72 h at 25 °C in yeast and mold (YM) medium containing 1.0% glucose, 0.5% peptone, and 1.0% yeast extract is more sensitive to alkali than the complex from other Mucoraceae. As a consequence, the chitosan can be isolated by boiling the biomass in 25% NaOH for 3 h, washing to neutrality, and freeze-drying. Typically, the chitosan is highly filmogenic and has a degree of acetylation of 0.05, free amine 0.86, pKa 6.2 ± 0.3, and average MW of 5×10^5 Da. It is poorly susceptible to the hydrolytic action of papain, lipase, and lysozyme due to the small degree of acetylation.

The *A. coerulea* material was poorly crystalline, showing a broad peak at 20° 2θ, but the spectrum for the alkali-treated material showed a broad peak at 10.72° and two peaks at 18.72° and 19.98° 2θ, with close similarity to the spectrum of authentic chitosan. Optical microscopy showed that the alkali-treated products, stained with Saphranine or with other stains, preserved the morphology of the fungus, with flattened and empty structures [30] (Fig. 1). This work introduced the concept that an extended surface area of the carbohydrate polymer leads to enhanced performance, as amply confirmed by most recent works dealing with chitin and chitosan nanofibrils. In fact, the partially re-acetylated chitosan (degree of acetylation 0.23) is promptly depolymerized by lysozyme, papain, and lipase thanks to the ideal degree of acetylation for maximum enzymatic activity. Remarkably, the re-acetylated

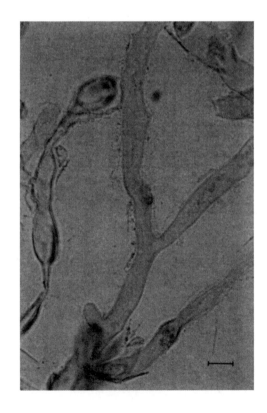

Fig. 1 *Absidia* chitosan after isolation in NaOH (250 g/kg), as observed at the optical microscope after staining with saphranine (*scale bar*: 10 μm). When re-acetylated to a degree of acetylation of 0.23, this chitosan, besides being soluble in the usual pH range for chitosans, is exceptionally soluble at pH values over 9. This work introduced the concept that an extended surface area of the carbohydrate polymer leads to enhanced performance. Reprinted from *Carbohydrate Polymers* 25 [29]. Copyright (1994) with permission from Elsevier

chitosan, besides being soluble in the usual pH range for chitosans, is exceptionally soluble at pH values over pH 9, a characteristic that should be taken into account instead of complaining that high MW chitosans have limited solubility.

High performance liquid chromatography (HPLC) data showed that the reacetylated chitosan was polydisperse, with fractions in the MW range $2 \times 10^5 – 1 \times 10^6$ Da (average 5×10^5 Da); after 10 min contact with papain, the average value was 43,000, and after 100 h was 600 Da. The HPLC and electrophoretic results showed that the *Absidia* chitosans were polydisperse due to the alkali treatment and, compared to the low MW chitosan from Fluka, contained a higher proportion of high MW fractions. Therefore, the alkaline extraction led to the same average MW of 5×10^5 Da, already reported by other authors for the acetic acid extraction.

The *Absidia* chitosans tested according to standard methods ASTM F813-83 and F619-79 with murine fibroblasts were found to be biocompatible in terms of cytotoxicity and lactate dehydrogenase activity, in agreement with Chung et al. [31]. By contrast, for solid-state fermentation, the chitosan production was higher (6.12 g/kg) but the MW was only 6.4 kDa [32].

3 Chitin and Chitosan Nanofibrils

Many significant scientific and technological advances have recently been made in the area of the isolation of nanofibrils (otherwise called chitin nanocrystals, or whiskers). In particular, articles have been published dealing with the following advances: (1) nanochitin isolated after hydrolysis with HCl; (2) nanochitin isolated mechanically in the presence of minor amounts of acetic acid; (3) nanochitosan obtained from partially deacetylated chitin; and (4) defibrillation of chitosan. These advances are of such importance that they overshadow the technology developed during the previous years, for reasons that will be apparent below [33].

3.1 Mechanically Isolated Nanofibrils in the Presence of Acetic Acid

α-Nanochitin has been isolated in the presence of acetic acid (pH 3) by the following process: the suspension was first blended, and then the slurry of 1% purified chitin was passed through a grinder at 1,500 rpm, with a clearance gauge of 0.15 mm shift, which was determined as the point of slight contact between the grinding stones. In principle, there is no direct contact between grinding stones thanks to the suspended chitin particles [34].

In a further work, the same team developed the concept that in order to fibrillate the chitin, it would be advantageous to enhance the cationic repulsion existing between chitin fibers with the aid of acetic acid at pH 3. In fact, Ifuku et al. [35]

showed that a protonation degree as small as 4% or less is sufficient to weaken the hydrogen bonds that protect chitin from fibrillation. One should keep in mind that all chitins are deacetylated to a minor extent in those positions where proteins were linked *ab origine*, and that this partial deacetylation (maximum 0.10) is large enough to protonate the fibers. Various industrial chitins, even in the alpha polymorphic form, under these conditions, lend themselves to the isolation of nanofibrils having a high degree of crystallinity and with 10–20 nm cross-section.

A very important extension of the work was the treatment of industrial chitin dry powders instead of "never dried" chitins. Thus, an important limitation that had prevented the large scale production of nanochitin in the past was overcome. By so doing, the strong acid treatment was abandoned, and the risks inherent to its use were avoided. This method provided a significant advantage for industrial application in terms of transportation costs, stable supply, shelf life, and storage space, since chitin nanofibers can be prepared from light, low volume, and non-perishable dry chitin. Chitin nanofibers from commercial pre-purified dry chitin are advantageous for laboratory-scale investigations because a large amount of chitin can be immediately and easily obtained by a simple fibrillation process without the purification processes that generally require 5 days for "never dried" chitin, namely removal of proteins, minerals, lipids, and pigments [36]. SEM images show that, in the absence of acetic acid, bundles of fibers are obtained. With acetic acid, nanofibrils are formed with a large area-to-volume ratio, which is of outstanding importance for adsorption of a wide range of drugs and other compounds. Finally, the Ifuku method does not require sonication, in contrast to the method of Fan et al. [37]. According to the latter, the two key factors for the preparation of the chitin nanofibers with a high aspect ratio (3–4 nm in cross-sectional width and at least a few microns in length) are as follows: (1) squid pen β-chitin is used as the starting material, and (2) ultrasonication of the β-chitin in water at pH 3–4 and 0.1–0.3% for a few minutes. No N-deacetylation occurs on the chitin during the nanofiber conversion, and the original crystal structure of β-chitin is maintained, although the crystallinity index decreases from 0.51 to 0.37. Cationization of the amino groups present on the crystallite surfaces of the squid pen β-chitin under acidic conditions is necessary for the preparation of the nanofibers.

The mechanical disintegration can be described as follows: the wet chitins are suspended in water at 0.1–0.3%. Several drops of acetic acid, a dilute hydrochloric acid solution, or a dilute NaOH solution are added to the chitin slurries to adjust their pH values from 3 to 8. Ultrasonication is applied to the slurries (15 mL each) for 2 min using an ultrasonic homogenizer at 19.5 kHz and 300 W output power (7 mm probe tip diameter). The temperature increase is kept below 5 °C during the ultrasonication [37].

The drawbacks of the previous preparation methods included low yield (ca. 50%), dangers from the use of boiling HCl, disposal of the black used HCl, disposal of enormous quantities of slightly acidic water, presence of HCl in the final product even after one week of dialysis or ultrafiltration, optional sonication, difficult adjustment of the pH value because of the strength of the HCl present, overall scaling-up difficulties, and excessive costs. All of these disadvantages were removed by the new technology.

Even though certain authors including Watthanaphanit et al. [38] used ultracentrifuges at 10,000 rpm for performing laboratory-scale preparations, the industrial centrifuges do not offer such performances and are precluded for HCl solutions. Nevertheless, Tzumaki et al. [39] used common laboratory centrifuges (3,400 rpm, 15 min) but had to sonicate for a long time (45 min) with the risk of overheating. Chang et al. [40] used both ultracentrifuge and ultrasonicator.

3.2 Mechanically Defibrillated Nanochitosans

Wet-grinding and high-pressure homogenization were combined by Liu et al. [41] to defibrillate chitosan particles into nanochitosan, which was made into a high strength liquid crystal film by self-organization at relatively low temperature. Raw chitosan powder was suspended in water to obtain a 0.1% slurry that was poured into a wet-grinding machine with a milling gap of about 0.2 mm. The chitosan slurry was forced to pass through the gap with a flow speed of 10 L/h and was then poured into the stainless-steel holding tank of a Microfluidizer (M-100P, Microfluidics, MA, USA) equipped with a pair of ceramic (200 μm) and diamond (87 μm) interaction chambers (Fig. 2). The slurry was cooled by passing through a stainless coil submerged in an ice bath, and then released back to the tank for the next cycle. Under the pressure of 207 MPa, the ground slurry passed through the interaction chambers at the rate of 133 mL/min for ten passes. The obtained homogenized chitosan slurry was subsequently centrifuged at 1,000 rpm for 5 min in a Sorvall RC-5B refrigerated centrifuge to remove the sediment and produce a homogeneous chitosan suspension. The latter was used to prepare a liquid crystal thin film 0.5 mm thick, at 10 °C.

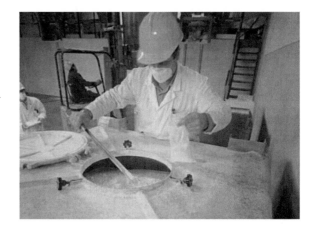

Fig. 2 Slurry in the stainless-steel holding tank of the Microfluidizer after continuous high shear fluid processing of chitosan powder for mechanical disassembly into nanofibrils. Scaleable results are produced for pilot and production purposes

The combination of wet-grinding and high-pressure homogenization resulted in the chitosan powder being defibrillated into small bundles of nanofibrils, which were uniform nanofibers with an average diameter of 50 nm and a length over 1 μm. These disassembled nanofibrils had a smaller diameter than the electrospun chitosan nanofibers, which usually have diameters in the order of several hundred micrometers. The large fibers were split apart side-by-side by the mechanical forces. The nanofibers, with various widths, consisted of bundles of parallel fibrils of only 1–5 nm diameter. When viewed between cross-polarizers, the chitosan liquid crystal film showed ordered patterns with colors of sepia and blue. The texture was composed of curled arcs, somewhat like the cholesteric arrangements of chitin, collagen, or cellulose nanofibers discovered in biological tissues. There was no pattern or fingerprint found in the control cast films, meaning that chitosan nanofibrils self-assembled into morphogenesis with cholesteric structure.

The chitosan cast film possessed high tensile strength (about 35.8 ± 7.6 MPa) and Young's modulus (about 580.0 ± 21.8 MPa). However, the chitosan liquid crystal film had a higher mechanical strength and Young's modulus, up to 100.5 ± 4.0 MPa and 2.2 ± 0.2 GPa, respectively, which are characteristic values for liquid crystalline polymers [42].

3.3 Nanochitosan Obtained from Partially Deacetylated Chitin or from Deacetylated Nanochitin

Watthanaphanit et al. [38] prepared nanochitosan by deacetylation with 50% NaOH and borohydride. As a consequence, the MW dropped to 59 kDa, much lower than that of chitosan from chitin powder under the same conditions (420 kDa). The degree of deacetylation was 0.50 and the suspensions were colloidal at 1–13%. Phongying et al. [43] completely destroyed their nanochitosan during their first attempt at deacetylating nanochitin. The new methods, however, opened new routes to a nanofibrillar product endowed with higher cationicity, i.e., chitosan, which is a more versatile polysaccharide than chitin. At the same time, Fan et al. [44] deacetylated the fine chitin powder in a relatively mild way, thus producing nanochitosan that underwent homogeneous dispersion at pH 3–4, with birefringence and high viscosity, whilst at pH 6–7 the dispersion was not homogeneous due to inadequate protonation.

The advantageous and characteristic features of the newly developed α-chitin nanofibrils include the following:

1. Commercially available pure α-chitins (originating from crab and shrimp shell) can be used as starting material.
2. Nanofibrils are obtained in high yields (85–90%).
3. The α-chitin nanofibril dispersions have high UV–vis transmittance, and hence high transparency, indicating that individualization of α-chitin fibrils can be achieved.

4. The rod-like morphology of the nanofibrils supports the high yields, because α-chitin nanofibrils prepared by acid hydrolysis from TEMPO-mediated oxidation have a spindle-like shape and a larger distribution range of widths.
5. The α-chitin nanofibrils have lesser safety issues than chemically modified materials such as TEMPO-oxidized α-chitins. As a consequence, potential applications can be expanded to functional foods, life sciences, and medical fields.

The α-chitin nanofibrils had an average width and length of 6.2 ± 1.1 and 250 ± 140 nm, respectively (ratio ca. 40). Because conversion to nanofibrils was achieved in water at pH 3–4, the protonation of the amino groups on the crystalline fibril surface, which means reciprocal repulsion, allows the individualization of α-chitin fibrils to be maintained for lasting periods [44].

Hariraksapitak and Supaphol [45] prepared functional bone scaffolds capable of enhanced physical, mechanical, and biological performances. The materials used to fabricate the porous scaffolds were hyaluronan and gelatin (1:1 w/w blend), and the reinforcing filler was nanochitin obtained from acid-hydrolyzed α-chitin. 1-Ethyl-3-(3-dimethylaminopropyl) carbodiimide was used as a crosslinker. The weight ratios of the nanochitin to the blend were up to 30%, the average pore size of the scaffolds ranged between 139 and 166 μm, regardless of the nanochitin content, but the incorporation of 2% nanochitin in the scaffolds doubled their tensile strength. According to TEM results, the as-prepared nanochitin was in the form of slender rods with sharp ends. The length and width of these rods were 255 ± 56 and 31 ± 6 nm, respectively, with a length:width aspect ratio of about 8. Although the addition of 20–30% nanochitin improved thermal stability and resistance to biodegradation, the scaffolds with 10% were the best for supporting the proliferation of cultured human osteosarcoma cells. The size of the pores for all of the scaffolds in both the transverse and the longitudinal sections ranged between 92 and 230 μm, with an average value between 139 and 166 μm. Variations in the content of nanochitin had no significant effect on the pore dimensions. It was concluded that a lower composition percentage of hyaluronan within the scaffolds would possibly establish a more favorable environment for cell growth.

Several applications were developed: melatonin was adsorbed on the nanofibrils by Hafner et al. [46] and Yerlikaya et al. [47]. Lipoic acid was likewise treated by Kofuji et al. [48]. More extended studies were made by Muzzarelli et al. [49] who incorporated chitin nanofibrils into wound dressings made of chitosan glycolate and dibutyryl chitin, and by other authors who prepared similar composites. Glycerol-plasticized potato starch was mixed with chitin nanofibrils to prepare fully natural nanocomposites by casting and evaporation. This led to improvements in tensile strength, storage modulus, glass transition temperature, and water vapor barrier properties of the composite. However, at >5 wt% loading, aggregation of the nanofibrils took place with negative effects [40]. On the other hand, Azeredo et al. [50] evaluated the effect of different concentrations of cellulose nanofibers and plasticizer (glycerol) on tensile properties, water vapor permeability, and glass transition temperature of chitosan edible films, and established a formulation to optimize their properties. The nanocomposite film with 15% cellulose nanofibers and 18%

glycerol was comparable to some synthetic polymers in terms of strength and stiffness. The incorporation of chitosan whiskers in alginate fibers was achieved by Watthanaphanit et al. [38], by mixing homogenized chitosan whisker colloidal suspension with 6% w/v sodium alginate aqueous solution, followed by wet spinning. The chitosan whiskers (length and width 309 and 64 nm, respectively, average aspect ratio ca. 4.8) were prepared by deacetylation of chitin whiskers obtained by acid hydrolysis of shrimp chitin. The noticeable improvement in the tensile strength of the nanocomposite yarns took place at the expense of the elongation at break. The chitosan whiskers imparted antibacterial activity against *Staphylococcus aureus* and *Escherichia coli* to the nanocomposite yarns.

Chitin nanofibrils were acetylated to modify the fiber surface; the acetylation degree could be controlled from 0.99 to 2.96 by changing the reaction time. In only 1 min of acetylation, the moisture content of the nanocomposite decreased from 4.0 to 2.2%. The nanofibril shape was maintained and the thickness of the nanofibrils increased linearly with the content of the bulky acetyl groups. Composites containing the acetylated chitin nanofibrils (25 wt%) were fabricated with acrylic resin [36].

Nanofibers based on poly(vinyl alcohol) as the matrix, and nanocrystals of α-chitin (ca. 31 nm in width and ca. 549 nm in length) as the nanofiller were prepared by Junkasem et al. [51]. The average diameters of the electrospun fibers ranged between 175 and 218 nm. The addition of increasing amounts of the whiskers caused the crystallinity of poly(vinyl alcohol) within the nanocomposite materials to decrease and the glass transition temperature to increase.

4 Electrospun Nanofibers

Electrospinning is a recent technique that is useful for production of chitin and chitosan nanofibers of indefinite length and some hundred nanometers in cross-section. At the present time, the manufacture of the nanofibers is laborious and time-consuming, and also presents safety issues. While the reader is referred to review articles on this matter [52], it should be said generally, that the manufacture of a ~300-μm thick, 30 × 15 cm mat from a solution of plain chitosan in methylene chloride plus trifluoroacetic acid requires ~4 h, compared to ~12 h for mats of the same size and ~20 μm thick by conventional electrospinning of chitosan/poly(ethylene oxide) in dilute acetic acid solution. This technique based on trifluoroacetic acid as an electrospinning solvent for chitosan yields a relatively high throughput. It relies on empirical knowledge, because varying the viscosity, temperature, electrical potential, geometry of the collector, and other parameters can cause the nanofibers to assume irregular forms (lack of uniformity, presence of beaded fibers) that prevent use. Several remedies such as neutralization with alkaline compounds or chemical crosslinking with glutaraldehyde have been tried with a view to stabilizing the chitosan nanofibers, but their neutralization in aqueous media results in undesirable contraction leading to partial or complete loss of their nanofeatures. It should also be kept in mind that the above-mentioned solvents are toxic, and therefore nanofiber manufacture at the present time is both slow and dangerous.

Scaling-up of chitosan nanofiber fabrication by electrospinning is problematic and challenging [53]. First of all, solutions with a high concentration of chitosan are not injectable, whereas those with a very low concentration result in a low output rate. On the other hand, the large quantity of organic solvents used during the electrospinning process alters or denatures the structure and properties of the natural chitosan. Furthermore, due to its polyelectrolyte nature, chitosan cannot be continuously spun because droplets persistently form. It is well known that the pore size and structure of a scaffold play vital roles in cell cultures because they are responsible not only for the adhesion, migration, and distribution of cells, but also for the exchange of nutrients and metabolic waste. Despite numerous efforts, issues relating to mechanical strength, uniformity, interconnections, and porosity of nanofiber mats have not yet been fully resolved.

A body of knowledge on the thermally driven formation of amide bonds between chitosans and the organic acids that dissolve them has been available since the late 1990s. In particular, Yao et al. [54] presented a protocol based on the use of lactic acid for the preparation of lactamidated chitosan in the form of films that, after purification with methanol and chloroform, were tested for biocompatibility toward fibroblasts. This matter was amply studied by Toffey et al. [55] with acetic acid and propionic acid, in the frame of projects concerning the regeneration of chitin from chitosan via amide bond formation, as well as by Qu et al. [56] who also used lactic acid. The topic has been discussed in review articles such as those by Kumar et al. [57] and Muzzarelli and Muzzarelli [33].

Therefore, one way to stabilize the nanofibers made of chitosan lactate salt is the thermal treatment that induces amide group formation and thus imparts water-insolubility to the product. In fact, chitosan lactate solutions of 3–6 wt% in methylene chloride and trifluoroacetic acid yielded stable, bead-free nanofibers with mean diameters of 50–350 nm [58]. A solution with 4.5 wt% chitosan lactate salt in methylene chloride plus trifluoroacetic acid resulted in the highest electrospinning rate. The residual solvent was removed from the as-spun nanofibers by incubation at 70 °C for 12 h. The conversion of the ionic bond between amino groups of chitosan and lactate groups to a covalent amide bond was accomplished by heating under vacuum at 100 °C for 3 h, which transformed some of the water-soluble chitosan lactate to water-insoluble chitosan lactamide. The amidation was confirmed by the absorption band at 1,790 cm^{-1} in the Fourier transform infrared spectra. The substitution degree was 0.165 ± 0.065, resulting in approximately 7.9 ± 3.1 wt% lactic acid in the form of amide in the nanofibers. It is possible that part of this lactic acid is in the form of a polylactide, but in any case this is an initial step towards the preservation of nanofibrous shape in physiological media [58].

An alternative to the experiments just described is the esterification of chitosan with the use of lactide or polylactide; for example, Skotak et al. [59] prepared chitosan derivatives following a "one pot" approach by grafting L-lactide oligomers via ring-opening polymerization. Chitosan (600 mg) was dissolved in 10 mL of methanesulfonic acid, followed by the addition of 3.05 g of the L-lactide monomer. This reaction mixture was stirred for 4 h at 40 °C under an argon atmosphere and then transferred to 100 mL of 0.2 M KH_2PO_4, 16 mL of 10 M NaOH, and comminuted ice. The side chain length had average values between 4.6 and 14 units. On average, there are two side chains of oligo-L-lactide per glucosamine ring, and their length depends on the initial reagents ratio. If this ratio increases, additional oligo-L-lactide grafts might be attached to hydroxyl groups located on carbons 1 or 4, generated in situ during degradation of chitosan when water content increases as a by-product of the main esterification reaction. Indeed, L-lactide-grafted chitosan samples display cytotoxicity over a range of substitution degree values, as demonstrated by fibroblast culture tests. These materials might be interesting for controlled release and drug delivery, where hydrolysis rate control is of key importance. This synthetic route renders the esterified chitosans soluble in a broad range of organic solvents, facilitating formation of ultrafine fibers via electrospinning [59].

Electrospinning was applied to fabricate biocompatible membranes made of poly(L-lactic acid) and chitosan. Thanks to their high porosity and interconnected structure, the electrospun mats were suitable scaffolds for cell or tissue growth. Injection rate, polymer concentration and applied voltage were varied to investigate their effects on electrospun fibers. The SEM microphotography indicated that the structures, including bead, bead-in-string and nanofibers with different diameters, would be controlled by adjusting the above variables. The diameter of strings was about 50 nm and the diameter of beads was 0.4–2 μm, depending on preparation conditions. There was a critical range in the above parameters for the formation of homogeneous nanofibers. Outside the critical range, the bead-on-a-string structures became significant instead of nanofibers. When the osteoblastic cells were cultured with nanofibrous membranes, the cell density was higher and the secretion of fibril was more significant compared with the cells cultured on dense films. The results indicated that the biocompatibility of poly(L-lactic acid) and chitosan would be improved by changing their topography from smooth surface into nanoscaled structures [60].

Chitosan-based, defect-free nanofibers with average diameters ranging from 62 ± 9 nm to 129 ± 16 nm were fabricated via electrospinning of blended solutions of chitosan and poly(ethylene oxide). Generally, SEM imaging demonstrated that, as total concentration of both polymers increased, the number of beads decreased, and as chitosan concentration increased, fiber diameter decreased. Chitosan/poly(ethylene oxide) solutions undergo phase separation over time. As a result, blended solutions could be electrospun with no trouble within 24 h of blending. The addition of NaCl stabilized these solutions for a longer time before and during electrospinning. Pure chitosan nanofibers with high degrees of deacetylation (about 80%) could not be produced: when attempting to electrospin chitosan from aqueous acetic acid at concentrations above the entanglement concentration. The electric field was insufficient to overcome the combined effect of the surface tension and viscosity of the solution. Therefore, the degree of deacetylation is a very important parameter that should be taken into account [53].

Chitosan, sodium chondroitin sulfate, and pectin-nanofibrous mats were prepared from the respective polysaccharide/poly(ethylene oxide) blend solutions by electrospray. Unblended polysaccharide solutions showed low processability, i.e., the solutions could not be electrosprayed. The addition of 500 kDa poly(ethylene oxide) to chitosan solutions enhanced the formation of a fibrous structure. Sodium chondroitin sulfate/poly(ethylene oxide) and pectin/poly(ethylene oxide) blend solutions were generally too viscous to be sprayed at 25 °C, but at 70 °C the fibrous structure was formed [61].

5 Supercritical Drying

A number of interesting properties are associated with the critical state. One of these is that the density of the liquid and of the vapor becomes identical, and for this reason the interface between the two phases disappears. Supercritical fluid technology is a relatively new approach to obtain micro- and nanoparticles. For pharmaceutical applications, supercritical carbon dioxide (sc-CO_2) is most widely used because of its low and easily accessible critical temperature and pressure (31.2 °C; 7.4 MPa), non-flammability, nontoxicity and inexpensiveness. Many drugs can be dissolved or liquefied in sc-CO_2 before being sprayed through a nozzle upon depressurization to produce fine drug particles. This can be achieved with solvent techniques such as the rapid expansion of supercritical solutions (RESS) and particles from gas-saturated solutions (PGSS). High supersaturation of drug in sc-CO_2, which contributes to the particle size reduction, is obtained by the RESS process. Alternatively, sc-CO_2 can be used as an antisolvent for the precipitation of drugs already dissolved in organic solvents [62].

Drying techniques have been explored for pharmaceutical biopolymer formulations: drying with the aid of a supercritical fluid is especially attractive for reasons of mild process conditions, cost-effectiveness, possible sterilizing properties of supercritical carbon dioxide, capability of producing microparticulate protein powders, and feasibility of scaling up.

Two concepts of using sc-fluid for the drying of proteins have been described in the literature. In the most important, the sc-fluid is used as an antisolvent for the protein, and as a means of water extraction. Three stages in the process can be distinguished: (1) the protein solution is concentrated due to the extraction of water by the sc-fluid; (2) the protein and other constituents are precipitated as a result of the increasing concentration in the solution; and (3) the particles formed are dried by extraction of the remaining solvent by the sc-fluid.

In the second concept, the SCF is dissolved at high pressure in the solution containing the protein and excipients and is sprayed to atmospheric conditions. The sc-fluid is used as propellant and/or effervescent agent during a low-temperature spray-drying process, enhancing the atomization process and thereby shortening the drying process. The sc-fluid drying processes for preparing protein- or polysaccharide-containing powders based on these concepts are described in more detail by Jovanovic et al. [63].

The formation of hydrophobic chitosan–silica hydrogels was accomplished in two ways by Ayers et al. [64]. Dried aerogels were exposed to hexamethyldisilazane vapors at 60 °C, or alternatively by soaking in the same compound diluted into ethanol. After supercritical drying, uncracked monoliths with very little shrinkage were obtained. When exposed to water, the aerogels adsorbed a small amount of liquid at their outer surface, but maintained their shape. The Brunauer–Emmett–Teller (BET) surface area of these aerogels was very large, in the range of 472–750 m^2/g, depending on the ratio of chitosan to silica [64].

Chitosan solution was prepared by dissolving chitosan (ranging between 5 and 50%, w/w) in 1% acetic acid solution; the solution was stirred at 100 rpm and heated at 50 °C until homogeneous. Then, the solution was poured into steel containers with an internal diameter of 2 cm and height of 1 cm and frozen at −20 °C for 5–24 h to obtain a hydrogel that was treated in four different ways:

1. Dried with air in a laboratory oven at 40 °C for 10 h
2. Put in a bath of acetone at ambient temperature for 24 h to allow the substitution of water with acetone and then dried with air in a laboratory oven at 40 °C for 8 h
3. Put in a bath of acetone at ambient temperature for 24 h and then dried by sc-CO$_2$
4. Put in a bath of acetone at −20 °C for 24 h and then dried by sc-CO$_2$

The sc-CO$_2$ drying procedure was as follows: Steel containers were loaded onto a metallic support that was put into the high-pressure vessel, which was then closed and filled from the bottom with sc-CO$_2$. When the required pressure and temperature were obtained (200 bar and 35 °C), drying was performed for 4 h with an sc-CO$_2$ flow rate of about 1 kg/h, which corresponded to a residence time inside the vessel of about 4 min. The depressurization time of 20 min was allocated to bring the system back to atmospheric pressure [65].

When preference was given to low temperature water substitution followed by supercritical gel drying to prevent the collapse of the chitosan gel (procedure 4), water substitution with acetone was performed at the same temperature as the gel formation (−20 °C, for 24 h). Subsequently, sc-CO$_2$ gel drying was performed at the same processing conditions. In this case, the 3D shape and the size of samples were preserved. Indeed, the SEM image reported in Fig. 3 shows the presence of a uniform nanonetwork with measured porosity higher than 91%; the mean diameter of the fibers was about 50 nm.

The obtained structures present a morphology very similar to the extracellular matrix, i.e., a finely interconnected nanoscale substructure, and could be suitable for scaffolding applications in tissue engineering. In fact, this kind of nanometric fibrous network is the ideal environment for cell adhesion and growth for various tissue engineering applications (bones, cartilages, blood vessels, skin, etc.) [65].

Materials of this kind are known as scaffolds, i.e., supports, either natural or artificial, that maintain tissue contour. Scaffolds must meet certain fundamental characteristics, such as high porosity, appropriate pore size, biocompatibility, biodegradability, and proper degradation rate. For example, a 1% chitosan solution

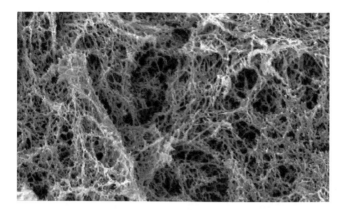

Fig. 3 SEM image of the chitosan structure obtained by low temperature water substitution followed by supercritical CO_2 hydrogel drying. Reprinted from *Journal of Supercritical Fluids* 54 [65]. Copyright (2010) with permission from Elsevier

was added slowly to aqueous formaldehyde and stirred until the chitosan solution turned into a more viscous hydrogel that was then subjected to solvent exchange into acetone. The chitosan–formaldehyde hydrogels were placed inside a sealed chamber of the sc-fluid reactor. Temperature and pressure were raised to 40 °C and 200 bar, respectively. The reaction was left for 2 h and a flow of CO_2 was then applied through the sample in order to replace all the organic solvent with CO_2. The pressure was then released slowly to the atmospheric value and the temperature was reduced to 20 °C [66].

In another more elaborated preparation, a 1% solution of chitosan was mixed with the crosslinker genipin solution (4% w/v) and stirring continued until the solution turned into viscous gel [2]. Then, the hydrogel was subjected to solvent exchange into acetone three times to remove water from the structure. After solvent exchange, the chitosan–genipin derivative was placed inside a sealed chamber of the sc-CO_2 extractor at 40 °C and 200 bar. The reaction was left for 2 h and a flow of CO_2 was then applied through the sample in order to replace all the organic solvent with CO_2. The pressure was then released slowly to the atmosphere and the temperature reduced to 20 °C. The chitosan derivative had a BET surface area of 49 m^2/g, with a monolayer volume of 11 cm^3/g. The porosimetry result showed that genipin-crosslinked chitosan scaffold had adequate surface area to provide cell adhesion and proliferation.

Cell attachment, proliferation, and differentiation over time on a material are indications of the cellular compatibility of the material and determine the suitability of the material for tissue engineering applications. Osteoblast proliferation on chitosan–genipin scaffolds was assessed using Almar Blue assay and found to be satisfactory considering that the number of cells attached to the genipin-crosslinked chitosan scaffolds after 1, 3, and 7 days of cell culture increased with time [67].

For the preparation of chitosan scaffolds loaded with dexamethasone, sc-fluid impregnation was carried out in the batch mode because preliminary experiments showed that this procedure gives more extended impregnation than the continuous process. The equipment consists basically in a high pressure reactor heated by means of a heating tape that maintains the temperature within ±1 °C. Carbon dioxide is liquefied through a cooling unit and compressed to the operating pressure. The fluid is preheated to the desired temperature in a heat exchanger before entering the high pressure vessel. The previously processed scaffold and the drug are loaded together but not in reciprocal contact, in the same vessel. The resulting dexamethasone-loaded chitosan scaffold was found suitable for sustained release of the drug in bone tissue engineering [68].

The surface area of chitin can be expanded to large values. Rapid expansion techniques with sc-CO_2 were used by Salinas-Hernandez et al. [69] to form chitin microstructures. Depending on the experimental conditions, they found that spherical microparticles with average diameters of 1.7–5.3 µm are obtained with expansion of supercritical solutions, whereas continuous microfibers with average diameters of 11.5–19.3 µm are obtained with expansion in a liquid solvent. Lower concentrations and smaller diameter nozzles favored the production of smaller diameter microstructures and narrow size distributions.

6 Conclusion

Controlled increase in the surface area of isolated chitins and chitosans certainly results in more convenient chemical and biochemical reactivity. Likewise, controlled porosity is a means for optimizing the growth of human or animal cells within scaffolds. The mechanical disassembly of animal chitins under controlled conditions represents an important step forward in the exploitation of nanochitins and nanochitosans. Along with supercritical carbon dioxide drying, mechanical disassembly exhibits practical advantages over electrospinning.

Acknowledgments The author is grateful to Marilena Falcone, Central Library, University, Ancona, Italy, for assistance in handling the bibliographic information, and to Maria Weckx for preparation of the manuscript.

References

1. Du JA, Yarema KJ (2010) Adv Drug Deliv Rev 62:671
2. Muzzarelli RAA (2009) Carbohydr Polym 76:167
3. Muzzarelli RAA (2011) Carbohydr Polym 83:1433
4. Muzzarelli RAA (1997) Cell Mol Life Sci 53:131
5. Muzzarelli RAA (2009) Carbohydr Polym 77:1
6. Baldrick P (2010) Reg Toxicol Pharmacol 56:290
7. Klokkevold PR, Fukayama H, Sung EC, Bertolami CN (1999) J Oral Maxillofac Surg 57:49

8. Scherer SS, Pietramaggiori G, Matthews J, Perry S, Assmann A, Carothers A, Demcheva M, Muise-Helmericks RC, Seth A, Vournakis JN, Valeri RC, Fischer TH, Hechtman HB, Orgill DP (2009) Ann Surg 250:322
9. Ivshina TN, Artamonova SD, Ivshin VP, Sharnina FF (2009) Appl Biochem Microbiol 45:313
10. Crestini C, Giovannozzi-Sermanni G (1996) In: Muzzarelli RAA (ed) Chitin enzymology, vol 2. Atec, Italy, p 595
11. Vetter J (2007) Food Chem 102:6
12. Chatterjee S, Adhya M, Guha AK, Chatterjee BP (2005) Process Biochem 40:395
13. Feofilova EP (2010) Microbiology 79:711
14. Muzzarelli RAA, Tanfani F, Emanuelli M (1981) J Appl Biochem 3:322
15. Smith JS, Berry DR (1977) The filamentous fungi, vols 1–3. Edward Arnold, London
16. Bento RA, Stamford TLM, Stamford TCM, de Andrade SAC, de Souza EL (2011) LWT-Food Science and Technology 44:588
17. Kuhlmann K, Czupala A, Haunhorst J, Weiss A, Prasch T, Schorken U (2000) Preparation and characterization of chitosan from Mucorales. In: Peter M, Domard A, Muzzarelli RAA (eds) Advances in Chitin Science, Druckhaus Schmergow Germany, pp 7–14
18. Rungsardthong V, Wonputtanakul N, Kongpien N, Chotiwaranon P (2006) Process Biochem 41:589
19. Niederhofer A, Muller BW (2004) Eur J Pharm Biopharm 57:101
20. Wu T, Zivanovic S, Draughon FA, Conway WS, Sams CE (2005) J Agric Food Chem 53:3888
21. Chatterjee S, Chatterjee S, Chatterjee BP, Guha AK (2009) Microbiol Res 164:347
22. Muzzarelli RAA, Tanfani F, Scarpini GF (1980) Biotechnol Bioeng 22:885
23. Vincendon M, Desbrieres J (2002) In: Muzzarelli RAA, Muzzarelli C (eds) Chitosan in pharmacy and chemistry. Atec, Italy, pp 511–518
24. Zamani A, Edebo L, Niklasson C, Taherzadeh MJ (2010) Int J Mol Sci 11:2976
25. Nwe N, Stevens WF, Tokura S, Tamura H (2008) Enzyme Microb Technol 42:242
26. Nwe N, Furuike T, Tamura H (2010) Chitin and chitosan from terrestrial organisms. In: Kim SK (ed) Chitin, chitosan, oligosaccharides and their derivatives: biological activities and applications. CRC, Boca Raton, pp 3–10
27. Berecochea-Lopez A, Decorde K, Ventura E, Godard M, Bornet A, Teissedre PL, Cristol JP, Rouanet JM (2009) J Agric Food Chem 57:1093
28. Neyrinck AM, Bindels LB, De Backer F, Pachikian BD, Cani PD, Delzenne NM (2009) Int Immunopharmacol 9:767
29. Muzzarelli RAA, Ilari P, Tarsi R, Dubini B, Xia W (1994) Chitosan from *Absidia coerulea*. Pp. 45–50
30. Muzzarelli RAA, Mattioli-Belmonte M, Pugnaloni A, Biagini G (1999) EXS 87:251
31. Chung LY, Schmidt RJ, Hamlyn PF, Sagar BF (1994) J Biomed Mater Res 28:463
32. Wang WP, Du YM, Qiu YL, Wang XY, Hu Y, Yang JH, Cai J, Kennedy JF (2008) Carbohydr Polym 74:127
33. Muzzarelli RAA, Muzzarelli C (2005) In: Dutta PK (ed) Chitin and chitosan: opportunities and challenges. SSM International, Contai, India, pp 129–146
34. Ifuku S, Nogi M, Abe K, Yoshioka M, Morimoto M, Saimoto H, Yano H (2009) Biomacromolecules 10:1584
35. Ifuku S, Nogi M, Yoshioka M, Morimoto M, Yano H, Saimoto H (2010) Carbohydr Polym 81:134
36. Ifuku S, Morooka S, Morimoto M, Saimoto H (2010) Biomacromolecules 11:1326
37. Fan YM, Saito T, Isogai A (2008) Biomacromolecules 9:1919
38. Watthanaphanit A, Supaphol P, Tamura H, Tokura S, Rujiravanit R (2010) Carbohydr Polym 79:738
39. Tzoumaki MV, Moschakis T, Biliaderis CG (2010) Biomacromolecules 11:175
40. Chang PR, Jian RJ, Yu JG, Ma XF (2010) Carbohydr Polym 80:420
41. Liu DG, Wu QL, Chang PR, Gao GZ (2011) Carbohydr Polym 84:686
42. Liu DG, Chang PR, Chen MD, Wu QL (2010) J Colloid Interface Sci 354:637

43. Phongying S, Aiba S, Chirachanchai S (2007) Polymer 48:393
44. Fan YM, Saito T, Isogai A (2010) Carbohydr Polym 79:1046
45. Hariraksapitak P, Supaphol P (2010) J Appl Polym Sci 117:3406
46. Hafner A, Lovric J, Voinovich D, Filipovic-Grcic J (2009) Int J Pharm 381:205
47. Yerlikaya F, Aktas Y, Capan Y (2010) LC-UV determination of melatonin from chitosan nanoparticles. Chromatographia 71:967
48. Kofuji K, Nakamura M, Isobe T, Murata Y, Kawashima S (2008) Food Chem 109:167
49. Muzzarelli RAA, Morganti P, Morganti G, Palombo P, Palombo M, Biagini G, Mattioli-Belmonte M, Giantomassi F, Orlandi F, Muzzarelli C (2007) Carbohydr Polym 70:274
50. Azeredo HMC, Mattoso LHC, Avena-Bustillos RJ, Ceotto G, Munford ML, Wood D, McHugh TH (2010) J Food Sci 75:N1
51. Junkasem J, Rujiravanit R, Supaphol P (2006) Nanotechnology 17:519
52. Jayakumar R, Prabaharan M, Nair SV, Tamura H (2010) Biotechnol Adv 28:142
53. Klossner RR, Queen HA, Coughlin AJ, Krause WE (2008) Biomacromolecules 9:2947
54. Yao FL, Chen W, Wang H, Liu HF, Yao KD, Sun PC, Lin H (2003) Polymer 44:6435
55. Toffey A, Glasser WG (1999) J Appl Polym Sci 73:1879
56. Qu X, Wirsen A, Albertsson AC (1999) J Appl Polym Sci 74:3186
57. Kumar MNVR, Muzzarelli RAA, Muzzarelli C, Sashiwa H, Domb AJ (2004) Chem Rev 104:6017
58. Cooper A, Bhattarai N, Kievit FM, Rossol M, Zhang M (2011) Phys Chem Chem Phys 13: 9969–9972
59. Skotak M, Leonov AP, Larsen G, Noriega S, Subramanian A (2008) Biomacromolecules 9: 1902
60. Chen JW, Tseng KF, Delimartin S, Lee CK, Ho MH (2008) Desalination 233:48
61. Seo H, Matsumoto H, Hara S, Minagawa M, Tanioka A, Yako H, Yamagata Y, Inoue K (2005) Polym J 37:391
62. Moribe K, Tozuka Y, Yamamoto K (2008) Adv Drug Deliv Rev 60:328
63. Jovanovic N, Bouchard A, Hofland GW, Witkamp GJ, Crommelin DJA, Jiskoot W (2004) Pharm Res 21:1955
64. Ayers MR, Hunt AJ (2001) J Non-Cryst Solids 285:123
65. Cardea S, Pisanti P, Reverchon E (2010) Generation of chitosan nanoporous structures for tissue engineering applications using a supercritical fluid assisted process, Pp. 290–295
66. Rinki K, Dutta PK, Hunt AJ, Clark JH, Macquarrie DJ (2009) Macromol Symp 277:36
67. Rinki K, Dutta PK (2010) Int J Biol Macromol 46:261
68. Duarte ARC, Mano JF, Reis RL (2009) Eur Polym J 45:141
69. Salinas-Hernandez R, Ruiz-Trevino FA, Ortiz-Estrada CH, Luna-Barcenas G, Prokhorov Y, Alvarado JFJ, Sanchez IC (2009) Ind Eng Chem Res 48:769

Production, Properties and Applications of Fungal Cell Wall Polysaccharides: Chitosan and Glucan

Nitar Nwe, Tetsuya Furuike, and Hiroshi Tamura

Abstract Chitosan and β-glucan have attracted increased interest for use in many pharmaceutical applications, especially in tissue engineering, medicine, and immunology. Commercially, chitosans are produced from the shells of shrimps and crabs and the bone plates of squids. In fungal cell walls, chitosan occurs in two forms, as free chitosan and covalently bounded to β-glucan. Low cost products of these two polymers could be produced using industrial waste mycelia and mycelia obtained from cultivation of fungus in medium obtained from industrial by-products. The quantity and quality of chitosan extracted from fungal mycelia depends on fungal strain, type of fermentation, fermentation medium composition such as trace metal content and concentration of nutrients, pH of fermentation medium, harvesting time of fungal mycelia, and chitosan extraction procedure. The growth of fungi in solid state/substrate and submerged fermentation, synthesis of chitosan and glucan in fungal cell walls, production of valuable products from fungi, production of chitosan and glucan from fungal mycelia, and applications of chitosan and glucan are discussed in this chapter.

Keywords Chitosan · Fungi · Glucan · Production · Properties

Contents

1 Introduction 188
2 Life Cycle of Fungi 189
3 Growth of Fungi in Solid State/Substrate and Submerged Fermentation 190

N. Nwe (✉), T. Furuike, and H. Tamura (✉)
Faculty of Chemistry, Materials and Bioengineering, Kansai University, Suita, Osaka 564-8680, Japan
e-mail: nitarnwe@gmail.com, nitarnwe@yahoo.com; tamura@kansai-u.ac.jp

4	Chitosan Metabolism in Fungi	194
5	Chitosan and Glucan in Cell Walls of Fungi	195
6	Production, Properties and Applications of Chitosan from Fungal Biomass	199
7	Production, Properties and Applications of Glucan from Fungal Biomass	202
References		203

1 Introduction

Fungi are eukaryotic organisms. In 1969, Whittaker placed fungi in a separate kingdom named fungi [1]. The growth of fungus starts from spores of fungus like a plant. However, they have no system to synthesize glucose from carbon dioxide like plants have. Fungi absorb nutrients and use the absorbed carbon and nitrogen compound to synthesize their cellular components. Fungi grow in terrestrial and aquatic environments. Depending on their nature, fungi have been grown in synthesis medium using solid state/substrate fermentation (SSF) or submerged fermentation (SMF) for manufacture of food products, medicine, enzymes and organic acids since ancient times. Several tons of waste mycelia of fungi remain at the end of the fermentation processes. To solve the solid waste disposal problem, the use of waste mycelia for production of valuable products such as chitosan/chitin and glucan has been considered since the end of the nineteenth century [2, 3]. Fermentation plants should agree to release their waste mycelia for production of chitosan instead of burning the waste mycelia [3].

Chitosan is a principal component of cell walls of certain fungi such as *Gongronella* spp., *Absidia* spp., *Aspergillus* spp., *Rhizopus* spp. [4–7]. These fungi belong to the class of Zygomycetes [1]. Therefore, fungi in the class of Zygomycetes have been considered as an alternative source for the production of a more consistent quality of chitosan. Moreover, extraction of chitosan from fungal sources is considered to have a number of advantages over crustacean sources. These include: (1) a raw material that is constant in composition and is available throughout the year [7], (2) the raw material is free from heavy metal contamination [8], (3) a demineralization step is not required for extraction of chitosan from fungal mycelia [9]. In addition, chitosan could be produced from fungi mycelia grown in SMF using industrial by-products and wastes such as barley–buckwheat-*shochu* distillery wastewater [10], sweet potato–*shochu* wastewater [10], apple pomace [11], soybean residue [12], and corn residue [12]. By using these materials to grow fungi, marine pollution could also be controlled by removal of nitrogen, protein, phosphorus, and other compounds from wastewater [10] and the cost for production of chitosan could be reduced. Using selected fungi, extracellular enzymes could be obtained as by-products from the fermentation medium, and glucan and chitosan–glucan complex also could be obtained as by-products during extraction of chitosan from fungal mycelia. These products have many medical and industrial applications.

Therefore, the production of chitosan from fungal mycelia is gaining increasing interest for large scale production. Production, properties and applications of chitosan and glucan from fungal mycelia are presented in this chapter.

2 Life Cycle of Fungi

Fungi are included in the plant kingdom if living organisms are divided into plant and animal kingdoms. In 1969, Whittaker placed fungi in a separate kingdom of a five-kingdom system (i.e., Plantae, Fungi, Animalia, Protista, and Monera) [1]. Fungi are heterotrophic, i.e., are unable to use carbon dioxide for their carbon source.

The growth of fungi starts with spores (Figs. 1 and 2) and they synthesize microscopic tubular filaments called hyphae (singular, hypha). The hypha grows by elongation in two directions: horizontal and vertical. The mass of hyphae is called mycelium (plural, mycelia). The undifferentiated or specialized hypha, named sporangiophore, is produced by mature hypha. Sporangiospores are formed in sporangium, which is borne on the tip of a sporangiophore. Fungi reproduce both asexually and sexually, as shown in Fig. 2a. Spores are the most common method of asexual reproduction in fungi. Two main types of asexual spores are sporangiospores and conidia [1].

Naturally, fungi grow on solid materials and in liquid medium. On solid material, fungi produce extracellular enzymes that convert the insoluble material into soluble form, and then fungi absorb the soluble material to their hyphae as their nutrient (Fig. 1). Fungi utilize the absorbed soluble materials to synthesize their cell wall materials such as glucan, chitin/chitosan, D-glucuronic acid, D-mannose, D-galactose, L-fucose, glycoproteins, glycopeptides, proteins, DNA, RNA and other cellular materials [1, 13]. Generally, fungal cell walls contain 80–90% carbohydrate, the remainder being proteins, lipids, and other compounds. The composition of fungal cell walls are variable, depending on their age and environmental factors.

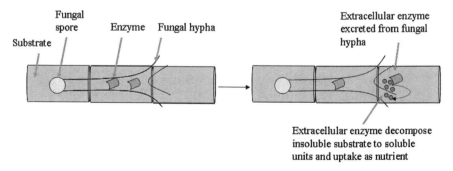

Fig. 1 Degradation of insoluble substrate by extracellular enzyme excreted from fungal hyphae and utilization of soluble materials for the growth of fungus

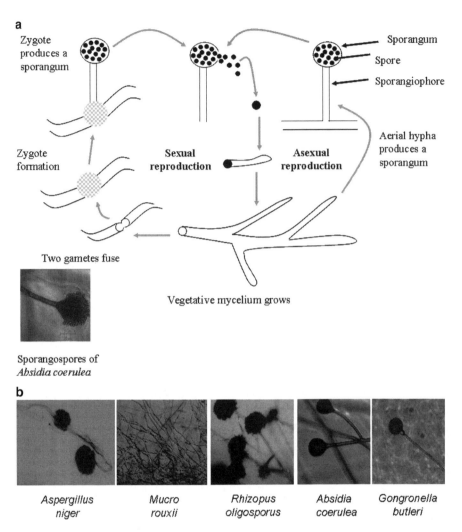

Fig. 2 (a) Life cycle of fungi, asexual and sexual reproduction of fungi. Most fungi in the class of Zygomycetes reproduce asexually. (b) Microscopic observation of *Aspergillus niger*, *Mucor rouxii*, *Rhizopus oligosporus*, *Absidia coerulea* and *Gongronella butleri*

3 Growth of Fungi in Solid State/Substrate and Submerged Fermentation

Fungal biomass cultivation can be accomplished by two approaches, namely SSF and SMF.

SSF is a microorganism-growing technique on and inside humidified particles (i.e., water content of solid substrate is maintained at a level corresponding to the growth and metabolism of fungi. But, the water content level should not exceed the maximal water holding capacity of the matrix) [14]. The SSF refers to two different processes: solid substrate fermentation and solid state fermentation [15]. Solid substrate fermentation should define only those processes in which the substrate itself acts as a carbon/energy source and solid support, and the fermentation process is carried out in the absence or near-absence of free water. Solid state fermentation should define any fermentation process in which the substrate acts as solid support,

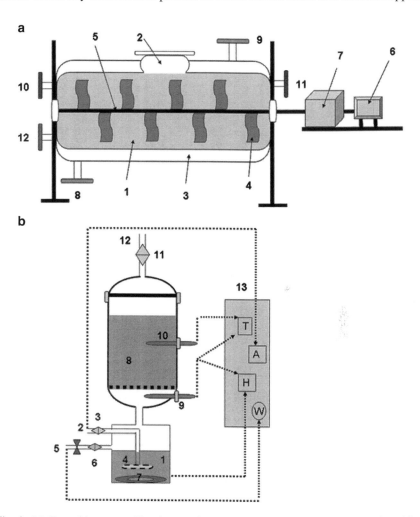

Fig. 3 (a) Drum bioreactor: (*1*) substrate chamber, (*2*) loading port, (*3*) jacket, (*4*) paddles, (*5*) central axis, (*6*) motor, (*7*) gear box, (*8*) water inlet, (*9*) water outlet (*10*) air inlet, (*11*) air outlet, (*12*) product. (**b**) Packed bed bioreactor (*1*) water-bath where humidification occurs, (*2*) air inlet, (*3, 11*) air filter, (*4*) sparger, (*5*) water input, (*6*) water filter, (*7*) heating coil, (*8*) basket with perforated bottom, (*9*) temperature probe for humidified air, (*10*) medium temperature probe; (*12*) air output, (*13*) controller and recorder, (*H*) relative humidity regulator; (*T*), temperature regulator; (*A*) airflow meter; (*W*) water supply

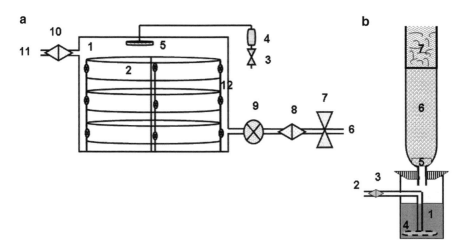

Fig. 4 (**a**) Try type bioreactor: (*1*) chamber, (*2*) trays (*3*) water valve, (*4*) UV tube, (*5*) humidifier, (*6*) air inlet, (*7*) air flow meter (*8*, *10*) air filter (*9*) air heater and humidifier, (*11*) air outlet, (*12*) tray holder. (**b**) Column bioreactor (*1*) water-bath where humidification occurs, (*2*) air inlet, (*3*) air filter, (*4*) sparger, (*5*) filter paper, (*6*) solid substrate, (*7*) cotton

and the fermentation process is carried out in the absence or near-absence of free water.

Solid substrate fermentation has been used for growth of fungi in most applications. The limiting factors in SSF are the unique sterilized conditions for fungal growth, limited accessibility and availability of substrate, unique conditions for mass transfer of oxygen, and the difficult regulation of physical factors such as mixing, pH, temperature, and moisture content [16].

Four basic types of SSF bioreactors have been developed (Figs. 3 and 4). These are: (1) drum bioreactor [16], (2) packed bed bioreactor [17, 18], (3) tray bioreactor [4, 16], (Ahmed et al. 1987; Hesseltine 1987; Pandey 1991 cited in [19]), and (4) column bioreactor (Raimbault and Germon 1976 cited in [20]). The structure and nature of the solid matrix used, type of microorganism involved, environmental conditions needed for the process, the type of use (research or industrial applications), and type of product should all be considered for the selection of appropriate design of bioreactor [19].

SMF has three main approaches: batch, fed-batch, and continuous cultivation. In all cultivations, the accretion of mycelia was observed on baffles, impellers, fermenter lid, and wall of fermenter (i.e., above the surface of medium). This problem has been solved by varying the inoculum size, changing the agitation speed, varying aeration, making the fermenter with hydrophobic materials, and changing the pH and medium composition. However, the results showed no more than minute improvements of the problem [21].

There are advantages and disadvantages in both fermentation methods. Although the SSF requires a longer fermentation period for microbial growth than the SMF, it reduces the volume of liquid effluents from the fermentation process (Raimbault

Production, Properties and Applications of Fungal Cell Wall Polysaccharides 193

and Germon 1976 cited in [20]). The SMF provides easier control of fermentation parameters than the SSF. In addition, the harvesting of biomass is easier for the SMF than the SSF.

Fungi have been used to produce a lot of valuable products such as enzymes, food products, organic acids, and medicines (Tables 1 and 2). Waste mycelia remain at the end of the fermentation processes and it has been proposed to transform them into valuable products such as chitosan and chitosan–glucan complex (Table 3).

Table 1 Valuable products from fungi

Fungi	Valuable products
Fungi in manufacturing of food	
Aspergillus oryzae [22]	Soy sauce and miso
Penicillium camemberti [22]	Cheese
Rhizopus oligosporus [22]	Tempe
Fungi in manufacturing of organic acid	
Aspergillus niger [23]	Citric acid, gluconic acid and oxalic acid
Aspergillus terreus [23]	Itaconic acid
Rhizopus oryzae [23]	L-lactic acid, fumaric acid and L-malic acid
Fungi in manufacturing of medicine	
Penicillium chrysogenum [24, 25]	Penicillin

Table 2 Production of enzymes from fungi

Fungus	Enzyme products from fungi
Aspergillus melleus [26]	Protease
Aspergillus niger [26, 27]	Xylanse, α-amylase, endoarabinase, glucoamylase, hemicellulase, pectinase, cellulase, catalase, phytase, protease, lipase, glucose oxidase
Aspergillus oryzae [26]	α-amylase, cellulase, glucoamylase, hemicellulase, pectinase, protease, lipase
Disporotrichum dimorphosporum [26]	Xylanse, glucanase, hemicellulase, cellulase
Endothia parasitica [26]	Milk-clotting enzymes
Humicola insolens [26]	Xylanse, hemicellulase, cellulase, pentosanase
Mortierella vinaceae [26]	α-Galactosidase
Mucor javanicus [26]	Lipase
Mucor meihei [26]	Milk-clotting enzymes, lipase-esterase
Mucor pusillus [26]	Milk-clotting enzymes, lipase
Penicillium emersonii [26]	Cellulase, glucanase, xylanase
Penicillium funiculosum [26]	Xylanse, glucoamylase, pectinase, cellulase, cellobiase, glucosidase, dextranase, glucanase
Penicillium lilacinum [26]	Dextranase
Penicillium simplicissimum [26]	Pectinase
Rhizopus niveus [26]	Glucoamylase
Rhizopus oryzae [26]	Carbohydrases
Trichoderma harzianum [26]	Xylanse, cellulase, glucosidase, glucanase, hemicellulase
Trichoderma longbranchiatum [26]	Xylanse, glucoamylase, pectinase, cellulase, glucanase, hemicellulase

Table 3 Production of valuable products using industrial waste mycelia from several industrial fermentation plants

Fungi	Industrial fermentation plants	Valuable products
Aspergillus niger [3, 24, 28]	Citric acid	Bioabsorbance, chitosan, chitosan–glucan complex
Penicillium chrysogenum [24, 25]	Penicillin	Bioabsorbance and chitosan
Claviceps paspali [24]	Ergotamine	Bioabsorbance

4 Chitosan Metabolism in Fungi

Fungi absorb carbon, nitrogen, and other materials from growth medium and use a large amount of carbon for biosynthesis of cell wall materials. Cell walls of fungi in the class of Zygomycetes such as *Gongronella* spp., *Absidia* spp., *Mucor* spp., *Rhizopus* spp., and *Aspergillus* spp. are composed of chitosan [4–7]. Chitosan has been easily extracted from mycelia of these fungi by treatment with 1 M NaOH and then with 2% acetic acid. According to most literature, the amount of chitosan in the cell wall of fungi depends on the species, fermentation medium composition, and conditions and type of fermentation. A lot of assumptions have been made about the synthesis of chitosan in the fungal cell wall. These include: (1) chitosan is synthesized directly by polymerization of unacetylated glucosaminyl residues from UDP-GlcN (uridine diphosphate D-glucosamine), (2) Chitin deacetylase and chitin synthetase are involved in the synthesis of chitosan in the cell wall of fungi, and (3) chitosan synthesis starts from the synthesis of chitin [8, 29–31].

Chitin biosynthesis starts with the conversion of glucose into *N*-acetylglucosamine-1-phosphate, which requires a series of reactions. "The *N*-acetylglucosamine-1-phosphate then reacts with UTP (the nucleotide uridine triphosphate) to form UDP-*N*-acetylglucosamine, which is the nucleotide diphosphate sugar. Finally, this sugar transfers the *N*-acetylglucosamine moiety to the growing chitin chain, functioning as a primer, and becomes one of its subunits. The enzyme chitin synthetase and Mg^{2+} ions are required for this polymerization step. The completed chitin molecule is a long chain of sugar subunits that are joined by β-1,4 links" [30]. According to the evidence from in-vitro experiments, chitin deacetylase converts the chitin chain to chitosan. Here, all chitin substrate could not be converted to chitosan by chitin deacetylase.

The possible pathway of the synthesis of chitosan in cell wall of fungus *Gongronella butleri* grown on sweet potato pieces supplemented with urea and mineral solution is shown in Fig. 5. In addition, the synthesis of chitosan occurs in the cell wall of fungi *G. butleri* and *Absidia coerulea* grown in SMF medium without glucose (authors' unpublished data). Therefore, the mechanism of the synthesis of chitosan in cell walls of fungi is not yet clear.

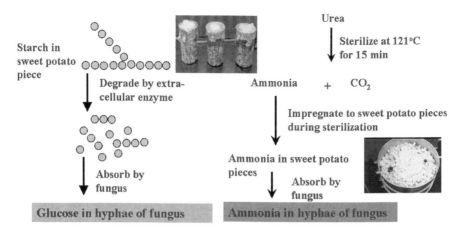

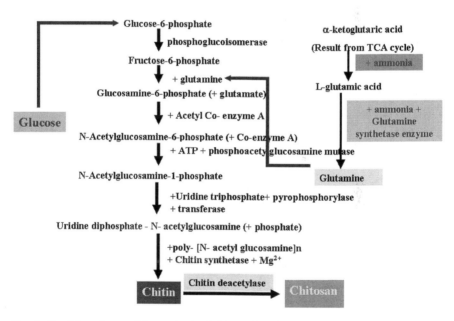

Fig. 5 Possible pathway of the synthesis of chitosan in cell wall of fungus *Gongronella butleri* grown in sweet potato pieces supplemented with urea and mineral solution

5 Chitosan and Glucan in Cell Walls of Fungi

Chitosan and glucan are the main components of the cell walls of fungi. In the cell walls, chitosan occurs in two forms, as free chitosan and covalently bonded to β-glucan [31–34].

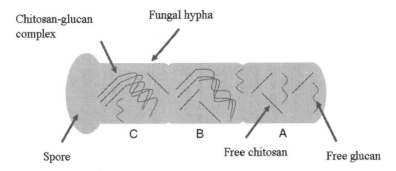

Fig. 6 Possible synthesis of chitosan chains (*straight lines*) and glucan chains (*wavy lines*) in various phases of fungal growth. (*A*) The individual chains of chitosan and glucan may be synthesized in the early stage of hyphae. (*B*, *C*) Linkage of glucan chains to chitosan chains may form in the later phase of hyphae growth

"These branched β-1,3-glucans are accompanied by varying amounts of glucans with β-1,6 links only, β-1,3 links only or alternating β-1,3 and β-1,6 links" (Wessels 1986, 1990 cited in [32]). "Together with hydrogen bonding among glucan chains this could result in a cross-linked network which confers rigidity to the wall" [35]. The individual chains of chitin/chitosan are aggregated into microfibrils with hydrogen bonds and this, together with the crosslinked network of glucan, results a very strong and rigid structure (Gooday 1979 cited in [32]), [35].

In 1990, Wessels et al. proposed that chitin and β-glucan chains initially accumulate individually in the fungal cell wall and thereafter form an interpolymer linkage [34]. A highly schematic view of β-glucan chains linked to chitosan is given in Fig. 6.

Chitosan could not be extracted directly from fungal mycelia by treatment with 2% acetic acid [36], but could be extracted from fungal mycelia after treatment with 1 M NaOH solution. In this process, protein and most of the soluble glucan are extracted out. Therefore it can be assumed that a basic pattern of organization of the cell walls of fungi includes an inner primary wall composed of free chitosan (a polymer of *N*-acetylglucosamine and glucosamine) and chitosan–glucan complex, and an outer wall composed largely of alkaline-soluble glucan, proteins, and other compounds (Fig. 7). The fungi with hyphae composed of chitin/chitosan were placed under the subclass Zygomycetes. In 1995, Gooday proposed that the chitin/chitosan microfibrils are in the innermost part of the Zygomycetes fungal wall, but they are probably a minor wall component in other groups of fungi [32].

The chitosan–glucan complex has been produced from fungal mycelia and has been tested for use in many applications. In 1980, Muzzarelli et al. produced a chitosan–glucan complex from waste mycelia of *Aspergillus niger* from a citric acid production plant [3]. They reported that the insoluble chitosan–glucan complex was obtained from the fungal mycelia by boiling with 30–40% NaOH for 4–6 h. Moreover, the chitosan–glucan complex was extracted easily from cell wall of the fungus *G. butleri* by treatment with 11 M NaOH at 45°C for 13 h [4, 37]. The

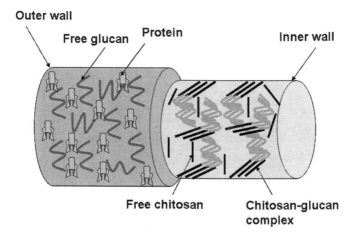

Fig. 7 Model of inner and outer wall of fungal hypha

resultant chitosan–glucan complexes have been used to prepare powders, scaffolds and membranes [3, 38] and these materials have been tested as flocculation agent [3] and as support for culture of mammalian cells [38]. Moreover Li et al., tested the chitosan–glucan complex for removal of several metal ions, such as Cr, Co, Ni, Cu, Cd, and Pb, from wastewater [39]. In addition, the carboxymethylated derivative of a chitosan–glucan complex with reduced molecular weight has antimutagenic activity [40].

On the other hand, the formation of the chitosan–glucan complex chains causes a considerable problem for the extraction of intact chitosan and glucan. It does not break down easily under mild extraction conditions [3, 36]. To extract the high quality and quantity of chitosan and glucan from fungal cell walls, the bond between chitosan and glucan must be investigated. Most researchers are trying to investigate the linkage between the chitosan and glucan in the fungal cell wall by digestion with glucanase, chitinase, and amylase. In 1979, Sietsma and Wessels reported that 90% of the β-glucan was obtained from the chitin–glucan complex by digestion with (1–3)-β-glucanase, and N-acetyl-glucosamine, lysine, and/or citrulline were identified as products after digestion of residue with chitinase [41]. Therefore, they suggested that the bridge linking the glucan chain with chitin contains lysine, citrulline, glucose, and N-acetyl-glucosamine. Similar evidence was obtained by Gopal et al., for the degradation of chitin–glucan complex by (1,3)-β- and (1,6)-β-glucanase, and subsequently by chitinase [42]. Carbohydrate expressed as glucose and N-acetyl-glucosamine monomers was detectable in equivalent amounts in the hydrolysate. The residue after chitinase treatment was further treated with α-amylase, but additional release of glucose could not be detected colorimetrically. Surarit et al. suggested a glycosidic linkage between position 6 of N-acetyl-glucosamine in chitin and position 1 of glucose in β-(1–6)-glucan in the cell wall of *Candida albicans* [43]. In 1990, Wessels et al. proposed a direct link between free amino groups in the glucosaminoglycan and the reducing end of the glucan chains forming the interpolymer linkages in the chitin–glucan complex [34]. Up to 1992, no clear evidence of the identity of the chemical link between the chitosan and glucan polymer chains had been uncovered [2]. After 1995, Kollar et al. and Fontaine et al. digested the cell wall of *Saccharomyces cerevisae* and *Aspergillus fumigatus* with 1% SDS and 1 M NaOH respectively and the insoluble fractions were digested with (1,3)-β-endoglucanase and chitinase [44, 45]. The soluble fractions were analyzed. On the basis of their results, they concluded that the terminal reducing residue of a chitin chain is attached to the nonreducing end of a β-(1,3)-glucan chain by a β-1,4 linkage. An insoluble residue remained at the end of both extraction processes.

Importantly, cell wall matrix must be broken down far enough in order to study the linkage between the chitosan and glucan in the fungal cell wall and to extract total chitosan (i.e., free chitosan plus chitosan bounded to glucan). In 1994, Muzzarelli et al. reported that the chitosan–glucan complex can be split by 25% NaOH [46].

The best decomposition conditions for the fungal mycelia was treatment with 11 M NaOH at 45°C for 13 h and then treatment with 0.35 M acetic acid at 95°C for 5 h [36]. Moreover the Termamyl treatment is obviously highly efficient at separating the chitosan from the glucan and offers possibilities for the isolation of purified chitosan [4, 36]. Based on these observations, it has been proved that these two polysaccharides, chitosan and glucan, are linked by α-(1–4)-glycosidic bond [4, 8, 37]. The IR spectra of alkaline-soluble and alkaline-insoluble glucan, and chitosan are shown in Fig. 8.

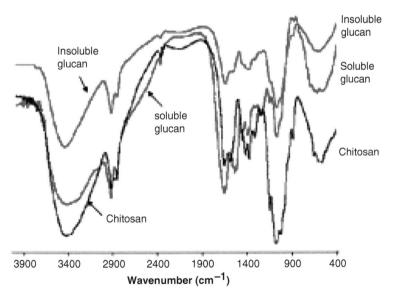

Fig. 8 Infrared spectra of soluble and insoluble glucan and chitosan from fungus *Gongronella butleri* USDB 0201. (Reproduced from [37])

6 Production, Properties and Applications of Chitosan from Fungal Biomass

Many researchers have evaluated the yield of chitosan from several fungi (*Absidia, Aspergillus, Cunninghame, Gongronella, Mucor, Penicillium, Phycomyces, Rhizopus* and *Zygorhyncus*) grown in SSF and SMF (Table 4). Firstly, a comparison was made between the yield of chitosan from mycelia of fungus *G. butleri* USDB 0201 grown in SSF and in SMF using various nitrogen sources [57]. We concluded that the production yield of chitosan from fungal mycelia grown in SSF is higher than that in SMF. Moreover, Crestini et al. reported that the yield of chitosan produced from *Lentinus edodes* grown in solid state fermentation (6.18 g/kg) was higher than that in SMF (0.12 g/L) [58]. Therefore, solid state fermentation is the best fermentation method for the production of chitosan from the fungal mycelia. The conditions for solid substrate fermentation have been optimized to improve the yield of chitosan from fungal mycelia grown in solid substrate fermentation. The chitosan yield was increased to a maximal 4.6 g/kg sweet potato under the fermentation conditions: inoculum size, 1.5×10^7 spores/kg solid substrate; inlet air flow rate, 1.2 L/[min (kg DM)]; humidity of inlet air, 95%; outside fermenter temperature, 29°C; and moisture content of the solid substrate 80% (Nwe and Stevens 2006 cited in [8]). The SSF offers numerous advantages over SMF. These include high volumetric productivity, relatively higher concentration of the products, less effluent generation, and simple fermentation equipment, etc. [15].

Table 4 Procedure for the extraction of fungal chitosan

Strain	Deproteination with NaOH solution			Extraction of chitosan with acetic acid			Chitosan yield
	Conc (M)	Temp. (°C)	Time (min)	Conc (%)	Temp. (°C)	Time (h)	
Absidia coerulea [12]	0.5	121	20	10	60	6	[a]6.12 g/kg of potato pieces
Gongronella butleri [47]	11	45	780	2	95	5	[a]4 g/kg of sweet potato
Gongronella butleri [47]	1	45	780	2	95	5	[a]0.8 g/kg of sweet potato
Rhizopus oryzae [48]	1	121	15	2	95	8	[a]4.3 g/kg of soybean residue
Rhizopus oryzae [49]	1	121	30	2	95	8	[a]5.63 g/kg of rice straw
Aspergillus niger [6]	1	121	15	2	95	8	[b]963 mg/L
Absidia atrospora [10]	0.5	115	60	2	RT	0.5	[b]296 mg/L
Absidia blakesleeana [50]	1	121	15	2	95	12	[b]280 mg/L
Absidia coerulea [47]	11	45	780	2	95	5	[b]500 mg/L
Absidia coerulea [47]	1	45	780	2	95	5	[b]450 mg/L

(*continued*)

Table 4 (continued)

Strain	Deproteination with NaOH solution			Extraction of chitosan with acetic acid			Chitosan yield
	Conc (M)	Temp. (°C)	Time (min)	Conc (%)	Temp. (°C)	Time (h)	
Absidia coerulea [50]	1	121	15	2	95	12	[b]480 mg/L
Absidia coerulea [51]	0.5	–	60	2	RT	24	[b]10 g/100 g mycelia
Absidia glauca [7]	1	121	15	2	25	1	[b]326 mg/L
Absidia glauca [52]	1	121	15	2	121	0.25	[b]7 g/100 g mycelia
Absidia glauca [52]	50% (w/w)	121	15	2	121	0.25	[b]8 g/100 g mycelia
Absidia orchidis [5]	1	121	10	1	–	–	[b]1.79 g/L
Absidia repens [53]	1	121	–	2	100	17	[b]2.8 g/L
Cunninghamella echinulata [7]	1	121	15	2	25	1	[b]398 mg/L
Gongronella butleri [47]	11	45	780	2	95	5	[b]800 mg/L
Gongronella butleri [47]	1	45	780	2	95	5	[b]360 mg/L
Gongronella butleri [7]	1	121	15	2	25	1	[b]467 mg/L
Gongronella butleri [50]	1	121	15	2	95	12	[b]250 mg/L
Gongronella butleri [10]	0.5	115	60	2	RT	0.5	[b]352 mg/L
Gongronella butleri [11]	0.5	90	120	10	60	6	[b]1.19 g/L
Mucor hiemalis [7]	1	121	15	2	25	1	[b]256 mg/L
Mucor rouxii [50]	1	121	15	2	95	12	[b]370 mg/L
Mucor rouxii [54]	1	121	15	2	95	–	[b]250 mg/L
Mucor rouxii [55]	1	121	15	1 M HCl	95	24	[b]4–8 g/100 g mycelia
Mucor spp. [7]	1	121	15	2	25	1	[b]252 mg/L
Penicillium chrysogenum [25]	0.5 9.5	70 130	3 1	2	100	5	[b]0.37 g/100 g mycelia
Phycomyces blakesleeanus [50]	1	121	15	2	95	12	[b]67 mg/L
Rhizopus arrhizus [7]	1	121	15	2	25	1	[b]234 mg/L
Rhizopus microsporus [7]	1	121	15	2	25	1	[b]149 mg/L
Rhizopus oligosporus [7]	1	121	15	2	25	1	[b]149 mg/L
Rhizopus oryzae [7]	1	121	15	2	25	1	[b]278 mg/L
Rhizopus oryzae [56]	0.5	121	15	2	95	12	[b]700 mg/L
Rhizopus oryzae [6]	1	121	15	2	95	8	[b]345 mg/L
Zygorhyncus moelleri [7]	1	121	15	2	25	1	[b]238 mg/L

– Not mentioned in the paper; *RT* room temperature
[a]Solid state fermentation
[b]Submerged fermentation

There are a few more data already published on the production of chitosan from fungal mycelia grown in the SSF. The solid substrates such as wheat straw [58], soybean and mungbean residues [48], sweet potato [4], rice straw [49], and potato pieces [12] have been used to grow fungi for production of chitosan. The conditions for separation of mycelia from solid matrix depend on the fungus species and nature of solid matrix. The separation of mycelia of *A. niger* grown on potato substrate was easier than that grown on sweet potato substrate [59]. However, mycelia of *G. butleri* could separate easily from both potato and sweet potato substrate [8]. The yield of chitosan obtained from the SSF depended on fungus species, solid matrix, incubation periods, and fermentation conditions.

In addition, Jaworska and Szewczyk reported the production of chitosan from fungus *Absidia orchids* in batch, repeated batch, and continuous fermentation [60]. They reported that the batch process is better than other fermentation methods since it is easy to operate and gave higher amount of chitosan.

Moreover, the chitosan extraction procedure is also one of the important factors for the production of chitosan from fungal mycelia. Various methods have been developed for the extraction of high yield pure chitosan from fungal cell walls (Table 4). The yield of chitosan depends on the extraction procedure used. The extraction of chitosan from mycelia of *Absidia glauca* using 1 M NaOH and 50% NaOH (w/w) gave chitosan yields of 7 and 8%, respectively (Table 4, [52]). However, both chitosans have 77% degree of deacetylation (DD) and molecular weight of 1×10^5 Da. This result pointed out that the deacetylation reaction could not occur under the treatment of mycelia with 50% NaOH at 121°C for 15 min and that this reaction helps to remove more protein and other cell wall components to obtain a higher yield of chitosan. Only free chitosan (i.e., chitosan unbound to other cell wall components) could be extracted under the treatment of mycelia with 1 M NaOH [4]. The total chitosan (free chitosan plus chitosan bounded to glucan) was extracted subsequently by 11 M NaOH at 45°C, and 0.35 M acetic acid at 95°C. The resulting extract was treated using a heat-stable, commercial α-amylase [4, 36]. The amount of free chitosan in the cell wall of *G. butleri* is lower than that in the cell wall of *A. coerulea*. However, the amount of chitosan bound to glucan in the cell wall of *G. butleri* is higher than that in the cell wall of *A. coerulea* [36].

The quality and quantity of chitosan extracted from the fungal mycelia (Tables 4 and 5) depend on the fungal strain: *Absidia*, *Gongronells*, *Rhizopus*, etc.; fermentation type: SSF and SMF (batch fermentation, fed batch fermentation and continuous fermentation); fermentation medium composition: carbon source and concentration, nitrogen source and concentration, and metal ions and their concentration; pH of the fermentation medium; fermentation conditions: inoculum size, harvesting time, fermentation temperature, inlet air flow rate; and chitosan extraction procedure [5, 7, 8, 50, 54, 58, 61]. Chitosans obtained from different species of fungi have been tested in various applications (Table 6).

Table 5 Properties of fungal chitosan from different species of fungi

Fungus species	%DD	MW (Da)	Viscosity (cP)
Absidia coerulea [51]	95	4.5×10^5	–
Absidia coerulea [50]	93	7×10^5	–
Absidia blakesleeana [50]	85	4×10^5	–
Absidia glauca [52]	77	1×10^5	–
Absidia coerulea [12]	85	6.4×10^3	
Absidia orchidis [5]	73	3×10^5	–
Aspergillus niger [6]	90	1.4×10^5	6.2
Aspergillus niger [49]	84	–	5.9
Cunnighamella blakesleeana [51]	65	1.4×10^5	–
Fusarium oxysporum [49]	73	–	2.7
Gongronella butleri [50]	90	5×10^5	–
Mortierella isabelina [51]	84	1×10^5	–
Mucor rouxii [54]	88	4.6×10^5	–
Mucor rouxii [51]	41	1.6×10^5	–
Mucor rouxii [50]	89	6×10^5	–
Penicillium chrysogenum [25]	84	3.6×10^4	–
Penicillium citrinum [49]	78	–	4.6
Phycomyces blakesleeanus [50]	88	4×10^5	–
Rhizopus delemar [51]	68	1.2×10^5	–
Rhizopus oryzae [6]	88	6.9×10^4	3.5
Rhizopus oryzae [49]	90	–	6.8

Table 6 Application of fungal chitosan

Source of chitosan	Application of chitosan
A. glauca var. paradoxa [62]	Clarification of apple juice
Rhizopus oryzae [49]	Antibacterial agent
Absidia coerulea [51]	Copper adsorption
Penicillium chrysogenum [25]	Sorption of heavy metal ion and controlled release of vitamin D2
Aspergillus niger [63]	Sorbent for chromatography
Gongronella butleri [64]	Tissue regeneration template
Gongronella butleri [65]	Plant growth stimulator

7 Production, Properties and Applications of Glucan from Fungal Biomass

Glucose joined through α-1,3-, α-1,4-, α-1,6-, β-1,3-, β-1,4- or β-1,6-linkages is called glucan [34, 66–71]. This polymer has been extracted from many fungi and the structure of the polymer has been studied by different analyses (Table 7). These analyses indicated that glucans in cell walls of fungi have a main chain of glucopyranosyl β-(1–3) linkages and branch chains of β-(1–6) linkages [30, 72–74]. The IR spectrum of glucans obtained from cell wall of fungus *G. butleri* is shown in Fig. 8.

Table 7 Analytical methods for determination of quality and quantity of glucans from cell walls of fungi

Parameters	Methods
Distinguishing glucan from other polysaccharides [70]	The reaction of D-glucan with iodine gave a faint blue color
Determination of linkage between monomer units [70, 71]	Methylation analysis, periodate oxidation, acetolysis, Smith degradation, enzymatic degradation
Determination of α- or β-configuration [70, 71]	IR and NMR spectroscopy
Determination of monomer units [70, 71]	Acid hydrolysis

"Extensive studies have demonstrated that (1–3)-β-D-glucans exhibit considerable immunomodulatory activity by binding specific macrophage receptors and activating macrophages, resulting in antitumor, antibacterial, and wound healing activings" (Müller et al. 2000; Ohno et al. 2001; Patchen et al. 1998; Sandula et al. 1999; Tsiapali et al. 2001 cited in [75]). Moreover, linear β-(1,3)-D glucan with β-(1,6)-D glucoside branches are increasingly attracting much attention owing to their substantial immunostimulating activity [76].

The solubility of glucan polymers depends on their degree of polymerization and degree of branching [75, 77]. Wang et al., assumed that "the abundance of –OH groups in glucan facilitates hydrogen bond formation, causing the natural glucan to exit as a compact triple stranded helix, which in turn contributes to poor glucan aqueous solubility" [75]. Therefore glucan polymer has been modified into its derivatives: (1–3)-β-D-glucan sulfate [75] and a carboxymethylated derivative [78]. Low molecular weight carboxymethylated derivative (90–100 kDa) has high mitogenic and comitogenic activities, as well as radioprotective and antimutagenic effects [78].

References

1. Dube HC (1990) Fungi, general characteristics. An introduction to fungi, 2nd revised edn. Vikas, New Delhi, pp 11–146
2. Roberts GAF (1992) Structure of chitin and chitosan. Chitin chemistry, 1st edn. Macmillan, London, pp 1–53
3. Muzzarelli RAA, Tanfani F, Scarpini G (1980) Chelating, film-forming, and coagulating ability of the chitosan–glucan complex from *Aspergillus niger* industrial wastes. Biotechnol Bioeng 22:885–896
4. Nwe N, Stevens WF (2002) Production of fungal chitosan by solid substrate fermentation followed by enzymatic extraction. Biotechnol Lett 24:131–134
5. Jaworska MM, Konieczna E (2001) The influence of supplemental components in nutrient medium on chitosan formation by the fungus *Absidia orchidis*. Appl Microbiol Biotechnol 56:220–224
6. Pochanavanich P, Suntornsuk W (2002) Fungal chitosan production and its characterization. Lett Appl Microbiol 35:17–21

7. Tan SC, Tan TK, Wong SM, Khor E (1996) The chitosan yield of zygomycetes at their optimum harvesting time. Carbohydr Polym 30:239–242
8. Nwe N, Furuike T, Tamura H (2010) Production of fungal chitosan by enzymatic method and applications in plant tissue culture and tissue engineering: 11 years of our progress, present situation and future prospects. In: Elnashar M (ed) Biopolymers, SCIYO Rijeka, chapter 7, pp 135–162
9. Nwe N, Furuike T, Tamura H (2011) Chitosan from aquatic and terrestrial organisms and microorganisms: production, properties and applications. In: Johnson BM, Berkel ZE (eds) Biodegradable materials: production, properties and applications. Nova Science, Hauppauge, NY, chapter 2, pp 29–50
10. Yokoi H, Aratake T, Nishio S, Hirose J, Hayashi S, Takasaki Y (1998) Chitosan production from *Shochu* distillery wastewater by funguses. J Ferment Bioeng 85:246–249
11. Streit F, Koch F, Mauro CML, Ninow JL (2009) Production of fungal chitosan in liquid cultivation using apple pomace as substrate. Braz J Microbiol 40:20–25
12. Wang W, Dua Y, Qiu Y, Wang X, Hu Y, Yang J, Cai J, John F, Kennedy JF (2008) A new green technology for direct production of low molecular weight chitosan. Carbohydr Polym 74:127–132
13. Dow JM, Rubery PH (1977) Chemical fractionation of the cell walls of mycelial and yeast-like forms of *Mucor rouxii*: a comparative study of the polysaccharide and glycoprotein components. J Gen Microbiol 99:29–41
14. Durand A, Blachere H (1988) Solid state fermentation. In: Raimbault M (ed) Solid state fermentation bioconversion of agro-industrial raw material. Proceedings of the seminar ORSTOM-Montpellier, France, pp 83–89
15. Pandey A, Soccol CR, Rodriguez-Leon JA, Nigam P (2001) Solid state fermentation in biotechnology: Fundamentals and application. Asiatech, New Delhi, pp 3–97
16. Laukevics JJ, Apsite AF, Viesturs UE (1984) Solid substrate fermentation of wheat straw to fungal protein. Biotechnol Bioeng 26:1465–1474
17. Durand A, de la Broise D, Blachere H (1988) Laboratory scale bioreactor for solid state process. J Biotechnol 8:59–66
18. Almanza S, Durand A, Renaud R, Maratray J, Diez M (1995) Laboratory scale reactor for aseptic solid state cultivation. Biotechnol Tech 9:395–400
19. Durand A, Renaud R, Maratray J, Almanza S, Diez M (1996) INRA-Dijion reactors for solid state fermentation: designs and applications. J Sci Ind Res 55:317–332
20. Araujo AADE, Lepilleur C, Delcourt S, Colavitti P, Roussos S (1997) Laboratory scale bioreactors for study of fungal physiology and metabolism in solid state fermentation system. In: Advances in solid state fermentation. Proceedings of the 2nd international symposium on solid state fermentation, FEMS-95, Montpellier, France, 27–28 February 1997. Kluwer, The Netherlands, pp 93–111
21. Davoust N, Hansson G (1992) Identifying the conditions for development beneficial mycelium morphology for chitosan-production *Absidia spp.* in submersed cultures. Appl Microbiol Biotechnol 36:618–620
22. Wong G (2003) Fungi in manufacturing of food. http://www.botany.hawaii.edu/faculty/wong/BOT135/Lect16.htm. Accessed 25 March 2011
23. Magnuson JK, Lasure LL (2004) Organic acid production by filamentous fungi. In: Tkacz J, Lange L (eds) Advances in fungal biotechnology for industry, agriculture, and medicine. Kluwer Academic/Plenum, New York, pp 307–340
24. Luef E, Prey T, Kubicek CP (1991) Biosorption of zinc by fungal mycelial wastes. Appl Microbiol Biotechnol 34:688–692
25. Tianwei T, Binwu W, Xinyuan S (2002) Separation of chitosan from *Penicillium chrysogenum* mycelium and its applications. J Bioact Compat Polym 17:173–182
26. Mathewson PR (1998) Enzymes. Eagan Press, Saint Paul, pp 93–95

27. Chen H, Liu L, Lv S, Liu X, Wang M, Song A, Jia X (2010) Immobilization of xylanase on chitosan using dialdehyde starch as a coupling agent. Appl Biochem Biotechnol 162:24–32
28. Cai J, Yang J, Du Y, Fan L, Qiu Y, Li J, Kennedy JF (2006) Enzymatic preparation of chitosan from the waste *Aspergillus niger* mycelium of citric acid production plant. Carbohydr Polym 64:151–157
29. Davis LL, Bartnicki-Garcia S (1984) Chitosan synthesis by the tandem action of chitin synthetase and chitin deacetylase from *Mucor rouxii*. Biochemistry 23:1065–1073
30. Moore-Landecker E (1996) Fundamentals of the fungi, 4th edn. Prentice Hall, Upper Saddle River, NJ, pp 251–278
31. Bartnicki-Garcia S (1968) Cell wall chemistry. Annu Rev Microbiol 22:87–108
32. Gooday GW (1995) Cell walls. In: Gow NAR, Gadd GM (eds) The growing fungus. Chapman & Hall, London, pp 3–62
33. Robson G (1999) Hyphal cell biology. In: Oliver RP, Schweizer M (eds) Molecular fungal biology. Cambridge University Press, Cambridge, pp 164–184
34. Wessels JGH, Mol PC, Sietsma JH, Vermeulen CA (1990) Wall structure, wall growth, and fungal cell morphogenesis. In: Kuhn PJ, Trinci APJ, Jung MJ, Goosey MW, Copping LG (eds) Biochemistry of cell walls and membranes in fungi. Springer, Berlin, pp 81–84
35. Sietsma JH, Vermeulen CA, Wessels JGH (1985) The role of chitin in hyphal morphogenesis. In: Muzzarelli R, Juniaux C, Gooday GW (eds) Chitin in nature and technology. Plenum, New York, pp 63–69
36. Nwe N, Stevens WF, Montet D, Tokura S, Tamura H (2008) Decomposition of myceliar matrix and extraction of chitosan from *Gongronella butleri* USDB 0201 and *Absidia coerulea* ATCC 14076. Int J Biol Macromol 43:2–7
37. Nwe N, Stevens WF, Tokura S, Tamura H (2008) Characterization of chitin and chitosan-glucan complex extracted from cell wall of fungus *Gongronella butleri* USDB 0201 by enzymatic method. Enzyme Microbial Technol 42:242–251
38. Nwe N, Stevens WF, Tamura H (2007) Extraction of the chitosan–glucan complex and chitosan from fungal cell wall and their application in tissue engineering. In: Abstracts of papers, 234th ACS national meeting, Boston, CARB-118
39. Li Q, Dunn ET, Grandmaison EW, Goosen MFA (1997) Applications and properties of chitosan. In: Goosen MFA (ed) Application of chitin and chitosan. Technomic Publishing Company, Lancaster, pp 3–29
40. Kogan G, Machova E, Chorvatovicova D, Sandula J (1998) Chitin–glucan complex of *Aspergillus Niger* and its derivatives: antimutagenic and antinfective activity. In: Chen RH, Chen HC (eds) Proceedings of the 3rd Asia Pacific chitin and chitosan symposium, Keelung, The National Taiwan Ocean University, Taiwan, pp 372–379
41. Sietma JH, Wessels JGH (1979) Evidence for covalent linkages between chitin and β-glucan in a fungal wall. J Gen Microbiol 114:99–108
42. Gopal P, Sullivan PA, Shepherd MG (1984) Isolation and structure of glucan from regenerating spheroplasts of *Candida albicans*. J Gen Microbiol 130:1217–1225
43. Surarit R, Gopal PK, Shepherd MG (1988) Evidence for a glycosidic linkage between chitin and glucan in the cell wall of *Candida albicans*. J Gen Microbiol 134:1723–1730
44. Kollar R, Petrakova E, Ashwell G, Robbins PW, Cabib E (1995) Architecture of the yeast cell wall, the linkage between chitin and β-1,3-glucan. J Biol Chem 270:1170–1178
45. Fontaine T, Simenel C, Dubreucq G, Adam O, Delepierre M, Lemoine J, Vorgias CE, Diaquin M, Latge JP (2000) Molecular organization of the alkali-insoluble fraction of *Aspergillus fumigatus* cell wall. J Biol Chem 275:27594–27607
46. Muzzarelli RAA, Ilari P, Tarsi R, Dubini B, Xia W (1994) Chitosan from *Absidia coerulea*. Carbohydr Polym 25:45–50
47. Nwe N, Furuike T, Osaka I, Fujimori H, Kawasaki H, Arakawa R, Tokura S, Stevens WF, Tamura H (2011) Laboratory scale production of ^{13}C labeled chitosan by fungi *Absidia*

coerulea and *Gongronella butleri* grown in solid substrate and submerged fermentation. Carbohydr Polym 84:743–750
48. Suntornsuk W, Pochanavanich P, Suntornsuk L (2002) Fungal chitosan production on food processing by-products. Process Biochem 37:727–729
49. Khalaf SA (2004) Production and characterization of fungal chitosan under solid-state fermentation conditions. Int J Agric Biol 6:1033–1036
50. Rane KD, Hoover DG (1993) Production of chitosan by fungi. Food Biotechnol 7:11–33
51. Miyoshi H, Shimura K, Watanabe K, Onodera K (1992) Characterization of some fungal chitosans. Biosci Biotechnol Biochem 56:1901–1905
52. Hu KJ, Yeung KW, Ho KP, Hu JL (1999) Rapid extraction of high-quality chitosan from mycelia of *Absida Glauca*. J Food Biochem 23:187–196
53. Davoust N, Persson A (1992) Effects of growth morphology and time of harvesting on the chitosan yield of *Absidia repens*. Appl Microbiol Biotechnol 37:572–575
54. Arcidiacono S, Kaplan DL (1992) Molecular weight distribution of chitosan isolated from *Mucor rouxii* under different culture and processing conditions. Biotechnol Bioeng 39:281–286
55. White SA, Farina PR, Fulton I (1979) Production and isolation of chitosan from *Mucor rouxii*. Appl Environ Microbiol 38:323–328
56. Hang YD (1990) Chitosan production from *Rhizopus* mycelia. Biotechnol Lett 12:911–913
57. Nwe N, Chandrkrachang S, Stevens WF, Maw T, Tan TK, Khor E, Wong SM (2002) Production of fungal chitosan by solid state and submerged fermentation. Carbohydr Polym 49:235–237
58. Crestini C, Kovac B, Giovannozzi-Sermanni G (1996) Production and isolation of chitosan by submerged and solid-state fermentation from *Lentinus edodes*. Biotechnol Bioeng 50:207–210
59. Prathumpai W (1998) Chitin and chitosan production by fungi in solid state and surface culture processes. Master thesis, Bioprocess Technology Program, Asian Institute of Technology, Bangkok, Thailand, pp 24–43
60. Jaworska MM, Szewczyk KW (2001) The continuous cultivation of *Absidia orchidis* fungi. In: Uragami T, Kurita K, Fukamizo T (eds) Proceedings of the 8th international chitin and chitosan conference and 4th Asia pacific chitin and chitosan symposium, Yamaguchi, Japan, Kodansha Scientific Ltd, Tokyo, pp 519–523
61. Rane KD, Hoover DG (1993) An evaluation of alkali and acid treatments for chitosan extraction from fungi. Process Biochem 28:115–118
62. Rungsardthong V, Wongvuttanakul N, Kongpien N, Chotiwaranon P (2006) Application of fungal chitosan for clarification of apple juice. Process Biochem 41:589–593
63. Kučera J (2004) Fungal mycelium – the source of chitosan for chromatography. J Chromatogr B 808:69–73
64. Nwe N, Furuike T, Tamura H (2009) The mechanical and biological properties of chitosan scaffolds for tissue regeneration templates are significantly enhanced by chitosan from *Gongronella butleri*. Materials 2:374–398
65. Nge KL, Nwe N, Chandrkrachang S, Stevens WF (2006) Chitosan as growth stimulator in orchid tissue culture. Plant Sci 170:1185–1190
66. Bartnicki-Garcia S (1999) Glucan, walls, and morphogenesis: on the contributions of J. G. H. Wessels to the golden decades of fungal physiology and beyond. Fungal Genet Biol 27:119–127
67. Carbonero ER, Montai AV, Mellinger CG, Eliasaro S, Sassaki GL, Gorin PAJ, Iacomini M (2005) Glucans of lichenized fungi: significance for taxonomy of the genera *Parmotrema* and *Rimelia*. Phytochemistry 66:929–934
68. Schmid E, Stone BA, McDougall BM, Bacic A, Martin KL, Brownlee RTC, Chai E, Seviour RJ (2001) Structure of epiglucan, a highly side-chain/branched $(1 \rightarrow 3; 1 \rightarrow 6)$-β-glucan from the micro fungus Epicoccum nigrum Ehrenb Ex Schlecht. Carbohydr Res 331:163–171

69. Hochstenbach F, Klis FM, Hvd E, Ev D, Peters PJ, Klausner RD (1998) Identification of a putative alpha-glucan synthase essential for cell wall construction and morphogenesis in fission yeast. Proc Natl Acad Sci 95:9161–9166
70. Wolski EA, Lima C, Agusti R, Daleo GR, Andreu AB, de Lederkremer RM (2005) An α glucan elicitor from the cell wall of a biocontrol binucleate *Rhizoctonia* isolate. Carbohydr Res 340:619–627
71. Marchessault H, Deslandes Y (1979) Fine structure of (1–3)-β-D-glucan: curdlan and paramylon. Carbohydr Res 75:231–242
72. Yalin W, Cuirong S, Yuanjiang P (2006) Studies on isolation and structural features of a polysaccharide from the mycelium of an Chinese edible fungus (*Cordyceps sinensis*). Carbohydr Polym 63:251–256
73. Rout D, Mondal S, Chakraborty I, Pramanik M, Islam SS (2005) Chemical analysis of a new (1 → 3)-, (1 → 6)-branched glucan from an eatable mushroom, *Pleurotus florida*. Carbohydr Res 340:2533–2539
74. Herrera JR (1991) Fungal glucans. In: Fungal cell wall: structure, synthesis, and assembly. CRC, Mexico, pp 59–88
75. Wang Y, Yao S, Guan Y, Wu T, Kennedy JF (2005) A novel process for preparation of (1 → 3)-β-D-glucan sulphate by a heterogeneous reaction and its structural elucidation. Carbohydr Polym 59:93–99
76. Ikeda N, Uno M, Harata M, Nishiyama Y, Kurita K (2001) Synthesis of branched polysaccharides from linear glucans. In: Uragami T, Kurita K, Fukamizo T (eds) Proceedings of the 8th international chitin and chitosan conference and 4th Asia pacific chitin and chitosan symposium, Yamaguchi, Japan, Kodansha Scientific Ltd, Tokyo, pp 368–369
77. Sietma JH, Wessels JGH (1981) Solubility of (1–3)-β-D/(1–6)-β-D-glucose in fungal walls: importance of presumed linkage between glucan and chitin. J Gen Microbiol 125:209–212
78. Sandula J, Kogan G, Kacurakova M, Machova E (1999) Microbial (1–3)-β-D-glucans, their preparation, physico-chemical characterization and immunomodulatory activity. Carbohydr Polym 38:247–253

Index

A
A99a 90
Absidia coerulea 167, 188, 190
Absidia glauca var. *paradoaxa* 170
Acetoxyethyl-triethoxysilane 134
N-Acetyl-L-cysteine (NAC) 36
N-Acetylglucosamine–1-phosphate 194
Acrylic acid-poly(ethylene glycol) methyl ether acrylate 14
Adipose-derived stem cells (ADSCs) 105
AG73 90
Alginate 5, 93
N-Alkyl chitosan 53
Alkyloxysilanes 135, 143
Aminopropyltriethoxysilane (APTES) 135, 143
Angiogenesis 48
Apatite–wollastonite/chitosan 154
Armillariella mellea 169
Asialoglycoprotein 91
Aspergillus niger 190, 196

B
Bilayer dermal equivalent (BDE) 110
Bioceramics 57
Biocompatibility 129
Biohybrid artificial liver 57
Biomaterials 81
Bionanocomposites 1
Bionanoparticles (BNPs) 11
Bioreactors 191
Bone 45, 117
Bone morphogenetic proteins (BMPs) 120, 145
Bone tissue 57
Brushite 150
Burns, skin tissue engineering 55

C
Calcium alginate 62
Calcium phosphate 48, 53, 58, 118, 130, 149
Calcium sulfate 156
Camptothecin 31
Carbon nanotubes (CNTs) 9
Cardiac tissue engineering 62
Cartilage 48, 53, 61, 112
  repair 13, 35, 112
  tissue engineering 57, 114
Chitin, deacetylation 21
Chitin–glucan 169
Chito-oligosaccharide (COS) 105
Chitosan 13, 19, 45, 81, 187
  amphiphilic 24
  cast film 176
  coatings 129, 141
  characterization 53
  crosslinkers 95
  degree of deacetylation (DD) 53, 84
  derivatives 19
  gel, multilayer 101
  membrane 109
  microspheres 108
  nanochitosan 167
  quaternization 22
  rods 100
  sulfated 85
  thiolated 87
Chitosan/alginate 93, 108
Chitosan/gelatin 92, 98
Chitosan/poly(butylene succinate) (CPBS) 113
Chitosan/poly(ethylene oxide) 178
Chitosan/poly(vinyl alcohol) (PVA) 14
Chitosan/silica xerogel hybrid membrane 119
Chitosan–apatite coatin 146
Chitosan–CaP 150

Chitosan–L-fucose 91
Chitosan–gelatin microspheres (CGMSs) 55
Chitosan–glucan 196
Chitosan–methacrylic acid–lactic acid (CML) 99
Chitosan-g-PCL-mPEG (CPP) 33
Chitosan-g-PEG-g-methacrylate 35
Chitosan–Pluronic hydrogel 36, 115
Chitosan-g-PNIPAAm 108
Chitosan-g-polyethyleneimine (PEI), mannosylated 91
Choanephora cucurbitarum 170
5β-Cholanic acid 26, 32
Cholesterol 26, 32
Cholic acid 32
Chondrocytes 30, 61, 99, 105, 112, 116
Chondroitin sulfate (CS) 93, 103, 132, 168, 181
Corneal tissue engineering 68, 96
Cow pea mosaic virus (CPMV)-co-P4VP 11
Crystal violet 14
CSO-SA 32
Cyclodextrin 95

D
Degree of deacetylation (DD) 53, 84, 131
Degree of quaternization (DQ) 86
Dental/craniofacial implants 129
Dextran 7
Dimethyl–3,3'-dithio-bis-propionimidate (DTBP) 95
3-(4,5-Dimethylthiazol–2-yl)–2,5-diphenyltetrazolium bromide (MTT) 11
DNA, release/delivery 5, 103
Doxorubicin 7, 31
Drug delivery 1ff
 triggered 14

E
Electrodeposition 129, 147
Electrospinning 51, 167, 178
Embryonic stem cells (ESCs) 105
Enhanced permeability and retention (EPR) 32
Ethylcellulose 35
1-Ethyl–3-(3-dimethylaminopropyl) carbodiimide 7, 24, 91, 95, 177
Extracellular matrix (ECM) 46, 82

F
F-actin fiber 106
Fatty acid derivatives 32

Fibroblast growth factor (bFGF) 55, 86, 93, 102, 116
Fungi 131, 169, 187, 194
 life cycle 189

G
Galactose 91
Galactosylated chitosan (GC) 91
Gas anti-solvent technique (GAS) 51
Gelatin 52, 92, 109, 168, 177
Gene-activated matrices 111
Gene delivery 29, 86
Gene silencing 29
Genipin 59, 94, 115, 167, 183
Gentamicin 142
Gibberellic acid 170
Glucan 170, 187, 195
Glucosamine 170
Glutaraldehyde (GA) crosslinking 110
β-Glycerophosphate 34
Glycolic acid (GA) 114
Glycosaminoglycans (GAGs) 84, 168
Gongronella butleri 171, 188
Grafting from/onto 27
Growth factors 57, 85, 102, 120, 131, 141

H
Hematopoietic stem cells (HSCs) 105
Heparin 67, 85, 103, 109, 118, 168
Hepatocyte grow factor (HGF) 102
Hepatocytes 57
Horseradish peroxidase (HRP) 114
Hyaluronan 132
Hyaluronic acid 93
Hydrogels 1, 3, 28, 98, 107, 110
 nanocomposites, magnetic 15
Hydrophobically modified glycol chitosan (HGC) 32
Hydroxyapatite (HA) 101, 150
 chitosan 28, 150
Hydroxybutyl chitosan (HBC) 13, 107
Hydroxyethyl cellulose 35
Hydroxyethyl methacrylate (HEMA) 9
N-(2-Hydroxyl) propyl–3-trimethyl ammonium chitosan chloride–carboxymethyl chitosan 14, 35
Hydroxypropylcellulose 3

I
Ibuprofen 6
Indoleacetic acid 170

Index 211

Iron oxide/microporous silica core–shell composite 16
Isocyantopropyltriethoxysilane (ICPTES) 135
N-Isopropylacrylamide (NIPAAm) 28
 grafted chitosan 13

L

Lactate dehydrogenase 173
Lactide 179
Lactose–chitosan 91
Lamivudine stearate 32
Laponite 14
Layer-by-layer 6, 157
Layered double hydroxide (LDH) biopolymer nanocomposites 6
Lentinus edodes 170, 199
Lineoic acid 26, 32
Liver tissue engineering 57

M

Macromolecules, modification 92
Magnesium aluminum silicate (MAS) 8
Magnetization 16
Mannose 91
Matrix–filler interaction 2
Membranes 109
Mesenchymal stem cells (MSCs) 105
Microspheres 118
Montmorillonite (MMT) 4
Morchella esculenta 169
N-mPEG-*N*-octyl-*O*-sulfate chitosan (mPEGOSC) 33
Mucoadhesiveness 87
Mucor rouxii 170, 190
Multiwalled carbon nanotubes (MWNTs) 9
Myocardial infarction 62
Mytomycin C 31

N

Nanochitin 167, 173
Nanochitosan 167
 defibrillated 175
Nanoclay 3
Nanofibrils 167, 173
Nerves 45
Nervous tissue engineering 68
Neural stem cells (NSCs) 70, 105
Neurospora crassa 170
NIPAAm/iron oxide-based hydrogel 15
Octacalcium phosphate (OCP) 151

N-Octyl-chitosan 25
N-Octyl-*O*-sulfate chitosan 86
N-Octyl-*N*-trimethyl chitosan chloride 25

O

Oleic acid 32
Oligo-L-lactide 180
Orthopedic implants 129
Osseointegration 133
Ovalbumin 86

P

Paclitaxel 9, 31
Paracetamol-loaded PEG 4
Particles from gas-saturated solutions (PGSS) 181
Passive targeting 32
PEO-PPO-PEO 100
Peptides 12, 16, 89, 106, 116
Phase separation 49
Phenol red 14
Phloretic acid (PA) 114
N-Phthaloylchitosan (PLC) 33
Phycomyces blakeesleanus 170
Plasmid DNA 6, 88, 103, 116
Platelet-derived growth factor (PDGF) 102
Polyanhydrides 48
Polydioxanone 48
Polyelectrolytes 13
Polyester fibers 118
Polyglycolic acid (PGA) 48
Polylactic acid (PLA) 48, 83
Polylactides 3, 179
Polymer–clay nanocomposites (PCNC) 8
Polymeric bionanocomposites (PBNCs) 1
Polyorthoesters 48
Polysiloxanes 134
Polyurethane (PU) 83, 137
Polyvinyl alcohol (PVA) 35, 83, 178
Poly(*N*-acetyl-D-glucosamine) 171
Poly(L-arginine) (PLR) 24
Poly(ε-caprolactone) (PCL) 3, 27, 33, 83
Poly(ethylene glycol) (PEG) 3, 25, 83
Poly(ethylene imine) (PEI) 23
Poly(ethylene oxide) (PEO) 3, 180
Poly(glycerol-sebacate) 62
Poly(α-hydroxy esters) 48
Poly(2-hydroxyethyl methacrylate) [poly(HEMA)] 9
Poly(3-hydroxybutyrate-*co*-3-hydroxyvalerate) (PHBV) 120

Poly(*N*-isopropyl acrylamide) (PNIPAAm) 28, 87
Poly(lactide-*co*-glycolic acid) (PLGA) 10, 12, 83
 chitosan/poly(vinyl alcohol) (PVA) 52
Poly(vinylidenefluoride) (PVDF) membranes 106
Poly(4-vinylpyrrolidone) (P4VP) 3
Porosity 47
Procainamide hydrochloride (PA) 4
Processability 48
Proteoglycans 168

Q
Quantum dots 1, 7

R
Rapid expansion of supercritical solutions (RESS) 51, 181
Regeneration 81
Repair 81
Replica molding 97
RGD 31, 89, 116
Rhizopus spp. 170, 188
Rods 100

S
Saccharomyces cerevisiae 170, 198
Salt leaching 49
Scaffolds 45, 47
 composite 109
 porous 96
Semi-interpenetrating polymer networks (semi-IPNs) 94
Silanes 133
 deposition/bonding 129
Silicates 4
Silk fibroin/chitosan 106
siRNA 29, 103
Skin 45, 54, 108
 damage 54
 tissue engineering 55
Solid freeform technique (SFF) 50
Solid state/substrate fermentation (SSF) 188
Solution casting 133

Stearic acid 26, 32
Stem cells 105
Steroid derivatives 26, 31, 32
Streptomyces spp. 170
Submerged fermentation (SMF) 188
N-Succinyl-chitosan 36, 114
Sugar–lectin 91
Sugars 91
Sulfonated carboxymethyl chitosan (SCC) 86
Supercritical drying 51, 181
Surface area 48, 97, 167, 182

T
Taylor cone 52
4-Thio-butylamidine (TBA) 87
Thioglycolic acid (TGA) 87
Three-dimensional environments 106
Tissue engineering 2, 13, 45, 182
Tissue regeneration 54, 81
Tissue repair 81, 85
Titanium, chitosan-coated 86, 130, 140
Transforming growth factor-beta (TGF-β) 102
Triethoxsilylbutyraldehyde (TESBA) 135, 144
Trimethyl chitosan (TMC) 23, 86
Two-dimensional environments 105

V
Vascular endothelial growth factor (VEGF) 86, 102
Vascular tissue engineering 62
Vitamin B_2 14
Vitamin B_{12} 14

W
Wound healing 35, 69, 110, 169
 skin 54, 91

Y
YIGSR 90

Z
Zein 6